D1662652

Nutraceuticals in Health and Disease Prevention

OXIDATIVE STRESS AND DISEASE

Series Editors

LESTER PACKER, PH.D.

ENRIQUE CADENAS, M.D., PH.D.

University of Southern California School of Pharmacy
Los Angeles, California

1. Oxidative Stress in Cancer, AIDS, and Neurodegenerative Diseases, *edited by Luc Montagnier, René Olivier, and Catherine Pasquier*
2. Understanding the Process of Aging: The Roles of Mitochondria, Free Radicals, and Antioxidants, *edited by Enrique Cadenas and Lester Packer*
3. Redox Regulation of Cell Signaling and Its Clinical Application, *edited by Lester Packer and Junji Yodoi*
4. Antioxidants in Diabetes Management, *edited by Lester Packer, Peter Rösen, Hans J. Tritschler, George L. King, and Angelo Azzi*
5. Free Radicals in Brain Pathophysiology, *edited by Giuseppe Poli, Enrique Cadenas, and Lester Packer*
6. Nutraceuticals in Health and Disease Prevention, *edited by Klaus Krämer, Peter-Paul Hoppe, and Lester Packer*

Additional Volumes in Preparation

Environmental Stressors in Health and Disease, *edited by Jürgen Fuchs*

Handbook of Antioxidants, Second Edition, Revised and Expanded, *edited by Enrique Cadenas and Lester Packer*

Related Volumes

Vitamin E in Health and Disease: Biochemistry and Clinical Applications, *edited by Lester Packer and Jürgen Fuchs*

Vitamin A in Health and Disease, *edited by Rune Blomhoff*

Free Radicals and Oxidation Phenomena in Biological Systems, *edited by Marcel Roberfroid and Pedro Buc Calderon*

Biothiols in Health and Disease, *edited by Lester Packer and Enrique Cadenas*

Handbook of Antioxidants, *edited by Enrique Cadenas and Lester Packer*

Handbook of Synthetic Antioxidants, *edited by Lester Packer and Enrique Cadenas*

Vitamin C in Health and Disease, *edited by Lester Packer and Jürgen Fuchs*

Lipoic Acid in Health and Disease, *edited by Jürgen Fuchs, Lester Packer, and Guido Zimmer*

Flavonoids in Health and Disease, *edited by Catherine Rice-Evans and Lester Packer*

Nutraceuticals in Health and Disease Prevention

edited by

KLAUS KRÄMER
BASF Aktiengesellschaft
Ludwigshafen, Germany

PETER-PAUL HOPPE
BASF Aktiengesellschaft
Offenbach/Queich, Germany

LESTER PACKER
University of Southern California School of Pharmacy
Los Angeles, California

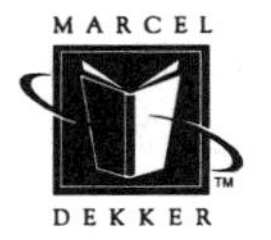

MARCEL DEKKER, INC. NEW YORK • BASEL

ISBN: 0-8247-0492-4

This book is printed on acid-free paper.

Headquarters
Marcel Dekker, Inc.
270 Madison Avenue, New York, NY 10016
tel: 212-696-9000; fax: 212-685-4540

Eastern Hemisphere Distribution
Marcel Dekker AG
Hutgasse 4, Postfach 812, CH-4001 Basel, Switzerland
tel: 41-61-261-8482; fax: 41-61-261-8896

World Wide Web
http://www.dekker.com

The publisher offers discounts on this book when ordered in bulk quantities. For more information, write to Special Sales/Professional Marketing at the headquarters address above.

Current printing (last digit):
10 9 8 7 6 5 4 3 2 1

PRINTED IN THE UNITED STATES OF AMERICA

Series Introduction

Oxygen is a dangerous friend. Overwhelming evidence indicates that oxidative stress can lead to cell and tissue injury. However, the same free radicals that are generated during oxidative stress are produced during normal metabolism and thus are involved in both human health and disease.

Free radicals are molecules with an odd number of electrons. The odd, or unpaired, electron is highly reactive as it seeks to pair with another free electron.

Free radicals are generated during oxidative metabolism and energy production in the body.

Free radicals are involved in:

- Enzyme-catalyzed reactions
- Electron transport in mitochondria
- Signal transduction and gene expression
- Activation of nuclear transcription factors
- Oxidative damage to molecules, cells, and tissues
- Antimicrobial action of neutrophils and macrophages
- Aging and disease

Normal metabolism is dependent upon oxygen, a free radical. Through evolution, oxygen was chosen as the terminal electron acceptor for respiration. The two unpaired electrons of oxygen spin in the same direction; thus, oxygen is a biradical, but is not a very dangerous free radical. Other oxygen-derived free radical species, such as superoxide or hydroxyl radicals, formed during metabolism or by ionizing radiation are stronger oxidants and are therefore more dangerous.

In addition to research on the biological effects of these reactive oxygen species, research on reactive nitrogen species has been gathering momentum. NO, or nitrogen monoxide (nitric oxide), is a free radical generated by NO synthase (NOS). This enzyme modulates physiological responses such as vasodilation or signaling in the brain. However, during inflammation, synthesis of NOS (iNOS) is induced. This iNOS can result in the overproduction of NO, causing damage. More worrisome, however, is the fact that excess NO can react with superoxide to produce the very toxic product peroxynitrite. Oxidation of lipids, proteins, and DNA can result, thereby increasing the likelihood of tissue injury.

Both reactive oxygen and nitrogen species are involved in normal cell regulation in which oxidants and redox status are important in signal transduction. Oxidative stress is increasingly seen as a major upstream component in the signaling cascade involved in inflammatory responses, stimulating adhesion molecule and chemoattractant production. Hydrogen peroxide, which breaks down to produce hydroxyl radicals, can also activate NF-κB, a transcription factor involved in stimulating inflammatory responses. Excess production of these reactive species is toxic, exerting cytostatic effects, causing membrane damage, and activating pathways of cell death (apoptosis and/or necrosis).

Virtually all diseases thus far examined involve free radicals. In most cases, free radicals are secondary to the disease process, but in some instances free radicals are causal. Thus, there is a delicate balance between oxidants and antioxidants in health and disease. Their proper balance is essential for ensuring healthy aging.

The term *oxidative stress* indicates that the antioxidant status of cells and tissues is altered by exposure to oxidants. The redox status is thus dependent upon the degree to which a cell's components are in the oxidized state. In general, the reducing environment inside cells helps to prevent oxidative damage. In this reducing environment, disulfide bonds (S—S) do not spontaneously form because sulfhydryl groups kept in the reduced state (SH) prevent protein misfolding or aggregation. This reducing environment is maintained by oxidative metabolism and by the action of antioxidant enzymes and substances, such as glutathione, thioredoxin, vitamins E and C, and enzymes such as superoxide dismutase (SOD), catalase, and the selenium-dependent glutathione and thioredoxin hydroperoxidases, which serve to remove reactive oxygen species.

Changes in the redox status and depletion of antioxidants occur during oxidative stress. The thiol redox status is a useful index of oxidative stress mainly because metabolism and NADPH-dependent enzymes maintain cell glutathione (GSH) almost completely in its reduced state. Oxidized glutathione (glutathione disulfide, GSSG) accumulates under conditions of oxidant exposure, and this changes the ratio of oxidized to reduced glutathione; an increased ratio indicates oxidative stress. Many tissues contain large amounts of glutathione, 2–4 mM in erythrocytes or neural tissues and up to 8 mM in hepatic tissues. Reactive oxygen and nitrogen species can directly react with glutathione to lower the levels of this substance, the cell's primary preventative antioxidant.

Current hypotheses favor the idea that lowering oxidative stress can have a clinical benefit. Free radicals can be overproduced or the natural antioxidant system defenses weakened, first resulting in oxidative stress, and then leading to oxidative injury and disease. Examples of this process include heart disease and cancer. Oxidation of human low-density lipoproteins is considered the first step in the progression and eventual development of atherosclerosis, leading to cardiovascular disease. Oxidative DNA damage initiates carcinogenesis.

Compelling support for the involvement of free radicals in disease development comes from epidemiological studies showing that an enhanced antioxidant status is associated with reduced risk of several diseases. Vitamin E and prevention of cardiovascular disease is a notable example. Elevated antioxidant status is also associated with decreased incidence of cataracts and cancer, and some recent reports have suggested an inverse correlation between antioxidant status and occurrence of rheumatoid arthritis and diabetes mellitus. Indeed, the number of indications in which antioxidants may be useful in the prevention and/or the treatment of disease is increasing.

Oxidative stress, rather than being the primary cause of disease, is more often a secondary complication in many disorders. Oxidative stress diseases include inflammatory bowel disease, retinal ischemia, cardiovascular disease and restenosis, AIDS, ARDS, and neurodegenerative diseases such as stroke, Parkinson's disease, and Alzheimer's disease. Such indications may prove amenable to antioxidant treatment because there is a clear involvement of oxidative injury in these disorders.

In this new series of books, the importance of oxidative stress in diseases associated with organ systems of the body will be highlighted by exploring the scientific evidence and the medical applications of this knowledge. The series will also highlight the major natural antioxidant enzymes and antioxidant substances such as vitamins E and C, flavonoids, polyphenols, carotenoids, lipoic acid, and other nutrients present in food and beverages.

Oxidative stress is an underlying factor in health and disease. More and more evidence is accumulating that a proper balance between oxidants and antioxidants is involved in maintaining health and longevity and that altering this balance in favor of oxidants may result in pathological responses causing functional disorders and disease. This series is intended for researchers in the basic biomedical sciences and clinicians. The potential for healthy aging and disease prevention necessitates gaining further knowledge about how oxidants and antioxidants affect biological systems.

As we move into the twenty-first century, new functions of nutrients encompassed by their involvement in cell-signaling cascades have been recognized. These functions are beyond their antioxidant activity and effects on the cellular balance between oxidants and antioxidants. The so-called functional foods, nutraceuticals, and optimal foods are under development and commercialization. The introduction of proteomics and genomics permits us to ascribe biological functions to food components. As might be expected, this has strengthened the development of ''designer foods'' aimed at improving health, promoting healthy aging, and preventing disease.

This volume in the Oxidative Stress and Disease series includes contributions and discussions of some food components and nutraceuticals, their putative mechanisms of action, and their implications for health and disease.

Lester Packer
Enrique Cadenas

Preface

The past decade has seen an enormous shift in our concept of nutrition. We have moved far beyond the goal of providing nutrition adequate to avoid the development of deficiency states to that of preventing or treating chronic diseases that have replaced infectious diseases as our major killers: cancer, heart disease, and diabetes. We have already made astonishing strides toward achieving this goal. For example, it is now accepted that supplementation with vitamin E, at levels impossible to achieve in the diet, can reduce the risk of heart disease.

The pace of research is constantly accelerating, and it has become difficult for the average health professional to keep up with the astounding achievements that have become almost routine. For this reason, ''The New Approach to a Healthy Life: Workshop on Nutraceuticals,'' a conference held on Dec. 3, 1998 in Ludwigshafen, Germany, was organized. The purpose of the meeting was to bring together the latest developments in research on nutritional substances used for disease prevention and therapy—substances that have been designated ''nutraceuticals.'' This volume includes the highlights reported at that meeting and will be of interest to health practitioners and researchers, as well as anyone interested in learning more about the studies that are quietly revolutionizing the field of nutrition.

During the first 85 years of the 20th century, the average human lifespan increased. This was mainly due to a 60% reduction in mortality. Major factors contributing to this remarkable occurrence were improved hygiene and nutrition, and medical advances, particularly the control of infectious diseases. We can forsee further improvements in the quality of life that will lead to the emergence of centenarians as a significant actuarial class, including more powerful means of maintaining the body's delicate balance between environmental stressors (oxidants) and our antioxidant defense system. Nutraceuticals, the so-called designer or functional foods, can be expected to provide the most significant improvements and developments.

A definition for nutraceuticals remains somewhat elusive. Simply put, they are ''foods specifically formulated to deliver health benefits.'' A more extensive definition states that a nutraceutical is a food, or any part of a food, that offers a health benefit above and beyond providing simple nutrition or basic fortification. Under this definition, the health benefit may include the prevention or treatment of disease or the enhancement of the body's functioning (Food Technology 1998; 52(6):44).

Perhaps the broadest definition of a nutraceutical has been formulated by Steven L. De Felice, M.D., as follows: ''A nutraceutical is any substance that is a food or part of a food and provides medical or health benefits, including the prevention and/or treatment of disease. Such products may range from isolated nutrients, dietary supplements, and diets to genetically engineered designer foods, herbal products, and processed foods such as cereals, soups, and beverages. It is important to note that this definition applies to all categories of foods and parts of food.''

Many organizations, including major corporations, research institutes, and university laboratories, are seeking to identify methods of optimizing nutrition that will produce healthy aging and a quality lifespan. This includes combinations of the approximately 40 micronutrients that have been identified, researched, and reported in the nutritional literature for years. But molecular nutrition is a relatively new field. The health consequences of deficiency of one or a combination of several micronutrients are largely unknown. On the other side of the coin are the beneficial effects that may be produced by intake of micronutrients at levels above the recommended daily allowance (RDA) or daily recommended intake (DRI). Added to the challenge are the varying needs of human beings of different genders, ages, and environments. The field is still in its infancy, and identifying the combinations of nutrients that may optimize health for the young, the elderly, men, women, various ethnic groups, and people in different areas of the world (or indeed different regions within a particular country) requires identification of the needs not only of the entire population in these regions, but also of subpopulations. At present, such detailed data are limited. Nevertheless, many exciting developments have occurred that show the promise of this young but rapidly emerging field of research and development.

In addition, genetic engineering of existing food sources is gaining momentum. One example are tomatoes engineered to enhance their lycopene content. Fortification with biofactors in amounts and forms far exceeding the levels in a diet composed of unmodified foodstuffs may someday be as routine for fruits and vegetables as it is now for fortified cereals.

We anticipate that new fields of research will be developed. Molecular nutrition and molecular biology will come together to identify food factors, and the lessons taught by traditional medicine will be updated using the tools of modern medicine.

To illustrate the unprecedented expansion of this field of research, this book includes a few examples of areas in which nutraceuticals have been developed and shown to be effective. The first several chapters are devoted to overviews and perspectives on this emerging field. Chapter 1 introduces the basic concepts relating nutraceuticals to both maintenance of health and prevention or treatment of pathology. Chapter 2 offers a perspective on nutraceuticals as they relate to our current theories of aging, especially concerning the health benefits of supplemental vitamin E and the concept of the antioxidant network. An exciting development in research on depression, arthritis, and inflammatory diseases is the emergence of S-adenosyl-L-methionine, a naturally occurring substance with few side effects. This is discussed from a general perspective in Chapter 3 and with respect to joint diseases in Chapter 4. One aspect of nutraceutical research is identifying the optimal form in which to provide a nutrient, as exemplified in Chapter 5 on methyltetrahydrofolate. We have now reached the second generation of carotenoid research, with the focus shifting away from beta-carotene to more balanced mixtures; Chapter 6 discusses lycopene and lutein, two carotenoids that are emerging as highly effective disease-preventing agents. An example of shifting nutritional balances to optimize intake of the more beneficial nutrients is the realization that polyunsaturated fatty acids (PUFAs) and, in particular, certain classes of PUFAs may be a key component of a healthy diet. This is discussed from a clinical perspective in Chapter 7. Lipoic (thioctic) acid has long been known as an essential cofactor in metabolism and is now recognized as a powerful antioxidant with great preventive and therapeutic potential. Chapter 8 provides a summary of the multiple uses of this powerful substance. Chapter 9 focuses on its metabolic aspects, in terms of both its function and its beneficial effects on cellular metabolism. Finally, Chapter 10 discusses creatine, which has been shown to be a safe and effective anabolic nutraceutical currently used by thousands of athletes and weekend warriors to promote strength. Other chapters (11–13) discuss the health effects of polyphenols, carnitine, and conjugated linoleic acid. Important research directions and regulatory issues are the topics covered in Chapters 14 and 15.

The first heyday in nutritional evolution came when most of the essential factors for prevention of acute nutritional disorders (such as scurvy and beri beri) were identified. The challenge that now awaits us is to go beyond the baseline requirements for survival to optimize nutrition, the major factor influencing our quality of life.

Nutraceuticals will be developed from established knowledge of caloric requirements for essential substances in the diet, and from elucidation of the many components in the food chain whose benefits are not yet fully known. Plants have survived through evolutionary adaptations that protect them from environmental stressors. These molecular adaptations often are also protective in human beings, but the analysis of the literally thousands of compounds contained in plant substances, and their effects on cellular, systemic, and organic biochemistry, has just begun.

In a field developing as quickly as that of nutraceuticals, one hesitates to recommend future areas for research for fear that the goals will be accomplished before the ink is dry. There are, however, several directions in which research may point. Literally thousands of phytochemicals exist and, no doubt, many thousands more are waiting to be discovered; classification and categorization are essential or researchers will be overwhelmed by the sheer numbers. We know very little about the bioavailability of even the most well studied of the nutraceutical compounds; plasma levels, although a good early indicator, can be misleading in terms of evaluation of tissue levels, and much research remains to be done in this area. The interactions of various food substances may provide synergistic benefits and this is an area of research that is almost untouched. To evaluate the efficacy of new nutraceuticals, it is critical to establish and validate early markers of pathology for chronic diseases such as cancer, heart disease, and diabetes. These conditions take decades to develop and in order to elucidate the effects of nutritional substances on their etiology in a timely manner, as well as to determine those at greatest risk, we must be able to detect alterations in early events. Genetic markers hold great promise in this area. In addition, although most nutraceuticals are known to be nontoxic, we must always keep safety and toxicity testing as top priorities—a ''natural'' substance is not necessarily a completely nontoxic substance.

In this, as in every area of research, each answer spawns several new questions. We hope that the present volume will serve as an early marker in the continuing development of the field of nutraceuticals.

Klaus Krämer
Peter-Paul Hoppe
Lester Packer

Contents

Series Introduction (Lester Packer and Enrique Cadenas) *iii*
Preface *vii*
Contributors *xiii*

1. Nutraceuticals: The Link Between Nutrition and Medicine 1
Hans K. Biesalski

2. The Role of Vitamin E in the Emerging Field of Nutraceuticals 27
Lester Packer and Stefan U. Weber

3. S-Adenosylmethionine (SAMe): Preclinical and Clinical Studies in Depression 47
Teodoro Bottiglieri

4. S-Adenosyl-L-Methionine: The Healthy Joint Product 63
Giorgio Stramentinoli

5. Methyltetrahydrofolate: The Superior Alternative to Folic Acid 75
John Scott

6. Lycopene and Lutein: The Next Steps to the Mixed Carotenoids 91
Robert M. Russell

7. n-3 Polyunsaturated Fatty Acids from Fish: Effects on Coronary Artery Disease 103
Erik Berg Schmidt and Jørn Dyerberg

8. Lipoic Acid: A Multifunctional Nutraceutical 113
Aalt Bast and Guido R. M. M. Haenen

9. R-α-Lipoic Acid 129
Klaus Krämer and Lester Packer

10. Creatine: Physiology and Exercise Performance 165
Klaus Krämer, Michael Weiss, and Heinz Liesen

11. Plant Phenols and Cardiovascular Disease: Antioxidants and Modulators of Cell Response 187
Fabio Virgili, Cristina Scaccini, Peter-Paul Hoppe, Klaus Krämer, and Lester Packer

12. L(−)-Carnitine and Its Precursor, γ-Butyrobetaine 217
Hermann Seim, Knut Eichler, and Hans-Peter Kleber

13. Conjugated Linoleic Acid 257
Werner G. Siems, Tilman Grune, Oliver Hasselwander, and Klaus Krämer

14. Contributions of Different Types of Evidence 289
Charles Hennekens

15. The Brave New World of Foods That Make Health-Related Claims 293
Stephen H. McNamara

Index *315*

Contributors

Aalt Bast, Ph.D. Department of Pharmacology and Toxicology, Universiteit Maastricht, Maastricht, The Netherlands

Hans K. Biesalski, M.D. Department of Biological Chemistry and Nutrition, University of Hohenheim, Stuttgart, Germany

Teodoro Bottiglieri, Ph.D. Department of Neuropharmacology, Baylor Institute of Metabolic Disease, Dallas, Texas

Jørn Dyerberg, M.D. Nova Medical Medi-Lab, Copenhagen, Denmark

Knut Eichler, Ph.D. Research, Fine Chemicals and Biotechnology, BASF Aktiengesellschaft, Ludwigshafen, Germany

Tilman Grune, M.D., Ph.D. Clinic for Physical Medicine and Rehabilitation, Humboldt University of Berlin, Berlin, Germany

Guido R. M. M. Haenen, Ph.D. Department of Pharmacology and Toxicology, Universiteit Maastricht, Maastricht, The Netherlands

Oliver Hasselwander New Business Development, Fine Chemicals, BASF Aktiengesellschaft, Ludwigshafen, Germany

Charles Hennekens, M.D. Department of Epidemiology and Public Health, University of Florida School of Medicine, Miami, Florida

Peter-Paul Hoppe, D.V.M. Department of Nutrition Research, BASF, Offenbach/Queich, Germany

Hans-Peter Kleber, M.D. Institute of Biochemistry, University of Leipzig, Leipzig, Germany

Klaus Krämer, Ph.D. Department of Human Nutrition, BASF Aktiengesellschaft, Ludwigshafen, Germany

Heinz Liesen, M.D. Institute of Sports Medicine, University of Paderborn, Paderborn, Germany

Stephen H. McNamara Hyman, Phelps & McNamara, P.C., Washington, D.C.

Lester Packer, Ph.D. Adjunct Professor, Department of Molecular Pharmacology and Toxicology, University of Southern California School of Pharmacy, Los Angeles, California

Robert M. Russell, M.D. Schools of Medicine and Nutrition, Tufts University, Boston, Massachusetts

Cristina Scaccini, Ph.D. National Institute for Food and Nutrition Research, Rome, Italy

Erik Berg Schmidt, M.D. Hjørring/Brønderslev Hospital, Copenhagen, Denmark

John Scott, Ph.D., Sc.D. Department of Biochemistry, Trinity College, Dublin, Ireland

Hermann Seim, Ph.D. Institute of Clinical Chemistry and Pathobiochemistry, University of Leipzig, Leipzig, Germany

Werner G. Siems, M.D., Ph.D. Department of Rheumatology and Orthopaedics, Herzog-Julius Hospital, Harzburg, Germany

Giorgio Stramentinoli, Ph.D. Crosspharma S.A., Milan, Italy

Fabio Virgili, Ph.D. National Institute for Food and Nutrition Research, Rome, Italy

Stefan U. Weber, M.D.* Department of Molecular and Cell Biology, University of California, Berkeley, California

Michael Weiss, M.D. Institute of Sports Medicine, University of Paderborn, Paderborn, Germany

*Present Address: Department of Anesthesiology and Critical Care Medicine, University of Bonn, Bonn, Germany

1

Nutraceuticals: The Link Between Nutrition and Medicine

Hans K. Biesalski
University of Hohenheim, Stuttgart, Germany

I. INTRODUCTION

Nutrition science during recent decades has been focused on the detection and understanding of deficiencies. With increasing knowledge of the existence and action of vitamins, specific recommendations were given with the aim of avoiding classical deficiency diseases such as xerophthalmia, beriberi, etc. A further step was the epidemiological evidence that diet contributes to the risk of certain diseases. The major finding was the correlation of a high fat intake with several kinds of cancer and cardiovascular disease. The consequences were special low-fat and low-cholesterol foods. However, the increasing knowledge about micronutrients including vitamins, minerals, and further compounds (carotenoids, flavonoids, anthocyans, etc.) on a molecular level together with results from epidemiological studies opens a new and exciting field of nutrition science, nutraceuticals (NC), as a link between nutrition and medicine.

Nutraceutical is a term coined in 1979 by Stephen DeFelice (1). According to DeFelice, it is defined "as a food or parts of food, that provide medical or health benefits, including the prevention and treatment of disease." Subsequently, several other terms (medical food, functional food, nutritional supplements) were used.

Nutraceuticals may range from isolated nutrients, dietary supplements, and diets to genetically engineered "designer" foods, herbal products, and processed products, such as cereals, soups, and beverages. The increasing interest in nutraceuticals reflects the fact that consumers hear about epidemiological studies indicating that a specific diet or component of the diet is associated with a lower risk for a certain disease (Table 1).

Table 1 Dietary Factors Linked to Diseases

	Total or saturated fat	Antioxidants	Folic acid	Calcium	Complex CHO, fiber	Omega-3 fatty acids
Cardiovascular disease	−	+	+	+	+	+
Cancer	−	+	+	+	+	+ (are used)
Diabetes	−	+			+	+
Cataract/AMD	−	+				
Obesity	−				+	
Osteoporosis				+		
Birth outcomes		+	+		+	+
Immune function	−	+	+		+	+

+ = Positive impact on health outcomes; − = negative impact on health outcomes.

Until recently, vitamins and other micronutrients were recommended only to avoid classical symptoms of deficiency. However, modern biology techniques have given us increasing insights into the molecular and cellular needs of the human organism. This has led to a more refined definition of the health benefits of and requirements for micronutrients (Table 2). Clinical symptoms of deficiencies are the end of a long-lasting pattern of low micronutrient intake. Long before these symptoms occur, the inadacquate delivery of micronutrients to their target tissue causes alterations that may be the basis for the development of chronic diseases. The compounds that have been studied most extensively are the antioxidants. Many potential benefits have been attributed to antioxidants in the form of dietary intake or supplementation. Antioxidants in general may be useful in the prevention of cancer and cerebrovascular disease. Supplementation with vitamin C may be beneficial in the management of asthma patients, and high dietary intake of vitamin E may prevent Parkinson's disease. Moreover, researchers have recently determined that the oxidized form of vitamin C, dehydroascorbic acid, readily crosses the blood-brain barrier (2). These findings have implications for affecting the uptake of antioxidants in the central nervous system (CNS); thus, it is assumed that this has the potential for improving the treatment of Alzheimer's disease.

The combination of vitamins E and C and β-carotene has been useful in reducing low-density lipoprotein (LDL) oxidation and subsequent atherosclerosis.

1. Vitamin C scavenges aqueous radicals and regenerates α-tocopherol from the tocopheroxyl radical species.

Table 2 Health Benefits of Vitamins, Minerals, and Trace Elements

Nutrient	Health benefits
Fat-soluble vitamins	
Vitamin A	Essential for growth and development; maintains healthy vision, skin, and mucous membranes; may aid in the prevention and treatment of certain cancers and in the treatment of certain skin disorders
Vitamin D (calciferol)	Essential for formation of bones and teeth; helps the body absorb and use calcium; prevents colon cancer
Vitamin E (tocopherol)	The most important fat-soluble antioxidant; boosts the immune system; prevents coronary heart disease
Vitamin K	Essential for blood clotting
Water-soluble vitamins	
Ascorbic acid (vitamin C)	Antioxidant; necessary for healthy bones, teeth, and skin; helps in wound healing; may prevent common cold
Thiamine (vitamin B_1)	Helps convert food into energy; essential in neurological function
Riboflavin (vitamin B_2)	Helps in energy production and other chemical processes in the body; helps maintain healthy eyes, skin, and nerve function
Niacin (vitamin B_3)	Helps convert food into energy; helps maintain proper brain function
Pyridoxine (vitamin B_6)	Helps produce essential proteins; helps convert protein into energy; lowers homocysteine
Folic acid	Necessary to produce the genetic materials of cells; essential in pregnancy for preventing birth defects; helps in red blood cell formation; protects against heart disease by lowering homocysteine
Pantothenic acid (in B-complex family)	Aids in synthesis of cholesterol, steroids, and fatty acids
Vitamin-like compounds	
Biotin (vitamin H)	Member of B-complex group of vitamins; required for various metabolic functions
L-Carnitine	Oxidation of fatty acids, promotion of certain organic acid excretions, and enhancement of the rate of oxidative phosphorylation
Choline	Lipotropic agents; have been used to treat fatty liver and disturbed fat metabolism

Table 2 Continued

Nutrient	Health benefits
Essential fatty acids (vitamin F)	Involved in proper development of various membranes and the synthesis of prostaglandins, leukotrienes, and various hydroxy fatty acids
Inositol	Necessary for amino acid transport and movement of potassium and sodium; lipotropic agent
Taurine (aminoethanesulfonate)	Aids in retinal photoreceptor activity, bile acid conjugation, white blood cell antioxidant activity; CNS neuromodulation, platelet aggregation, cardiac contractility, sperm motility, growth, and insulin activity
Minerals	
Calcium	Essential for building bones and teeth and maintaining bone strength; prevents colon cancer
Iron	Helps in energy production; helps to carry oxygen in the bloodstream and to transfer oxygen to muscles
Magnesium	Essential for healthy nerve and muscle function and bone formation; may help prevent premenstrual syndrome (PMS); may help to prevent coronary heart disease
Phosphorus	Essential for building strong bones and teeth; helps in formation of genetic material; helps in energy production and storage
Trace elements	
Chromium	Works with insulin to convert carbohydrates and fat into energy
Cobalt	Essential component of vitamin B_{12}, but ingested cobalt is metabolized in vivo to form the B_{12} coenzymes
Copper	Essential for making hemoglobin and collagen; essential for healthy functioning of the heart; helps in energy production; helps in absorption of iron from digestive tract; essential for antioxidative function of SOD
Fluorine	Presumably makes enamel resistant to erosive action of acids produced by bacteria in the oral cavity
Iodine	Essential for proper functioning of the thyroid
Manganese	Required for glucose utilization, synthesis of the mucopolysaccharides of cartilage, biosynthesis of steroids

Table 2 Continued

Nutrient	Health benefits
Molybdenum	May function as an enzyme cofactor
Nickel	Involved in specific metalloenzymes
Selenium	Antioxidant cofactor essential for healthy functioning of the heart muscle
Silicone	Functions in the development and maintenance of connective tissue
Tin	May be involved in growth and reproductive functions
Vanadium	May be involved in functions related to growth and reproduction
Zinc	Essential for cell reproduction, normal growth and development in children, wound healing, and production of sperm and the hormone testosterone

2. Vitamin E in the form of α-tocopherol protects polyunsaturated fatty acids (PUFA) within the membranes and the LDL particle, reduces platelet adhesion, and inhibits smooth muscle cell proliferation and protein kinase C activity.
3. β-Carotene provides antioxidant activity, especially in the skin and in the arterial wall, where low partial pressures of oxygen are found.

The combination of different antioxidants allows us to mimic the antioxidant network.

Increased intake of antioxidants is associated with a lower risk for cancer, coronary heart disease (CHD), and other degenerative diseases. However, it must be noted that while the correlation exists between increased nutrient uptake and specific diseases, the response of any given individual is quite variable. These individual variations in dietary responsiveness are likely due to the different genetic composition of each individual. Numerous genetic factors are involved in determining responsiveness to specific dietary nutrients. These include genes important for nutrient absorption as well as those important for the metabolism and processing of the nutrient in the diet. Additionally, the amount of each nutrient in the diet also has an impact on the level of specific gene expression. Such regulatory mechanisms may also account for individual differences in susceptibility to diet-induced diseases. There is evidence that groups exist with a high risk for diseases like cancer or CHD despite normal or even optimum intake of micronutrients. These are individuals who have a mutation in an enzyme involved in either metabolism or distribution of micronutrients. This ''polymorphism'' results in inadequate function or low tissue concentration of the micronutrient.

For example, elevated plasma homocysteine has emerged as a new independent risk factor for coronary artery disease. There is evidence from several studies that a mild to moderate rise in plasma homocysteine is strongly associated with the development of atherosclerosis (3). The major determinants of plasma homocysteine concentrations are nutritional and genetic factors. A common single base pair exchange of cytosine to thymidine at nucleotide 677 of the methylene tetrahydrofolate reductase (MTHFR) gene leads to thermolabile MTHFR with reduced enzyme activity, resulting in raised plasma homocysteine concentrations (4). It has been reported that this mutation is associated with the development of coronary artery disease (5). An intake exceeding the usual recommendation may help to protect from CHD in cases of high homocysteine in groups with the above-mentioned mutation or due to low folate intake.

Those genetically predisposed to pancreatic cancer have low serum levels of selenium. Thus, it is assumed that supplementation with selenium may help to prevent this condition (6).

It must be considered that the effect of a high intake of selected micronutrients as is described in epidemiological studies might only appear in groups with specific polymorphisms. However, if the intake of one or more micronutrients is low in genetically normal people, this situation is similar to the above-described polymorphism. So at least more people than those with genetic polymorphism will benefit from specific NC. A genetic polymorphism which influences micronutrient metabolism and associated increased risk for a specific disease is indeed a very good model for studying the effectiveness of NC.

In addition to increasing knowledge about the importance of micronutrients in the prevention of diseases, new compounds, so-called phytochemicals, entered the stage in recent years. Over the past decade, medical and scientific knowledge of the role of phytochemicals in specific disease processes has advanced at an accelerating pace. Many different classes of phytochemicals have been implicated as having preventive effects against different diseases mainly, at very early stages of disease development (Table 3). Phytochemicals with anticancer effects were detected, and the fact that these compounds occur mainly in vegetables seem to confirm the epidemiological evidence that a high intake of vegetable protects against different kinds of cancer (Table 4). At the same time, revolutionary technologies—including biotechnology—have created a new age in which nutritional discoveries, product innovations, and mass production are possible as never before. These medical and scientific developments have spawned an important and explosive new area of research, resulting in increasing numbers of potential nutritional products with medical and health benefits.

Science and technology are increasing the possibility of modifying traditional foods and developing new food sources to meet these newly defined health

Table 3 Potential Biological Activities of Phytochemicals

Mode of action	Examples
Antioxidants	Carotenoids, tocopherol, flavonoids, catechins
Protection against hormone-dependent cancers	Isoflavones, lignans
Hypocholesterolemic effects	Saponins, tocotrienols
Inducers of DNA repair	Vanillin, cinnamaldehyde, coumarin, anisaldehyde
Antimetastatic agents	Tangeretin, catechin, retinoside
Inhibitors of cell proliferation	Quercetin, kaempferol, genistein, daidzein

needs. Using modern genetics, chemistry, and molecular biology, the scientific community for the first time is able to design and construct foods having specially desired characteristics.

The products themselves represent a major departure from contemporary foods, in part because they are based on the new approach to nutrition as a way to reduce risk for disease. Modern nutritional thought is beginning to slowly reflect a fundamental change in our understanding of health. Increased knowledge of the impact of diet on regulation at the genetic and molecular level will lead to a rethinking of health goals, resulting in dietary strategies targeted on whole body rather than specific factors.

Evidence for potential protective effects of selected phytochemicals is generally based on experiments demonstrating a biological activity in a relevant in vitro bioassay or experiments using animal models. In some cases this is supported by both epidemiological studies and a limited number of intervention experiments in humans.

Table 5 summarizes herbals and phytochemicals and their relation to specific diseases. Herbs and phytochemicals claimed effective for treatment of different diseases entered the market in many cases without a scientific basis for their claims of efficacy or safety. Herbal extracts are composed of several components, each having a possible effect on a cellular level. Consequently, it has not been clear which compound is the effective one or whether a specific combination is necessary. It cannot be excluded that, in addition to more or less beneficial phytochemicals, including other micronutrients, harmful components also exist in herbal products. Consequently, the health benefit of phytochemicals should be elucidated with isolated compounds in selected in vitro and in vivo systems. This includes bioavailability, dose effect levels in target tissues, and the definition of biological markers (biomarkers) that indicate the effect of a phytochemical at a very early stage of disease development.

Biomarkers that may serve to define the effect of nutraceuticals in the chemoprevention of certain diseases, such as cancer, coronary heart disease (CHD),

Table 4 Foods Containing Compounds Claimed to Prevent Cancer

Action	Food source	Chemopreventive agent	Tumor site
Modification of carcinogen activation	Alliums (e.g., garlic and onions)	Alkyl sulfides and disulfides	Esophagus, colon, lung
	Crucifers (e.g., cauliflower, broccoli, cabbage)	Isothiocyanates	Liver, lung, mammary
	Citrus	Monoterpenes	Mammary, pancreas
	Turmeric	Flavonoids	Colon, skin
	Teas	Polyphenols	Colon, lung, skin
Modulation of carcinogen detoxification	Alliums	Sulfide volatiles, alkylcysteines	Esophagus, colon, lung
	Crucifers	Isothiocyanates	Liver, lung, mammary
Interception of DNA-reactive species	Green tea	Polyphenol fractions	Colon, lung, skin
	Green tea	Epigallocatechin gallate (EGCG)	Duodenum, skin
	Green tea	Tea infusion	Esophagus, forestomach, lung, skin
	Ellagic acid (found in a variety of fruits and nuts)	Polyphenolics	Esophagus
		Curcumin	Skin, mammary, colon, forestomach (nonhuman)
Reversal of abnormal proliferation	Citrus	Monoterpenes	General
		Calcium	Colon
		Vitamin A and its precursors and metabolites	General

Table 5 Diseases Treated with Herbal and Phytochemical Products

Diseases and compounds	Activity claimed
Digestive system disorders	
Chamomile	Oral: anti-inflammatory; spasmolitic; antimicrobial topical; wound healing, anti-inflammatory; antimicrobial
Ginger	Carminative, antiemetic, cholagogue, positive inotrophic; treatment of dizziness
Licorice	Expectorant, secretalytic; treatment of peptic ulcers
Milk thistle	Prophylaxis and treatment of chronic hepatoxicity
Peppermint	Leaf: carminative, choleretic
	Oil: reduces symptoms of irritable bowel syndrome (IBS)
Plantago seed/Psyllium seed	Cathartic
Senna	Cathartic
Kidney, urinary tract, and prostate disorders	
Beaberry	Antibacterial for urinary tract infection (UTI), diuretic
Cranberry	Bacteriostatic for treatment of UTIs
Goldenrod	Prophylaxis and treatment of urinary calculi and kidney and kidney stones
Saw palmetto	Antiadrenergic, anti-inflammatory; treat symptoms of benign prostatic hyperplasia (BPH)
Performance and endurance enhancer	
Echinacea	Oral: immunostimulant; treatment of cold and flu symptoms
	Topical: treatment of hard-to-heal wounds, eczema, burns, psoriasis, herpes, herpes simplex, etc.
Elcuthero	Adaptogen (facilitating resistance to various kinds of stress)
Ginseng	Adaptogen
Nervous system disorders	
Feverfew	Treatment of headaches, fever, and menstrual problems; prophylactic to reduce frequency, severity, and duration of migraine headaches
St. John's wort	Anxiolytic, anti-inflammatory, antidepressant, monoamine oxidase inhibitor
Valerian	Spasmolytic, mild sedative, sleep aid
Willow bark	Anti-inflammatory, analgesic, antipyretic, astringent; treatment of rheumatic and arthritic conditions, mild headache, and gout
Metabolic and endocrine disorders	
Black cohosh	Emmenagogue; treatment of premenstrual discomfort and dysmenorrhea

Table 5 Continued

Diseases and compounds	Activity claimed
Black currant seed oil	Dietary source of linoleic acid; treatment of atopic eczema
Borage seed oil	Dietary source of linoleic acid; treatment of atopic eczema
Chaste tree berry	Treatment of menstrual disorders
Evening primrose oil	Dietary source of linoleic acid; treatment of atopic eczema
Respiratory tract disorders	
Ephedra	Bronchodilator, vasoconstrictor, reduces bronchial edema, appetite suppressant (note: FDA has restricted use of ephedra-containing products)
Horehound	Expectorant, antitussive, cholerectic
Slippery elm	Mucilaginous demulcent, emollient, and nutrient; used to sooth irritated mucous membranes or ulcerations of the digestive tract
Cardiovascular system disorders	
Garlic	Antibacterial, antifungal, antithrombotic, hypotensive, fibrinolytic, anti-inflammatory, antihyperlipidemic
Ginkgo	Increases vasodilation and peripheral blood flow rate in capillary vessels and end arteries; treatment post-thrombotic syndrome, chronic cerebral vascular insufficiency, short-term memory loss, cognitive disorders secondary to depression, dementia tinnitus, vertigo
Grapeseed	Antioxidant; treatment of hypoxia from atherosclerosis, inflammation, and cardiac or cerebral infarction
Hawthorne	Sleep aid; treatment of diminished cardiac performance
Pine bark	Antioxidant; treatment of hypoxia form atherosclerosis, inflammation, and cardiac or cerebral infarction
Disorders of the skin, mucous membranes, and gingiva	
Aloe vera gel	Dilates capillaries, anti-inflammatory; emollient and wound-healing properties when applied topically
Goldenseal	Antimicrobial, astringent, antihemorrhagic; treatment of mucosal inflammation, dyspepsia, and gastritis
Melissa, lemon balm	Topical antibacterial and antiviral
Tea tree oil	Topical bacteriostatic and germicidal
Witch hazel	Topical treatment of local inflammation of skin and mucous membranes; astringent, anti-inflammatory, and local hemostyptic for minor skin injuries, hemorrhoids, and varicose veins

Source: Adapted from Ref. 51.

Table 6 Selected Biomarkers to Describe Relationship Between Nutrition and Disease Prevention

Biomarker	Nutraceutical	Disease
Bone density	Calcium	Osteoporosis
Homocysteine	Folic acid	CHD
ODC	Carotenoids	Cancer
MMP	Carotenoids/Retinoids	Photoaging
DNA damage	Antioxidants	Cancer
LDL oxidation	Vitamin E	CHD
Visual acuity (ERG)	Carotenoids	AMD

adult macular degeneration (AMD), etc. can be taken to determine dose effect levels, bioavailability, and safety of selected nutraceuticals in specific cells and tissues (Table 6).

A biomaker should be correlated to the disease process and to the NC tested under in vitro and in vivo conditions. The following examples demonstrate approaches for determining the effectiveness of nutraceuticals using different biomarkers.

II. β-CAROTENE AND SKIN PROTECTION

Acute and chronic exposure to nonphysiological high doses of ultraviolet (UV) light leads to a variety of changes in the epidermis, dermis, and the adnexal organs of the skin. The most significant changes are premature aging of the skin (photoaging), UV-induced hyperkeratosis or atrophy, provocation of skin diseases, and, finally, precancerous lesions (actinic keratoses) and neoplasms of the skin, such as squamous cell carcinoma, basal cell carcinoma, and possibly malignant melanoma (7–9). Furthermore, the local and systemic immune response can be negatively modulated (10,11).

It is well known that exposure to UV rays can initiate free radicals, especially in the epidermis, which participate in the development of the above-mentioned pathological skin changes (12). UV irradiation at physiological doses representative of the UVA (1–20 J/cm^2 at a fluence of 3.3 mW/cm^2) in natural sunlight is an efficient inducer of lipid peroxidation, while UVB irradiation at physiological doses (5–50 mJ/cm^2, fluence: 0.4 mW/cm^2) does not induce lipid peroxidation. Only at very high nonphysiological UVB doses (500 mJ/cm^2) was a significant TBARS production (marker for lipid peroxidation) observed.

Consequently, researchers are looking for substances that can either suppress the damaging effects of free radicals or block the UV-induced initiation of free radicals. One substance that fulfills those needs is β-carotene (BC) (13–15). Studies have shown that the level of BC in the blood and retinol in skin (16,17) can decrease after exposure to natural sun and artificial UV light; therefore, the provision of the epidermis with adequate amounts of β-carotene either from cutaneous storage or from the blood may not be sufficient.

Recently it was documented that UVA irradiation substantially reduces the two major retinoid receptors, RAR-γ and RAR-α, in RNA and protein in human skin in vivo (18). This will result in a loss of transcriptional control of AP-1–dependent target genes, some of which are involved in skin cancer genesis and aging.

We demonstrated an effect of retinoic acid on UV induced lipid peroxidation (19) in human skin fibroblasts (Fig. 1). Cells were irradiated with UVA (1–20 J/cm^2) or UVB (5–500 mJ/cm^2). As indicator of lipid peroxidation, TBARS in medium supernatant, and as a marker of DNA damage, ornithine decarboxylase (ODC) activity were determined, 1 hour postirradiation (p.i.) with 20 J/cm^2 UVA. TBARS production was enhanced by 3 μM atRA treatment (121% of vehicle-treated cells) and decreased by 10 μM atRA treatment (75% of vehicle-treated cells) and was not significantly altered in UVB irradiated cells. ODC activity peaked in vehicle-treated cells 24 hours p.i. with 50 mJ/cm^2 UVB to 738% of sham irradiated control cells, and was reduced to 493% by 3 μM atRA (Fig. 2). Treatment with 10 μM atRA further decreased ODC activity (366%), and this activity peak occurred at 36 hours p.i. ODC activity was not significantly enhanced by UVA irradiation.

These results suggest that in normal human skin fibroblasts atRA and/or its metabolites influence the UVA generation of reactive oxygen species (ROS) by at least two distinct antagonistic mechanisms, while the ODC response to UVB-induced DNA damage involves a ROS-independent, retinoid-sensitive regulatory pathway.

The overexpression of ornithine decarboxylase is critical with respect to carcinogenesis (20). The polyamines putrescine, spermidine, and spermine have been shown to be essential for mammalian cell growth and function. Intracellular polyamine concentrations are highly regulated by the enzyme ODC (EC 4.1.1.17), which catalyzes the conversion of ornithine to putrescine, the initial and often rate-limiting step in polyamine biosynthesis. The level of ODC activity in quiescent cells is extremely low but readily induced by a wide variety of growth-promoting agents or UV light (21,22). Rapidly proliferating cells and neoplastic cells express elevated levels of ODC. Inhibition of ODC results in a depletion of putrescine and spermidine pools with the consequence of growth arrest of normal and neoplastic cells in vitro and in vivo (23,24).

Incubation of human skin fibroblasts with β-carotene and UVB irradiation as described above completely abolished the UVB-induced ODC increase

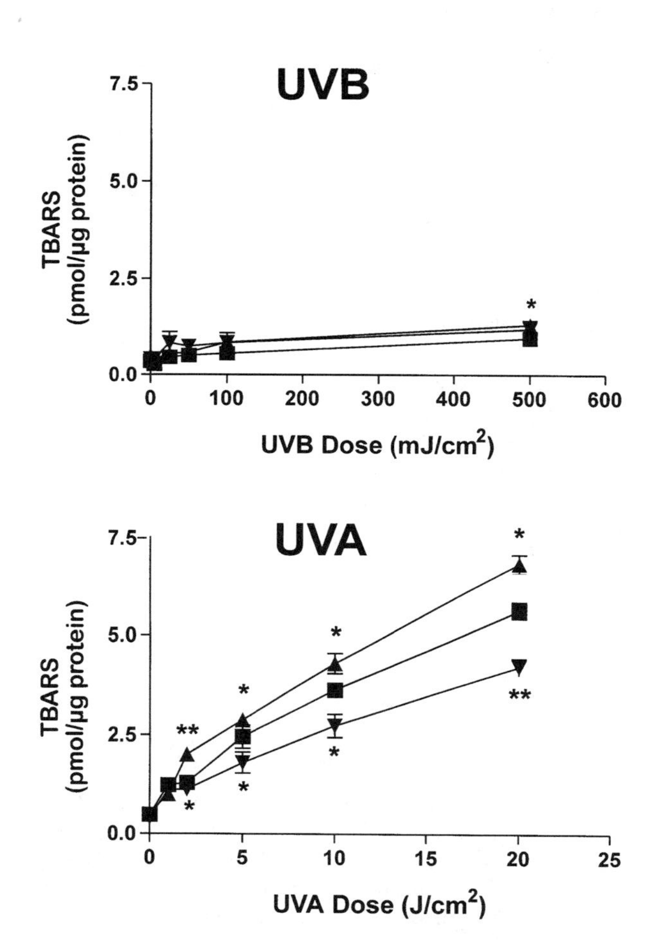

Figure 1 Effect of atRA treatment on UV-induced TBARS accumulation in cell culture supernatant. HFP-1 cells were treated for 16 hours with vehicle alone (■), 3 µm (▲), or 10 µm atRA (▼) before irradiation with different doses of UVA or UVB. TBARS in cell culture supernatant were analyzed 1 hour postirradiation as described (41) and measured with a microplate fluorescence reader. TBARS is expressed as pmol TBARS per µg cell protein. Data shown represent mean ±SEM of two independent experiments with three determinations in each. Statistical significance of the difference between vehicle-treated and atRA-treated cells at the confidence level $p < 0.05$ (*) or $p < 0.01$ (**).

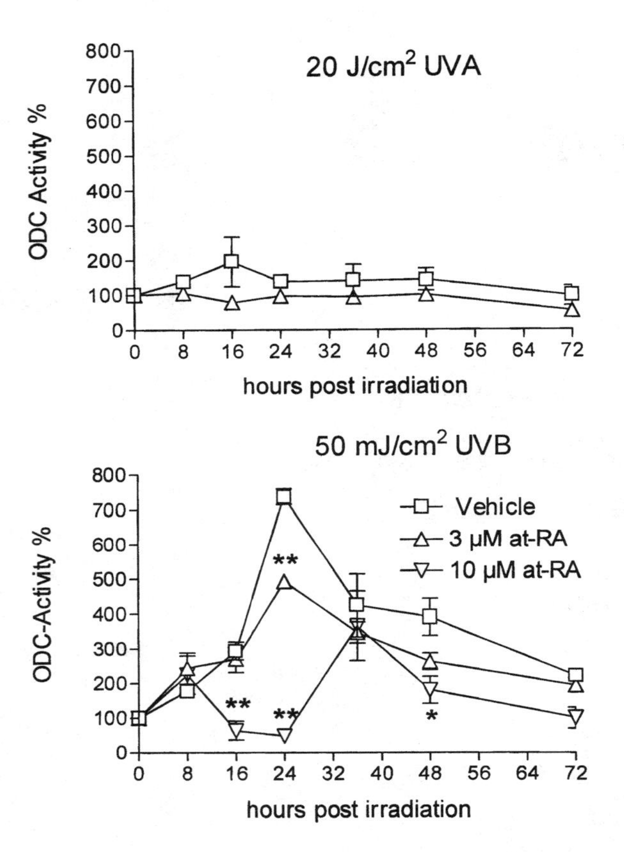

Figure 2 Effect of atRA on UV-induced ornithine decarboxylase response in HFP-1 cells. Cells were treated for 16 hours with vehicle alone (■); 3 μm (▲) or 10 μm atRA (▼) before irradiation with 20 J/cm² UVA or 50 mJ/m² UVB and ODC activity (liberation of $^{14}CO_2$ from L-[1-^{14}C]-ornithine) determined at the time points postirradiation indicated. Data given are from one representative experiment with three determinations (mean ± SEM) per treatment and time point. ODC activity is expressed as percent activity, with the activity of vehicle-treated, sham-irradiated cells set as 100%. Statistical significance of the difference between vehicle-treated and atRA-treated cells at the confidence level $p < 0.05$ (*) or $p < 0.01$ (**).

(Fig. 3). A similar effect was documented in the colonic mucosa following a 3-month dietary intake of β-carotene. This at least shows that the effect of β-carotene on ODC expression is not only due to UV light–mediated effects. A low level of β-carotene or other carotenoids in blood or tissues may increase the risk for neoplastic transformation of cells. Indeed, natural sunlight (12 days) decreases

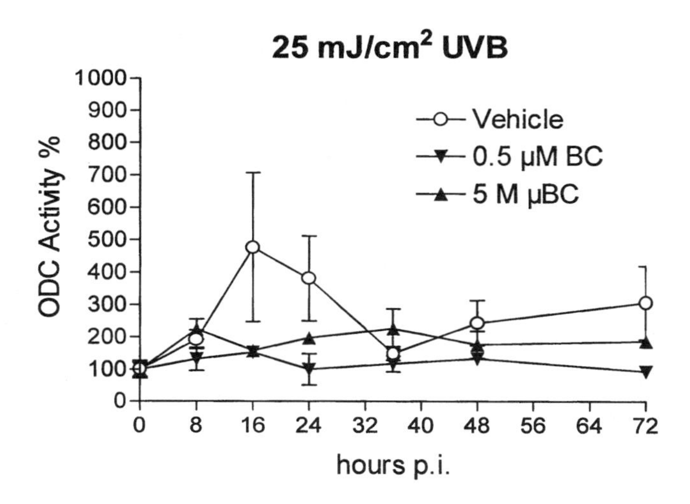

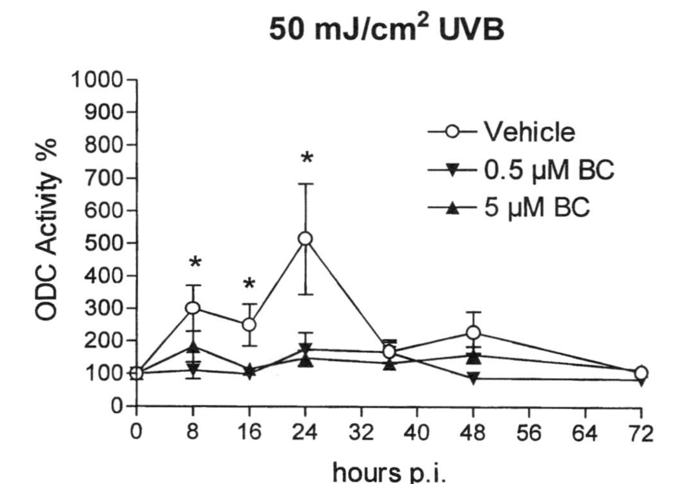

Figure 3 Effect of at β-carotene on UV-induced ODC-response in HFP-1 cells. Cells were treated for 7 days with vehicle alone (○); 0.5 μm at β-carotene (▲) or 5 μm at β-carotene (▼) before irradiation with 25 mJ/cm² UVB or 50 mJ/m² UVB and ODC activity (liberation of $^{14}CO_2$ from L-[1-^{14}C]-ornithine) determined at the time points postirradiation indicated. Data given are from one representative experiment with three determinations (mean ± SEM) per treatment and time point. ODC activity is expressed as percent activity, with the activity of vehicle-treated, sham-irradiated cells set as 100%. Statistical significance of the difference between vehicle-treated and at β-carotene–treated cells at the confidence level $p < 0.05$ (*) or $p < 0.01$ (**).

cutaneous β-carotene to more than 50% (25). Whether this contributes to the increased cancer risk following UV exposure remains to be further elucidated. In addition, it is not known whether β-carotene might prevent the above-mentioned UVA-induced RAR/RXR downregulation.

In recent preliminary studies we found a suppressive effect of β-carotene on MMP-1 expression. Solar UV irradiation results in premature skin aging, thought to be an initiating event of skin carcinogenesis (26,27). One reason for premature skin aging, UVB-induced expression of matrix-degrading metalloproteinases (MMP), has been recently demonstrated in vivo (28). Within minutes, low-dose UVB upregulated the stimulators of the metalloproteinase genes, the transcription factors AP-1 and NF-κB. Retinoic acid (RA), a transrepressor of AP-1, topically applied to the skin prior to UVB irradiation, substantially reduced the UVB-induced AP-1 activation and subsequently metalloproteinase expression.

Following a 7-day incubation we were able to show that in β-carotene–supplemented human skin fibroblasts the UVB-induced increase of MMP-1 was nearly completely abolished. These results are consistent with a recent in vivo observation that β-carotene prevents the increase of MMP-1 following irradiation with a solar light imitator, compared with a placebo-treated control group (Fig. 4). β-Carotene was without any effect on MMP concentration during the 8-week supplementation period. Irradiation with a solar light simulator results in a sig-

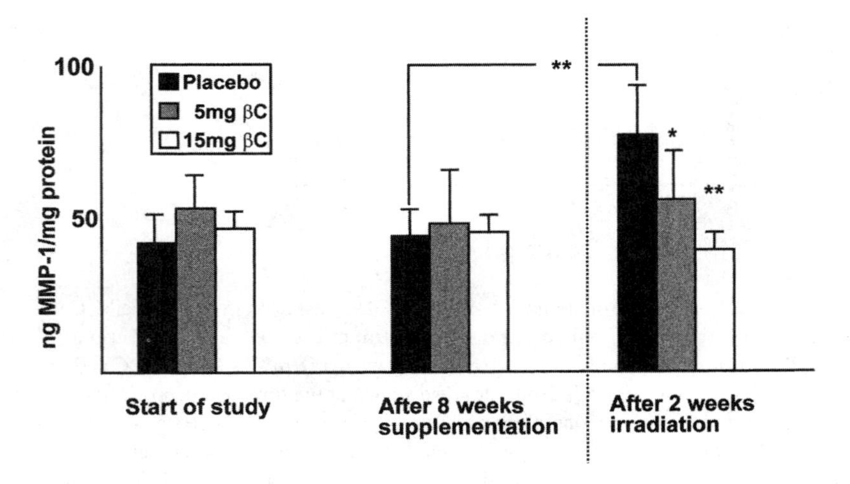

Figure 4 MMP-1 was measured in skin biopsies of 36 female volunteers in three groups (12 each) before supplementation with 5 or 15 mg β-carotene or placebo (start of study) 8 weeks after supplementation and 2 weeks after irradiation (solar light simulator).

nificant increase of MMP-1 in the placebo group. In contrast, in the treated groups the MMP-1 levels remained unchanged. These data clearly show that β-carotene is involved in the protection of the skin against deleterious effects of sunlight.

MMP and ODC may serve as (AP-1–controlled) biomarkers, which allow study of the effects of β-carotene or other carotenoids on different cells and tissues and, with respect to MMP, are also useful for human intervention studies.

III. EFFECTS OF VITAMIN C AND E IN SMOKERS

Data have been published showing a harmful effect of vitamin C on DNA oxidation (29). Supplementation of volunteers with 500 mg of vitamin C resulted in an increase of 8-oxoadenine. Despite a decrease of 8-oxoguanine, which positively correlates with plasma vitamin C (30), this DNA oxidation was claimed to be a harmful effect of vitamin C. One reason for such a pro-oxidative effect of vitamin C could be the vitamin C radical that results from the antioxidative action of vitamin C. To further elucidate whether vitamin C elicits such pro-oxidative effects, we measured the occurrence of vitamin C radical in smokers and the effect on DNA damage (31).

There is increasing evidence that oxidative stress induced by cigarette smoke is an important early event in several diseases, including lung cancer and atherosclerosis. The gas phase of cigarette smoke contains numerous compounds of free radicals, which have been shown to be involved in oxidation processes. Epidemiological studies have shown a positive correlation between serum copper and iron levels and risk of cardiovascular disease, supporting the theory that LDL oxidation may be mediated by cigarette smoke. Physiological concentrations of ascorbic acid can protect lipids in plasma and LDL against peroxidative damage in vitro and preserve the endogenous antioxidant α-tocopherol in LDL. Harats et al. (38) found significantly higher TBARS concentrations in plasma and LDL 90 minutes after acute smoking of 5–7 cigarettes. Increased oxidizability of LDL was not seen when subjects were supplemented for 4 weeks with vitamins C or E. Because oxidative modification of nucleic acid can lead to genetic damage, the protective role of antioxidants may play a major role at the initiation stage. Mutagenic effects of smoking are well documented in the literature by counting sister-chromatid exchanges as well as micronuclei in circulating human lymphocytes. The cytokinesis-block micronuclei assay can be used as a marker of DNA damage induced by oxidative stress.

We studied the effects of vitamin C and E intake on the signal intensity of semihydroascorbate radical used as a marker of oxidative stress in human plasma. Twelve smokers and 12 nonsmokers followed a 14-day supplementation with 1000 mg ascorbic acid daily during the first week and 1000 mg ascorbic acid and 335.5 mg α-tocopherol daily during the second week. Measurement of these antioxidants showed significant lower plasma concentrations in smokers than in nonsmokers. After 7-day intake of vitamin C, the group of smokers had a significant increase in the electron paramagnetic resonance signal intensity ($p < 0.05$) and plasma ascorbic acid ($p < 0.001$). Nonsmokers had no such increase (Fig. 5). To further evaluate the association of the ascorbate radical concentration with the amount of ascorbic acid in blood plasma, it was essential to compare both parameters. A correlation with significant increases in smokers can be seen

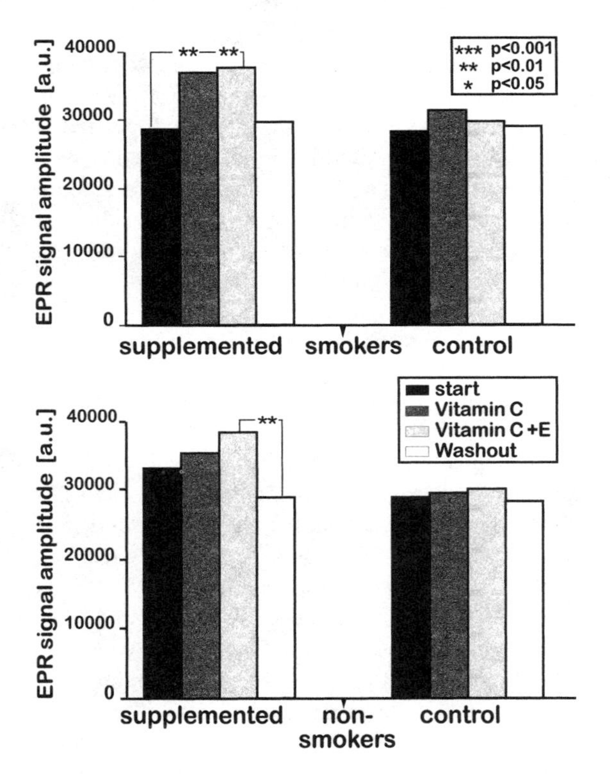

Figure 5 EPR spectroscopic measurements of the semihydroascorbate radicals in human plasma of smokers and nonsmokers on day 0, day 7, day 14, and day 21. Data represent the mean values (X ± SEM, $n = 6$) of the signal height of the spectral lines. 6 smokers and 6 nonsmokers received 1000 mg ascorbic acid daily during the first week and 1000 mg ascorbic acid and 335.5 mg α-tocopherol daily during the second week. Control groups (6 donors) received no vitamins. Bars represent mean values (X ± SEM, $n = 6$) obtained from 6 donors. p-values relate to comparisons of a given parameter versus the same parameter one week before within one group: $p < 0.05$; ** $p < 0.01$; *** $p < 0.001$; **** $p < 0.0001$.

after 7-day intake of vitamin C. In nonsmokers this effect was not as pronounced, but a significant decline in plasma concentration of ascorbate and ascorbate radical formation was observed after washout of the supplements. The fact that the initial ascorbate radical intensity is directly proportional to the overall rate of ascorbate oxidation demonstrates an increase in ongoing oxidative stress in smokers, whereas nonsmokers did not show such effects after intake of vitamin C and E. In addition, the significant decrease of the ratio of ascorbate radical to ascorbic acid, which was only evident in smokers after one-week supplementation with vitamin C, indicates the demand of antioxidants. Further treatment for 7 days with vitamin E revealed no effects on ascorbate radical formation in either group, but a substantial ($p < 0.0001$) decline was observed in nonsmokers after washout of the supplements. The micronuclei (MN) test performed by the cytokinesis-block method as an indicator of mutagenic effects showed appreciably higher values of micronuclei in smokers compared to nonsmokers (Fig. 6). During supplementation with vitamins C and E, a reduction in micronuclei frequency was evident in smokers and nonsmokers. However, the decrease was significant only in smokers ($p < 0.05$) after administration of both vitamins. To understand the mechanism of protection provided by supplementation with antioxidants, it is important to test the vitamins in vivo. Therefore, we used the micronuclei and sister-chromatial exchange (SCE) assay as different indicators of mutagenic effects induced by oxidative stress. The SCE frequency is especially increased by genotoxic agents disturbing DNA synthesis, while the number of micronuclei responds to a broad variety of mutagens causing clastogenic and aneugenic effects. In our study the number of SCE was significantly higher in smokers than in nonsmokers. However, vitamin supplementation did not change the SCE frequencies significantly. This result probably indicates that S-phase–dependent DNA damage is not influenced by the vitamins C and E. Our findings are consistent with data published by van Rensburg et al. (39). The frequencies of MN had significantly higher levels at the beginning in smokers as compared to nonsmokers. Following vitamin C treatment the mean values decreased slightly but not significantly in both groups. However, the combined vitamin C and E treatment induced a further MN reduction in both groups with a significant minimum in smokers. These data differ from findings of Podmore et al. (29), who used levels of 8-oxoguanine and 8-oxoadenine in peripheral blood lymphocytes as markers of DNA damage. Supplementation of 500 mg of vitamin C per day induced a significant increase in 8-oxoadenine. These somewhat conflicting results of vitamin C supplementation may be explained by the very different mutagenic assays used in our study. Furthermore, Levine et al. and Poulsen et al. mentioned that artefactual oxidation may have occurred during lymphocyte isolation and DNA extraction in the study of Podmore et al. (29). In the present report (31), in vitro effects can be excluded due to the fact that spontaneous occurrence of MN in human lymphocytes are generally rare. In addition, we measured TBARS as a

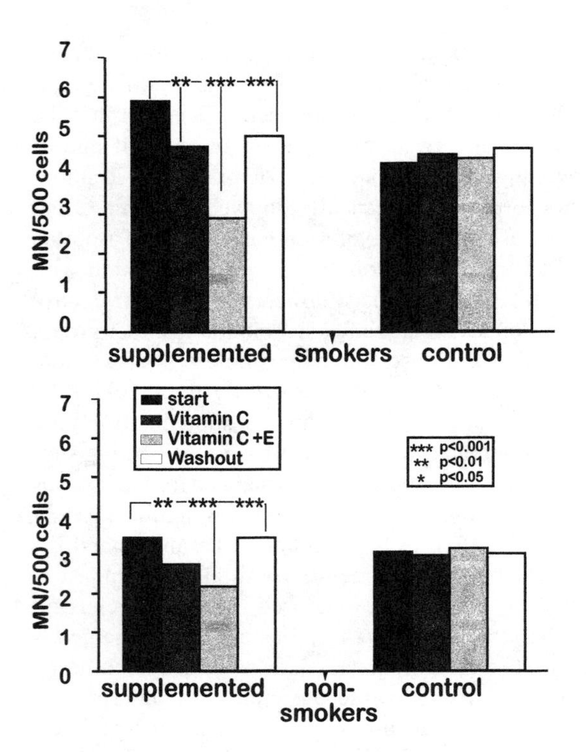

Figure 6 The frequency of micronuclei in peripheral blood lymphocytes of smokers and nonsmokers on day 0, day 7, day 14, and day 21. Bars represent mean values of MN per 500 BN cells (X ± SEM, $n = 6$). Conditions of study design are as given in the legend to Fig. 5.

marker of lipid peroxides, which are potential contributors to the background genetic damage. Similar to the results of the CBMN assay, rates of TBARS were reduced after intake of ascorbic acid and α-tocopherol, indicating a correlation of both parameters.

The results document that despite normal dietary intake of antioxidants in smokers and nonsmokers, supplementation can substantially reduce oxidative damage. However, the effect of these vitamins is greater in nonsmokers, underlining the health benefit of smoking cessation.

IV. SAFETY ASPECTS

NC either as supplements or added value (in a functional food) are offered to the general population as safe and healthy. As long as NC are components of the traditional diet and their daily intake does not exceed the usual (physiological) level, i.e., the level (range) to which we are evolutionary adapted, these NC can be claimed as safe. Whether NC elicit a benefit at physiological concentrations with respect to disease prevention is still unknown. However, if the intake exceeds the physiological level, concerns have been raised as to whether NC blur the line between foods and drugs. The latter implies that side effects might occur following a long and high intake of a NC. The results of the ATBC (32) and CARET (33) studies which show an increasing risk for lung cancers in smokers taking either 30 mg of β-carotene or 20 mg of β-carotene plus 25,000 IU of vitamin A for a period of 5 or 4 years, respectively, document that even generally recognized as safe (GRAS) nutraceuticals might be harmful. The intake level of β-carotene in both studies exceeded the reported maximum intake from a normal diet two- to threefold. Nevertheless, a higher intake of vitamin E might be beneficial, but we do not know whether an intake of 400 mg (25 times the normal dietary intake) might have side effects after a longer time period. In addition, modification of the micronutrient pattern in functional foods might cause problems. Altered intakes of dietary amino acids, for example, modulate the activity of a variety of major metabolic systems, not the least of which is the kinetics of amino acids oxidation (34). This regulation occurs at very low intakes, and the precise mechanism and system involved depend on the specific amino acid. Young and Marchini (34) were able to demonstrate that these effects occurred at every level of protein metabolism, ranging from transcription to posttranslational and degradation. It seems clear that any modification of absorption and digestion of amino acids or any other nutrient could result in profound regulatory changes. As a result, dietary recommendations should take into account not only what foods should be eaten but also the optimal nutrient pattern in relation to the totality of the diet and lifestyle. In the transition from the molecular to the systemic, the univariable experiments so popular with nutrition scientists will have to be replaced by much more complex experiments in which a variety of variables and specific biomarkers must be considered simultaneously (35).

The research on NC offers a fascinating and promising link between nutrition and medicine. For the first time there will be a chance to prevent diseases before clinical symptoms occur. Overall, it is important to understand the role of food (both its nutrient and nonnutrient components) in modulating expression and risk of diseases and to ensure that food products designed to prevent or treat diseases are indeed safe (Table 7).

The research priorities reflect this approach but rely on a body of basic research that elucidates the underlying genetic, biochemical, and pathophysiological mechanisms. While the general relationship of diet to the major chronic diseases is now recognized, further research is needed to identify and characterize the specific dietary factors and their roles. The products mentioned in Table 7 claim health benefits that have not been scientifically validated or contain pharmaceutical ingredients, as is the case with Cholestin.

Table 7 Nutraceuticals Currently Under Development or on the Market

Type	Product description	Claims
Dietary supplement	Cardia; salt alternative	Lowers blood pressure
Dietary supplement	Cholestin; lovastatin from red rice yeast	Lowers cholesterol
Dietary supplement	Lactoferrin; cactoferrin sequesters iron, hampering microbial growth	Antimicrobial for use in immunocompromised patients or premature infants
	Lysozyme; an antibacterial enzyme that attacks cell walls	Antimicrobial for use in immunocompromised patients or premature infants
Dietary supplement	Neuromins; contains DHA	Lowers heart disease risk
Functional food	Formulaid; infant formula supplement contains algae- and fungi-derived fatty acids DHA and ARA	Enhances neurological and visual development in infants
Dietary supplement	SeaGold; contains DHA.	Lowers heart disease risk
Functional food	Laurical; canola oil engineered to be high in laurate	Lowers cholesterol
Functional food	Ostar; beta-glucan derived from oat	Aids in control of blood glucose
Functional food	Soybean and canola oils engineered without *trans* fatty acids	Lowers heart disease risk
Functional food	Phytrol; plant-derived sterol FCP	Lowers heart disease risk
Functional food	Proventra; kefir supplemented with bovine polyclonal antibodies	Boosts immune function
Functional food	PMS Escape; a candy bar	Boosts serotonin levels in brain, with benefit in premenstrual syndrome
Functional food	Benecol margarine; contains stanol	Reduces absorption of cholesterol in gut
Medical food	NiteBite; time-release glucose snack bar for diabetics	Prevents nocturnal hypoglycemia
Medical food	Nutritional drink for diabetics; plant-derived insulin	Potentiating factor that aids insulin
Medical food	Bile-salt stimulated lipase; breaks down lipids in gut	For CF patients and newborns

Perhaps more important, it seems clear that, given the nature of the product to be tested, human evaluations will have to be made prior to the approval of these products for general distribution. One of the important virtues of the modern food distribution system is that within a few days virtually all segments of the population of industrialized countries can be exposed to new products. On the other hand, this efficient distribution system presents a special problem: it does not provide an opportunity for limited human experience prior to widespread distribution. As a result, some kind of controlled human exposure will have to be included as part of the testing program. In turn, this will place more pressure on studies designed to determine the metabolism of nutrients and other materials in new food products to provide a basis for designing the protocols for human studies, since the kind of testing that can be done on people is severely limited.

What this suggests is that the most important scientific questions today and in the future will be not in the classical, separable areas of toxicology, nutrition, and food science, but rather in the interface among toxicology and nutrition, genetics, molecular biology, and food science.

Biomarker studies with intermediate endpoints reflecting the efficacy of an NC in preventing a disease process will be needed. A disease-related valid biomarker will allow us to control and compare epidemiological and intervention studies. Because of the complexity of the products that contain phytochemicals and the analytical procedures involved, future research should consider standardization of experimental design, test substances, availability of standards, appropriate development, and choice of analytical procedures. Consideration should also be given to the characterization of the test substance after it is incorporated into complex food matrices and to the prevention of the formation of artefacts during the extraction process. Acceleration of and improved access to the latest and most complete scientific information available about functional foods and more useful databases on phytochemicals will also be needed. Support for information technology and allocation of adequate resources will be essential for continued relevant research on NC (36). Individual need depends on many different variables, including individual diseases, genetic polymorphism, or environmental factors.

Nutraceuticals that are based on clear scientific data demonstrating efficacy and safety will indeed be a good and beneficial link between nutrition and medicine.

REFERENCES

1. DeFelice SL. Nutraceuticals: Opportunities in an Emerging Market. Scrip Mag 9; 1992.
2. Agus DB, Gambhir SS, Pardridge WM. Vitamin C crosses the blood-brain barrier

in the oxidized form through the glucose transporters. J Clin Invest 100(11):2842–2848, 1997.
3. Boushey CJ, Beresford SA, Omenn GS. A quantitative assessment of plasma homocysteine as a risk factor for vascular disease probable benefits of increasing folic acid intakes. JAMA 274:1049–1057, 1995.
4. Kang SS, Wong PW, Susmeno A. Thermolabile methylene tetrahydrofolate reductase: an inherited risk factor for coronary artery disease. Am J Hum Gene 48:536–545, 1991.
5. Monta H, Taguchi J, Kurihara H. Genetic polymorphism of 5, 10-methylene tetrahydrofolate reductase as a risk factor for coronary artery disease. Circulation 95:2032–2036, 1997.
6. Mathew P, Wylli R, Van Lente F, Steffen RM, Kay MH. Antioxidants in hereditary pancreatitis. Am J Gastroenterol 91(8):1558–1562, 1996.
7. Glass AG, Hoover RN. The emerging epidemic of melanoma and squamous cell skin cancer. JAMA 262:2097–2100, 1989.
8. Jung EG. Photocarcinogenesis of the skin. J Dermatol 18:1–10, 1991.
9. Moan J, Dahlback A. The relationship between skin cancers, solar radiation and ozone depletion. Br J Cancer 65:916–921, 1992.
10. Kripke ML. Immunology and photocarcinogenesis. J Am Acad Dermatol 14:149–155, 1986.
11. Baadsgaard O. In vivo ultraviolet irradiation of human skin results in profound perturbation of the immune system. Arch Dermatol 127:99–109, 1991.
12. Kochevar IE, Pathak MA, Parish JA. Photophysics, photochemistry and photobiology. In: Dermatology in General Medicine. New York: McGraw-Hill, 1987, pp 1441–1451.
13. Mathews-Roth MM. Photoprotection by carotenoids. Fed Proc 46:1890–1893, 1987.
14. Mathews-Roth MM, Krinsky NI. Carotenoids affect development of UV-B induced skin cancer. Photochem Photobiol 46:507–509, 1987.
15. Krinsky N. Antioxidant functions of carotenoids. Free Rad Biol Med 7:617–635, 1988.
16. White WS, Kim C, Kalkwarf HJ, Bustos P, Roe DA. Ultraviolet light-induced reductions in plasma carotenoid levels. Am J Clin Nutr 47:879–883, 1988.
17. Berne B, Nilsson M, Vahlquist A. UV irradiation and cutaneous vitamin A: an experimental study in rabbit and human skin. J Invest Dermatol 83:401–404, 1984.
18. Wang Z, Boudjelal M, Kang S, Voorhees JJ, Fisher GJ. Ultraviolet irradiation of human skin causes functional vitamin A deficiency, preventable by all-trans retinoic acid pre-treatment. Nature Med 5:418–422, 1999.
19. Francz PI, Conrad J, Biesalski HK. Effect of retinoic acid on UVA/B-induced gene expression and lipid peroxidation in human skin fibroblasts in vitro. Biol Chem 379: 1263–1269, 1998.
20. Russell DH. Ornithine decarboxylase as a marker of carcinogenesis. In: Milman HA, Weisburger EK, eds. Handbook of Carcinogen Testing. Park Ridge, NJ: Noyes Publishers, 1985:464–481.
21. Pegg AE. Polyamine metabolism and its importance in neoplastic growth and as target for chemotherapy. Cancer Res 48:759–774, 1988.

22. Niggli HJ, Francz PI. May ultraviolet light-induced ornithine decarboxylase response in mitotic and postmitotic human skin fibroblasts serve as a marker of aging and differentiation? Age 15:55–60, 1992.
23. Pegg AE. Recent advances in the biochemistry of polyamines in eukaryotes. Biochem J 234:249–262, 1986.
24. McCann PP, Pegg AE, Sjoerdsma A. Inhibition of polyamine metabolism. In: Biological Significance and Basis for New Therapies. Orlando, FL: Academic Press, 1987, pp 1–371.
25. Biesalski HK, Hemmes C, Hopfenmuller W, Schmid C, Gollnick HP. Effects of controlled exposure of sunlight on plasma and skin levels of beta-carotene. Free Radic Res 24:215–224, 1996.
26. Talwar HS, Griffiths CEM, Fisher GJ, Hamilton TA, Voorhees J. Reduced type I and type III procollagens in photodamaged adult human skin. J Invest Dermatol 105: 285–290, 1995.
27. Van Weelden H, De Gruijl FR, Van der Leun JC. In: The Biological Effects of UV-A Radiation. Urbach F, Gange RW, eds. New York: Praeger, 1986, pp 137–146.
28. Fisher GJ, Datta SC, Talwar HS, Wang ZQ, Varani J, Kang S, Vorhees J. Molecular basis of sun-induced premature skin ageing and retinoid antagonism. Nature 379: 335–339, 1996.
29. Podmore ID, Griffiths HR, Herbert KE, Mistry N, Mistry P, Lunec J. Vitamin C exhibits pro-oxidant properties. Nature 392:559, 1998.
30. Cooke MS, Evans MD, Posmore ID, Herbert KE, Mistry N, Mistry P, Hickenbotham PT, Hussieni A, Griffiths HR, Lunec J. Novel repair action of vitamin C upon in vivo oxidative DNA damage. FEBS Lett 439(3):363–367, 1998.
31. Schneider M, Diemer K, Engelhart K, Zankl H, Trommer WE, Biesalski HK. Protective effects of vitamins C and E in smokers monitored by the semidehydroascorbate radical formation in plasma and the frequency of micronuclei in lymphocytes. Free Rad Res (in press).
32. Albanes D, Heinonen OP, Huttunen JK. Effects of α-tocopherol and β-carotene supplements on cancer incidence in the Alpha-Tocopherol Beta-Carotene Cancer Prevention Study. Am J Clin Nutr 62:1427S–1430S, 1995.
33. Omenn GS, Goodman GE, Thornquist MD. Effects of a combination of beta carotene and vitamin A on lung cancer and cardiovascular disease. N Engl J Med 334:1150–1155, 1996.
34. Young VR, Marchini JS. Mechanisms and nutritional significance of metabolic responses to altered intakes of protein and amino acids with reference to nutritional adaptation in humans. Am J Clin Nutr 51:270, 1990.
35. Miller SA, Stephenson MG. Scientific and public health rationale for the dietary guidelines. Am J Clin Nutr 42:739, 1985.
36. Kaaks R, Riboli E, Sinha R. Biochemical markers of dietary intake. In: Tonilio P, ed. Application of Biomarkers in Cancer Epidemiology. Lyon: IARC-Scientific Publications, 1997, pp. 103–126.
37. Church DF, Burkey TJ, Pryor WA. Preparation of human lung tissue from cigarette smokers for analysis by electron spin resonance spectroscopy. Methods Enzymol 186:665–669, 1990.

38. Harats D, Ben-Naim M, Dabach Y, Hollander G, Havivi E, Stein O, Stein Y. Effect of vitamin C and E supplementation on suceptibility of plasma lipoproteins to peroxidation induced by acute smoking. Atherosclerosis 85(1):47–54, 1990.
39. van Rensburg CE, Theron A, Richards GA, van der Merwe CA, Anderson R. Investigation of the relationships between plasma levels of ascorbate, vitamin E and β-carotene and the frequency of sister-chromatid exchanges and release of reactive oxidants by blood leucocytes from cigarette smokers. Mutat Res 215(2):167–172, 1989.
40. Duke JA. The Green Pharmacy. Emmaus, PA: Rodale Press, 1997.
41. Jentzsch AM, Bachmann H, Fürst P, Biesalski HK. Improved analysis of malondialdehyde in human body fluids. Free Radic Biol Med 20:251–256, 1996.

2

The Role of Vitamin E in the Emerging Field of Nutraceuticals

Lester Packer
University of Southern California School of Pharmacy, Los Angeles, California

Stefan U. Weber
University of California, Berkeley, California

The aim of this chapter is to review the role of nutraceuticals in oxidative stress and healthy aging. The first part is an introduction to life span, oxidative stress, antioxidants, and the concept of nutraceuticals. In the second part, the results of large-scale epidemiological studies on health risks and antioxidants are discussed, showing beneficial effects of the main lipophilic antioxidant vitamin E. Vitamin E, its isoforms, and their potential as nutraceuticals are the focus of the remainder of the chapter.

I. THE CHANGING LIFE SPAN

From 1900 to 1985 there was a drastic change in life span throughout the world. At every stage of life, life span was extended. When comparing the percentage of surviving females in the United States in 1900 and 1985 (1) (Fig. 1), a considerable shift in curve occurred, indicating a longer life expectancy. This shift is attributed primarily to three factors: advances in medicine, particularly in the ability to control infectious diseases, better hygiene, and better nutrition. These factors have led to a remarkable 65% reduction in mortality. Although another 65% reduction in mortality cannot be expected in the next 85 years, extending the average human life span may continue at a slower rate in the future by manip-

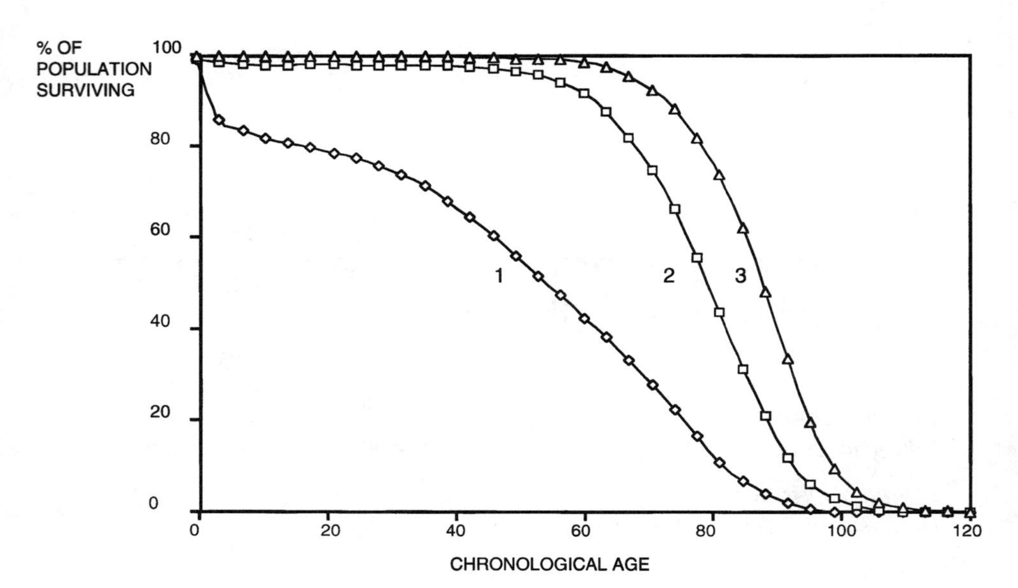

Figure 1 Survival curves displaying the average life expectancy for U.S. females. Curve 1 displays the survival for a person born in 1900, curve 2 the survival for people born in 1985, and curve 3 the survival if a similar reduction in the death rate as the one from curve 1 to 2 occurs again. (From Ref. 1.)

ulating the delicate balance between the environment and the body's antioxidants and other defense mechanisms.

The increasing number of centenarians through the years reflects this drastic reduction in mortality. Between 1980 and 1990, there were a total of 126,752 female and 27,669 male centenarians recorded in 13 countries in which reliable birth and death registries exist. In particular, 55,761 females and 13,066 males reached 100, resulting in a 4:1 ratio, while 57 females and 7 males reached 110 or older, resulting in an 8:1 ratio (2,3) (Fig. 2). All of the centenarians examined had remarkably good immune system function. Therefore it is thought that the key to controlling life span is linked to the processes essential to the body's maintenance. Besides having a healthy immune system, the ability to repair DNA, the presence of antioxidants and stress proteins, accurate DNA replication, accurate protein synthesis, and tumor suppression also play an essential role in healthy aging according to the predictions of the disposable soma theory of aging (3). Among these, antioxidants are the only factor that can be manipulated by diet. Antioxidants prevent oxidation of important biomolecules. Oxidative stress and the role antioxidants play will be discussed in the following sections.

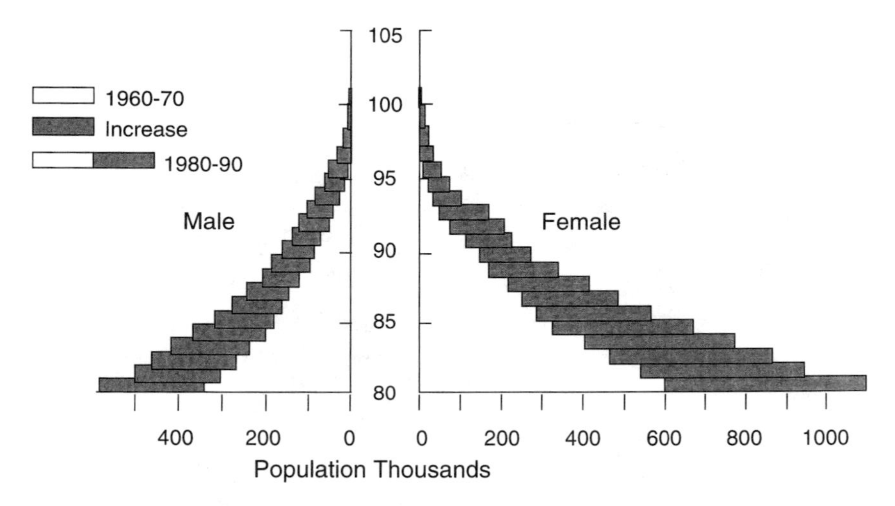

Figure 2 Growth of the oldest old population from 13 European countries with good demographic data. The white part of the graph displays the situation from 1960 to 1970. The largest increases in population have occurred for ages just over 80 years, but the population of centenarians has increased explosively. (From Ref. 63.)

II. FREE RADICALS AND OXIDATIVE STRESS

All through our lives, we have a fire burning inside of us fueled by our metabolism, which is constantly generating free radicals as a byproduct. These free radicals, generated mainly by mitochondria, cause chronic oxidative stress. Using Helmut Sies's definition, oxidative stress is ''a change in the prooxidant-antioxidant balance in favor of the former, potentially leading to biological damage'' (4). Given this definition, molecular markers are expected to be generated during oxidative stress. Free radicals are direct indicators of oxidative processes. There are many sources of free radicals from both the external and internal environments. An important source is our own body's metabolism. It follows that more free radicals are generated during strenuous exercise than during sedentary activity. Alcohol as an ingredient in beverages also increases the formation of free radicals by oxidative metabolism (5). In the body, free radicals play an essential role in enzyme-catalyzed reactions, activation of nuclear transcription factors (6), and gene expression (7). In fact, many systems involving signal transduction seem to include steps that require oxidative processes (8). Also, reactive oxygen species (ROS) are a part of the defense mechanism used by our immune system to generate free radicals to target tumor cells and microbial infections (9–11).

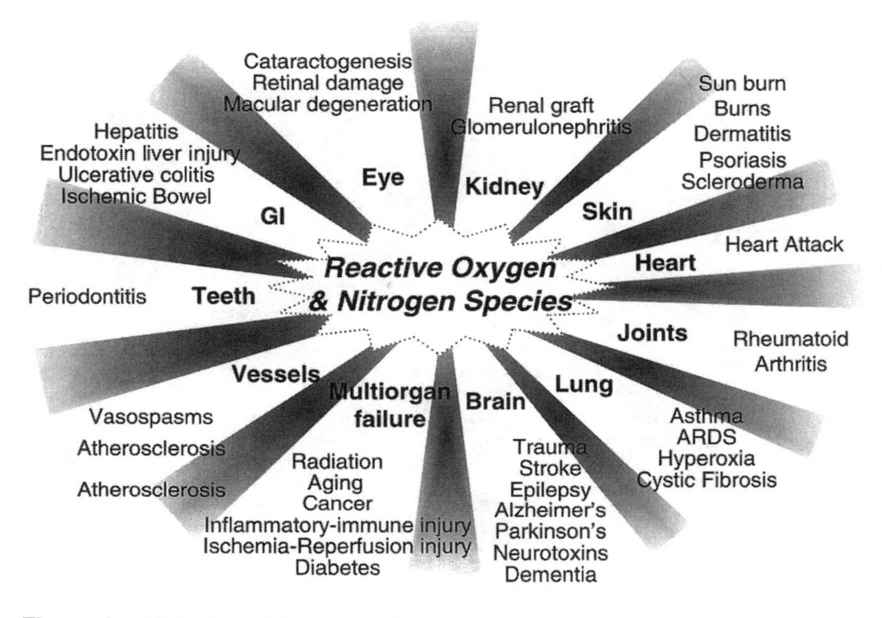

Figure 3 Clinical conditions involving free radicals.

Although free radicals are essential to the body, in excess they may lead to cytotoxicity and oxidative damage to healthy tissue that may lead to disorders. Most clinical conditions show evidence of free radical damage (12,13) (Fig. 3). There is evidence of free radical damage to major organs and the brain caused by the chronic diseases of aging and by neurological diseases (14). For example, the formation of cataracts in the eye is a result of oxidative damage and is associated with aging (15)—everyone will get a cataract if he or she lives long enough. In many such disorders, supplementation with antioxidants has been shown to be beneficial (16,17).

III. ANTIOXIDANTS

Antioxidants have been defined in many different ways. For the purposes of this chapter, an antioxidant is any substance that, following absorption from the gastrointestinal tract, participates in physiological, biochemical, and cellular processes that inactivate free radicals or prevent free radical–initiated chemical reactions. It possesses the attributes of nutrients that may be either directly affected

Table 1 Proteins in the Body with Antioxidant Properties

Proteins	Function
Superoxide dismutases (copper/zinc, manganese)	Superoxide removal
Catalase (iron), thioredoxin, glutathione peroxidases (Se)(cytosolic and phospholipid), thioredoxin peroxidase	Hydroperoxide removal
Thioredoxin	Protein disulfide reduction
Glutathione disulfide reductase	Oxidized glutathione reduction
Thioredoxin disulfide reductase	Oxidized thioredoxin reduction
Glutathione-S-transferase hydroperoxide	Toxic metabolite removal
Methionine sulfoxide reductase	Repair oxidized methionine residues
Transferrin ferro-oxidase	Iron transport
Ferritin	Iron storage
Ceruloplasm	Copper storage

by antioxidants and free radicals or indirectly affected by changing the redox balance.

Many different enzymes and proteins have antioxidant functions (Table 1). Some proteins bind transition metals like iron and copper in such a way that they cannot participate in free radical reactions during delivery to tissues. New proteins and enzymes with antioxidant function are still being discovered. For example, ferro-oxidase is an enzyme that will deliver iron into mitochondrial ferritin so that the iron is not able to generate free radical reactions (18). Also, many familiar substances found in the diet have been identified as antioxidants. Fruits and vegetables provide important substances, such as vitamin C, vitamin E, carotenes, bioflavonoids, lipoic acid, and ubiquinone, which are part of the antioxidant defense system (19).

IV. THE ANTIOXIDANT NETWORK

A metabolic antioxidant is a substance that protects biological tissue from free radical damage due to its ability to recycle or regenerate biological reductants. Most antioxidants are redox-active substances such as vitamins E and C, lipoic acids, bioflavonoids, and other polyphenols. The exceptions are the carotenoids, which act as sinks for singlet oxygen and other free radical reactions. Other antioxidants act as reductants that exist in different environments. It is well accepted that these metabolic antioxidants act together to create what is now called the

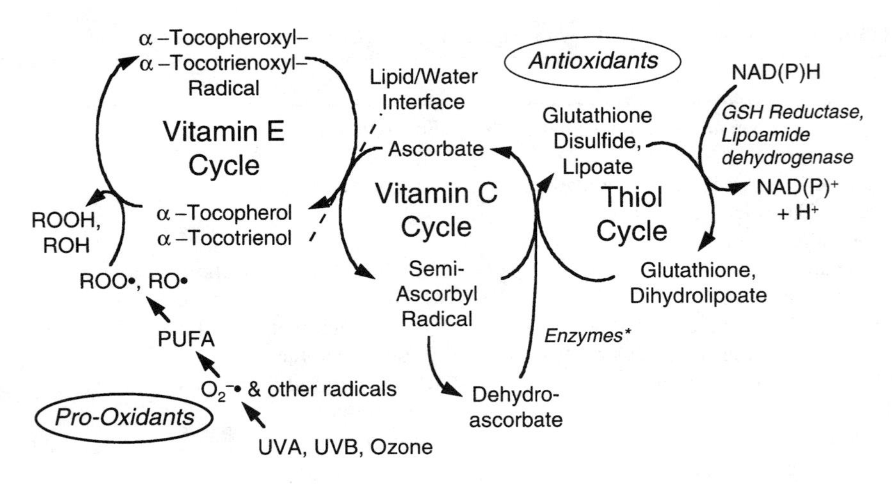

Figure 4 The redox antioxidant network.

antioxidant network (Fig. 4). This term refers to the ability of different antioxidants to interact with one another and to regenerate each other. When membrane-bound tocopherol protects the biomembrane from oxidation, it reacts with a radical to form a tocopheroxyl radical. This radical is more stable than the scavenged one. At the lipid/water interface, ascorbate can react nonenzymatically with the vitamin E radical in order to regenerate tocopherol (20). In this reaction ascorbate becomes the semiascorbyl radical, which in turn can be recycled to ascorbate by glutathione using different enzymes such as glutaredoxin, protein disulfide isomerase, and thioredoxin reductase. If vitamin C is further oxidized to dehydroascorbate, ascorbate can be regenerated by glutathione-dependent dehydroascorbate reductase. Oxidized glutathione can be reduced by enzymes like glutathione reductase consuming metabolic energy in the form of NADPH. In summary, metabolic energy feeds into the thiol cycle, which enzymatically feeds into the vitamin C cycle, which finally regenerates vitamin E nonenzymatically in the vitamin E cycle (21). Other redox-active substances can participate in the antioxidant network, e.g., lipoic acid can nonenzymatically regenerate vitamin C (22).

Experimental evidence for the recycling of vitamin E can be obtained by electron spin resonance (ESR) analysis of the tocopheroxyl and the semiascorbyl radical in human low-density lipoprotein (LDL) (23). If vitamin E is oxidized by radical reactions, the tocopheroxyl radical appears. If, however, vitamin C is present during the reaction, it will regenerate vitamin E by undergoing oxidation to the semiascorbyl radical, which is detectable in ESR. Under these experimental conditions the vitamin E radical signal will disappear until all of the vitamin C is consumed. There is a linear relationship between the lag period of the return of the tocopheroxyl radical and the concentration of vitamin E. Since many small molecule antioxidants occur naturally and are part of our diet, they are ideal candidates to be nutraceuticals.

V. NUTRACEUTICALS

There are many different yet similar definitions of nutraceuticals:

1. Any substance that may be considered a food or part of a food and provides medical or health benefits, including the prevention and treatment of disease (24).
2. A food or any part of a food that offers a health benefit above and beyond providing simple nutritional or basic fortification (25). Under this definition, the health benefit may include the prevention or treatment of disease or the enhancement of the body's functioning.
3. Any substance that is a food or part of a food that provides medical or health benefits including the prevention and/or treatment of disease. Such products may range from isolated nutrients, dietary supplements, and diets to genetically engineered designer foods, herbal products, and processed foods such as cereals, soups, and beverages (26). It is important to note that this definition applies to all categories of foods and parts of food.

Nutraceuticals are the "active" ingredients of so-called functional foods. For example, orange juice containing extra fiber as well as manufactured foods packed with nutrients are considered functional foods. Unlike Japan, the United States does not have an official definition of a functional food, but many in the U.S. food industry agree that functional foods are foods specifically formulated to deliver health benefits. Functional foods defined as conventional foods with added health benefits are novel and are increasing in popularity in most industrialized countries. Individual products are subject to heated debate because of the controversial marketing of their proposed health benefits. Scientific evidence is required to support the claims for individual products.

VI. VITAMIN E AND THE PREVENTION OF DISEASE

Vitamin E has been identified as a substance with important antioxidant qualities. Numerous studies have identified the benefits of vitamin E in health and disease. It has been linked to a reduction in the risk for heart disease, delay of disease progression in Alzheimer's patients, and it may be important in cancer prevention

(27,28). A cross-cultural study involving 20 different study populations in Europe produced very interesting results regarding the activity of vitamin E as an antioxidant. This study looked at the number of people who died of ischemic heart disease in different parts of Europe. When comparing the average deaths per 100,000 for six populations in northern Europe (355) to the average for the population in southern Europe (99), a significant 3.5-fold difference was observed (29).

High cholesterol, which is correlated with ischemic heart disease mortality, accounted for the difference in 12 study populations. For the other 8 study populations, there was no difference in cholesterol and heart disease mortality, but there was an inverse correlation between the plasma level of vitamin E α-tocopherol level and death. A higher concentration of vitamin E resulted in lower mortality. After normalizing the data from the other 12 populations and examining it again, there was still a high correlation between the plasma vitamin E level and ischemic heart disease mortality.

The 88,000 nurses study was another investigation which correlated vitamin E concentrations with lowering the risk for major coronary heart disease. This study showed that participants who took 200 IU or more of vitamin E a day in their diet for at least 2 years benefited by a 41% reduction in relative risk for major coronary disease (30) (Fig. 5). Many risk factors such as smoking, blood pressure, menopause, etc., were taken into account, but not one factor could be singled out as a cause. A similar study carried out with 29,000 male physicians

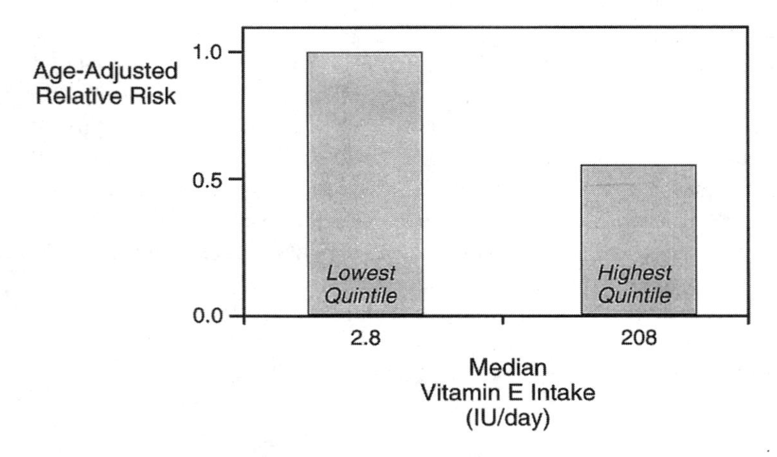

Figure 5 In the 88,000 Nurses Study, dietary vitamin E greater than 200 IU (mg/day) was associated with a 41% decreased risk for major coronary heart disease.

also produced almost the same results reducing the risk for major coronary heart disease by 37% (31).

Although 200 IU of vitamin E is 20 times the recommended daily allowance in the United States, another study, the Cambridge Heart Antioxidant Study (CHAOS), increased the amount of supplementation and still obtained positive results (32). In this study, 2002 men and women who had had one heart attack were separated into two groups who were given either 400 or 800 IU of vitamin E a day for a period of 510 days. Those people who were given the supplementation had a 77% decrease in the occurrence of a second heart attack (nonfatal myocardial infarction) (Fig. 6). This study shows that vitamin E is not only preventative but is in a way a treatment for disease, and we may see more and more disease treated using nutritional antioxidants in conjunction with established medicinal management strategies.

Besides lowering the risk for cardiovascular disease, vitamin E supplementation has also shown benefits in Alzheimer's patients. Mary Sano and her colleagues at Columbia University carried out a study in which 2000 IU of vitamin E in the form of α-tocopherol, 200 times the daily allowance, was given to 347 Alzheimer's disease patients. Event-free survival was remarkably delayed in the patients with supplementation (33). Since Alzheimer's is not as widespread as atherosclerosis, the study population was rather small, but currently a follow-up study is being carried out involving 720 patients.

Vitamin E has also been linked to cancer prevention. Paul Knekt (34) ana-

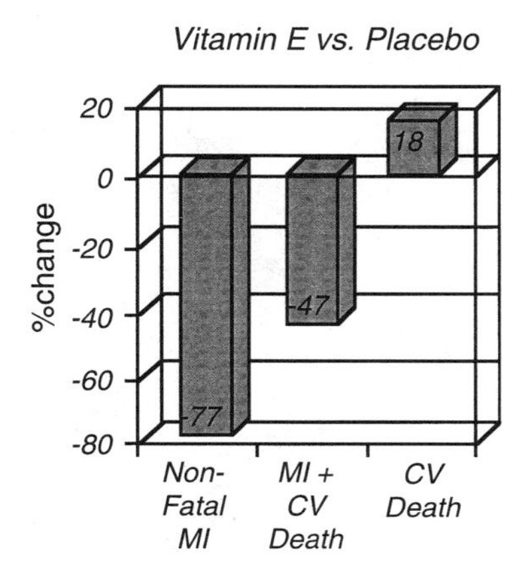

Figure 6 Results of the Cambridge Heart Antioxidant Study (CHAOS): vitamin E supplementation (controlled by placebo treatment) decreased the risk for nonfatal myocardial infarction.

Table 2 Dietary Sources of Vitamin E

Vegetable oil	Caloric intake for vitamin E levels	
	200 mg	2000 mg
Wheat germ	1,353	13,530
Soybean/Corn	2,250	22,500
Sunflower	3,674	36,735
Safflower	5,294	52,940

lyzed more than 100 studies regarding vitamin E. Most of the studies analyzed were case-controlled or nested studies and often relied on dietary questionnaires. Also very few of the studies were intervention studies that involved introducing an exact amount of vitamin E into the study population. Nevertheless, in these 100 studies, most of the cases showed a beneficial effect correlated with higher plasma levels of vitamin E, and Knekt's analysis suggests that vitamin E has important cancer-prevention activity (34).

Epidemiological evidence demonstrates that vitamin E has a remarkable effect of decreasing the risk of cardiovascular disease, and it also has important implications for Alzheimer's and cancer patients. All of these studies used amounts of vitamin E that are virtually impossible to obtain through natural sources. In order to obtain the 200 mg of vitamin E used in the 88,000 nurses study through wheat germ oil—the vegetable oil that is the richest source of vitamin E—1300 calories would have to be consumed in a day. It follows that 13,000 calories would have to be consumed in order to reach the levels of the Alzheimer's study. Because the recommended average caloric intake per day is 2,000 calories, all of the calories in the diet would have to come from the oil (Table 2).

VII. MOLECULAR BASIS FOR VITAMIN E ACTION

Multiple studies of the health and biological effects of vitamin E have been carried out. We know that human lipoproteins, particularly LDL, are carriers of vitamin E to peripheral tissues. A typical LDL particle consists of about 2500 molecules, 7 of which are vitamin E: 6.5 molecules of α-tocopherol, 0.5 molecule of γ-tocopherol. No other vitamin E molecules are generally found in LDL. Vitamin E molecules in LDL proteins have been found to remarkably suppress the severity of coronary artery disease. There was a significant negative correlation between the stenosis score (the blood flow score) and the LDL vitamin E concentration, which showed that the higher the vitamin E level in the LDL (not the plasma), the lower the stenosis score (35).

It is known that LDL, which is easily susceptible to oxidation, is one of the many risk factors for atherosclerosis. Herman Esterbauer, a pioneer of research on LDL oxidation, described the process of LDL oxidation (36). It was shown that the first antioxidant that disappeared in LDL subjected to oxidative stress was vitamin E, followed by carotenoids at different rates. After the lipophilic antioxidants are completely consumed, oxidative damage accumulates and conjugated dienes are formed in the lipid components of the LDL. This was monitored by following the absorbance of a suspension of LDL at 234 nm. Esterbauer studied the effects of the addition of α-tocopherol to a human LDL suspension in vitro on the lag time—the time required for the initiation of the accumulation of lipid damage in LDL. There was a linear positive correlation between the amount of tocotrienol that was added to the LDL and the length of lag time, in which the higher the concentration of the tocotrienol that was administered to the suspension of LDL, the longer the lag time. These data point toward the idea that vitamin E serves as protection against LDL oxidation.

Vitamin E consists of a family of eight different molecules consisting of four different tocopherols—α, β, δ, γ (Fig. 7). Each tocopherol is different depending on the substitutions of different methyl groups around the aromatic ring. Vitamin E contains a phenolic hydroxyl group that is the active portion of the molecule. It quenches free radicals similar to lipid peroxyl radicals using hydrogen and/or electron donation (27). Tocotrienols are another naturally occurring form of vitamin E that differs only with respect to the tail of the molecule, with three unsaturated double bonds in an isoprenoid fashion (37). This structural difference allows these molecules to be more mobile within the biological membrane than the tocopherols (38,39). There is some experimental evidence that tocotrienols may by more efficient in protecting LDL from oxidation than tocopherol. If the above-described experiment is carried out with tocotrienol instead of tocopherol, the lag time is increased, which indicates that α-tocotrienol may be more effective in protecting LDL from in vitro oxidation than α-tocopherol (23). All forms of both tocopherols and tocotrienols are potential nutraceuticals and therefore are a major focus of research.

VIII. RECENT STUDIES ON TOCOTRIENOLS

Together with our collaborators, an in vivo study was carried out looking at tocotrienol supplementation in humans (40). The subjects received 250 mg of either α-tocotrienyl acetate, β-tocotrienyl acetate, γ-tocotrienyl acetate, or the placebo supplements per day. Before the study began, tocotrienols were not detectable in plasma. After 8 weeks of supplementation, there was only a small

RRR-α-Tocopherol

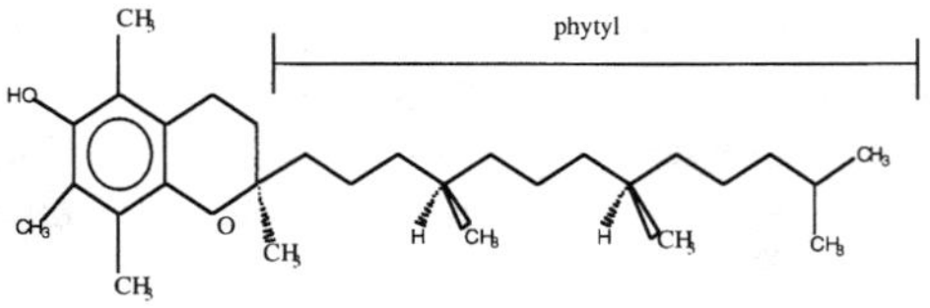

RRR -β-Tocopherol

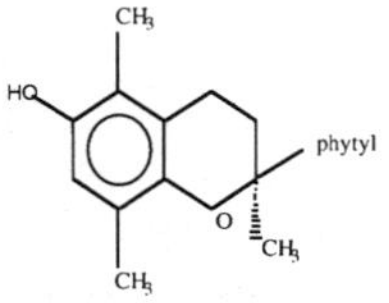

RRR -γ-Tocopherol

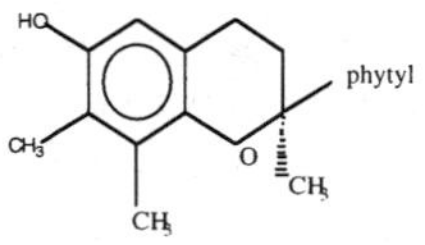

RRR -δ-Tocopherol

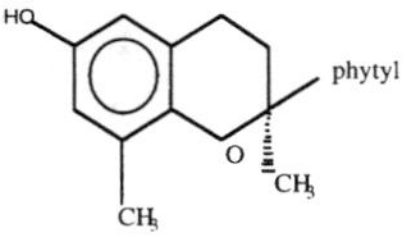

R-α- Tocotrienol

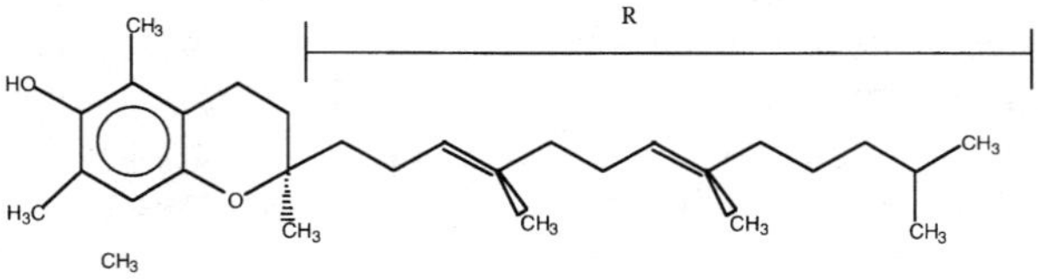

R-β- Tocotrienol

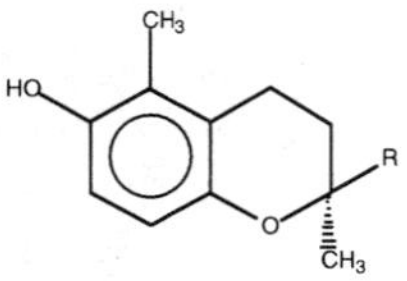

R-γ- Tocotrienol

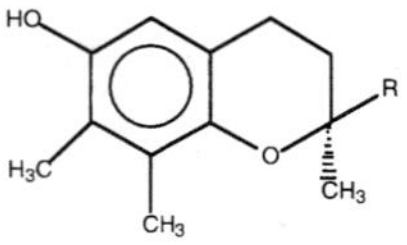

R-δ- Tocotrienol

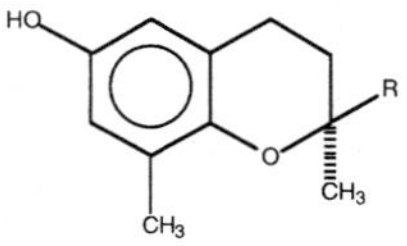

Figure 7 Naturally occurring forms of vitamin E: (a) tocopherols; (b) tocotrienols.

Table 3 Effects of Tocotrienyl Acetate Supplementation

	Group size (N)	Plasma tocotrienols[a] (μM)
α-Tocotrienol acetate	13	0.98 + 0.8
β-Tocotrienol acetate	13	0.09 + 0.07
γ-Tocotrienol acetate	12	0.54 + 0.45
Placebo	13	N.D.

[a] Values after 8 weeks supplementation; N.D. initially.

increase in the free plasma tocotrienol levels. The most apparent increase was slightly less than 1 μM in magnitude using α-tocotrienol supplementation (Table 3). Taking into consideration the basic level of other forms of vitamin E in human plasma, which is on average between 22 and 32 μM, the results of this study showed that less than 5% of the total vitamin E was influenced by tocotrienol supplementation. The LDL was then isolated and subjected to oxidation by copper. Two hundred μg of LDL protein was incubated with 2.5 μM of copper for 5 hours at 37°C. During this time, the susceptibility of LDL to oxidation was followed using the 234 nm absorbance and the lag time recorded and analyzed. After 8 weeks of supplementation at 250 mg/day, α-tocotrienol increased the resistance of LDL oxidation by over 22% in concentrations less than 1 μM increase in the plasma (Fig. 8). This resistance may afford protection in cardiovascular diseases.

α-Tocotrienol has more potent antioxidant actions in biological systems relative to α-tocopherol because of its unique molecular structure. Because the structure of α-tocotrienol allows for greater mobility and a greater ability to seek out targets and lipid oxidation, it has more recycling activity and more inhibition of liver peroxidation (38,39). Tocotrienols may prevent human LDL oxidation both in vitro and in vivo. Most of the studies done thus far have used α-tocopherol and equate vitamin E with tocopherol, but this will change soon.

Vitamin E has been implicated in many different systems as an important part of signal transduction. It has been shown to modulate the activation of redox-sensitive transcription factors like NF-kB (41) and AP-1 (42), mainly due to its antioxidant function. There are also cases where the action of vitamin E may exceed a mere antioxidant effect (43). Even though all isoforms of tocopherol have the same antioxidant capacity, α-tocopherol is the only isoform that inhibits protein kinase C (44). Recently the effects of vitamin E isoforms on glutamate-induced stress in a neuronal cell model (HT4 hippocampal cells) has been investigated. Usually glutamate treatment results in cell death, but the addition of vitamin E mitigates the glutamate toxicity. Interestingly, α-tocotrienol may be more protective than α-tocopherol (44a). Further studies are currently in progress to dissect the mechanism involved.

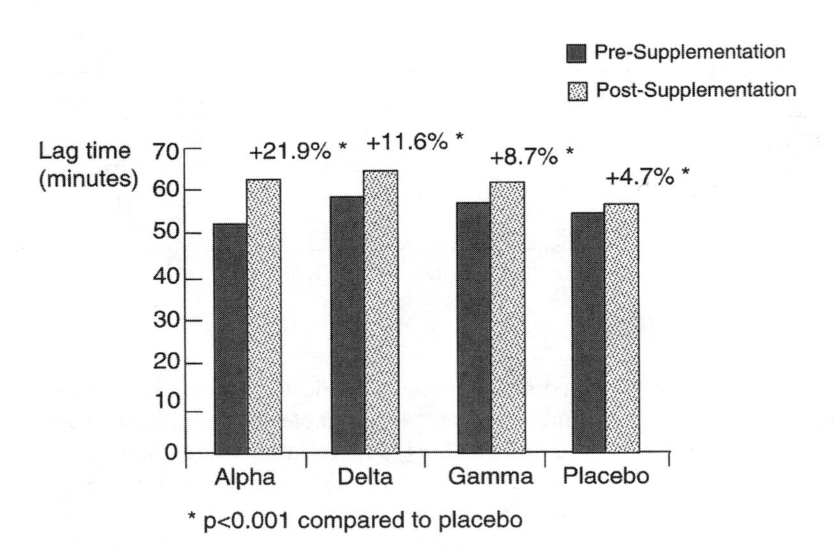

Figure 8 Effects of supplementation with tocotrienols on LDL oxidative susceptibility.

IX. ANTIOXIDANTS IN THE SKIN

According to the philosopher Wittgenstein, the body is the best picture of the soul. In other words, the way we think and feel is mirrored in our body. Reciprocally, there is an intimate relationship between the way we look and the way we feel about ourselves. Since the skin is the most visible part of our body, skin aging and its prevention is a focus of public interest as well as of research efforts.

The human skin is composed of different layers: the epidermis, the dermis, and the subcutis. The epidermis consists mostly of keratinocytes that undergo a program of terminal differentiation into enucleated corneocytes. These form the stratum corneum (SC), a protective layer of 20–30 sheets of dead cells (45), which protects against exogenous physical and chemical stressors as well as limits the transepidermal water loss. The dermis contains fibroblasts embedded in an extracellular matrix of collagen and elastic fibers, which play a pivotal role in skin aging.

Since the skin is a constant target of environmental oxidative stress, it is important to analyze its antioxidant defense capacity. The epidermis and dermis were found to be equipped with all of the endogenous small molecule antioxidants and antioxidant enzymes described above. In general, the concentrations of antioxidants were higher in the epidermis than in the dermis (46). Recently, antioxidants have also been discovered in the SC. Different layers of the SC can be analyzed by sequential removal by tape strips, from which the compound of interest can be extracted and assayed (47,48). Using this noninvasive method it was discovered, that vitamin E in the form of α- and γ-tocopherol forms gradients with rising concentrations from the skin surface toward deeper SC layers (49). Also, the hydrophilic antioxidants vitamin C, glutathione, and uric acid were found to be distributed in logarithmic or exponentially shaped gradients in the SC (50). Exposure to minimal doses of ultraviolet radiation (UV) radiation, which were not even enough to cause a slight reddening of the skin after 24 hours, depleted up to 50% of vitamin E in human SC (Fig. 9). The environmental oxidant ozone (O_3) depleted vitamin E and C as well as glutathione and uric acid in a single dose of 1 ppm for 2 hours in murine SC (49,51). Repeated exposure to this dose for 5 days increased the damage and induced lipid peroxidation as measured by the formation of malondialdehyde. Analysis of protein oxidation revealed that both UV light and O_3 caused dose-dependent protein carbonyl formation in murine or human SC (52). Recently, different isoforms of vitamin E, tocotrienols, were discovered in mouse skin. Surprisingly, up to 13% of total vitamin E in skin consists of tocotrienols, a percentage at least one order of mag-

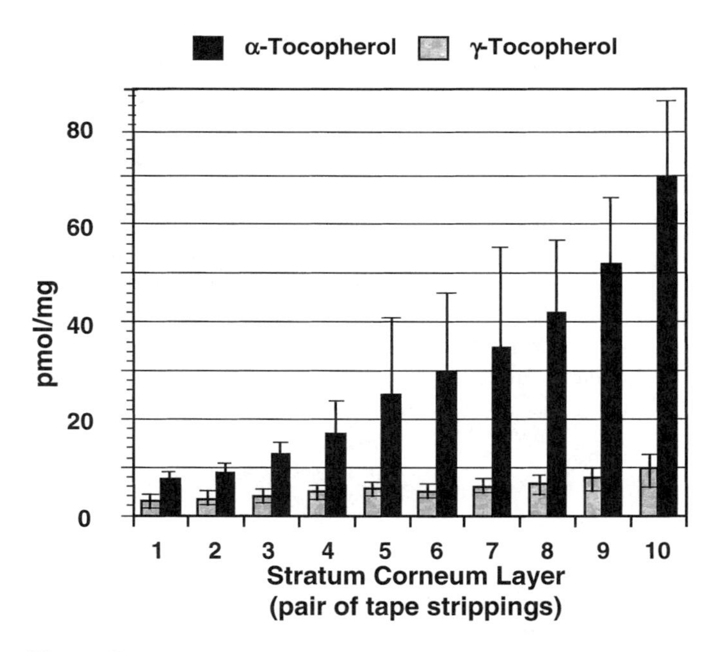

Figure 9 Distribution of α-tocopherol in the human stratum corneum. Low-dose UV irradiation significantly depleted vitamin E.

Table 4 Tissue Distribution of Vitamin E Forms (% total vitamin E)

	α-Tocopherol	γ-Tocopherol	α-Tocotrienol	γ-Tocotrienol
Brain	99.8 ± 0.4	0.2 ± 0.4	—	—
Heart	98.1 ± 0.2	0.8 ± 0.2	0.3 ± 0.0	0.8 ± 0.2
Kidney	97.5 ± 0.6	1.6 ± 0.3	0.3 ± 0.2	0.6 ± 0.3
Liver	97.2 ± 1.5	1.4 ± 0.3	0.5 ± 0.3	0.9 ± 0.9
Skin	85.6 ± 7.2	0.6 ± 0.3	3.4 ± 1.5	10.4 ± 6.0
Skin + subcutis	90.8 ± 1.4	0.5 ± 0.2	2.2 ± 0.3	6.5 ± 1.3

nitude higher than in other tissues (53). Topical application of tocotrienols greatly enriched murine skin with vitamin E, which was partially depleted by oxidative stressors such as UV light and O_3 (54,55).

Antioxidants, predominantly vitamins E and C, are used frequently in topical formulations to boost the skin's antioxidants defenses and to protect it against environmental stressors. Vitamin E has been shown to protect the skin from lipid peroxidation (56), DNA damage (57), sunburn reaction (58), skin inflammation (13), and immunosupression (59,60). To preserve the antioxidant capacity of vitamin E in formulations, its hydroxyl group on the chromanol nucleus must be esterified (61). After penetration into the skin, the acetate must be hydrolyzed by unspecific esterases to regain the antioxidant function of vitamin E (45). To test if tocotrienyl acetates are hydrolyzed in vivo, they were applied to the back of hairless mice (Table 4). Significant hydrolysis was observed after 5 days of application, concomitant with a multifold increase in free α-tocotrienol. This may open up the way for large-scale use of tocotrienols as topical antioxidants (62).

It may also be possible to boost skin antioxidants by oral administration, which would replenish antioxidants such as vitamin E evenly throughout the whole skin. Indeed, initial experiments from our laboratory indicate that oral supplementation of antioxidants increases the skin's antioxidant capacity. This opens up new dimensions for the use of nutraceuticals.

X. CONCLUSION

Tocotrienols are potentially the nutraceutical of the twenty-first century. Their antioxidant properties are remarkable. They may even exhibit beneficial effects beyond their mere antioxidant function. Via oral application they may benefit different systems of the body and the human body as a whole. Investigations into how to maintain the delicate balance between oxidants and antioxidants is a promising area of research. Maintaining this balance is necessary to shift the human life span further to healthy aging and longevity. In the long run, nutraceutical antioxidants will be able to tip the balance in the right direction and help people lead longer and healthier lives.

ACKNOWLEDGMENTS

The authors would like to thank Pauline Kim for valuable assistance with the manuscript and Krisnadi Poedjosoedarmo for preparing the figures and tables.

REFERENCES

1. Olshansky SJ. Practical limits to life expectancy in France. In: Robine JM, Vaupel JW, Jeune B, Allard M, eds. Longevity: To the Limits and Beyond. Heidelberg: Springer, 1997.
2. Jeune B, Kannisto V. In: Robine JM et al., eds. Longevity: To the Limits and Beyond. Heidelberg: Springer, 1997.
3. Kirkwood TBL. Is there a biological limit to the human life span? In: Robine JM, Vaupel JW, Jeune B, Allard M, eds. Longevity: To the Limits and Beyond. Heidelberg: Springer, 1997.
4. Sies H. Oxidative Stress. New York: Academic Press, 1985.
5. Aleynik SI, Leo MA, Aleynik MK, Lieber CS. Alcohol-induced pancreatic oxidative stress: protection by phospholipid repletion. Free Radic Biol Med 26:609–619, 1999.
6. Flohé L, Brigelius-Flohé R, Saliou C, Traber MG, Packer L. Redox regulation of NF-kappa B activation. Free Radic Biol Med 22:1115–1126, 1997.
7. Saliou C, Kitazawa M, McLaughlin L, Yang JP, Lodge JK, Tetsuka T, Iwasaki K, Cillard J, Okamoto T, Packer L. Antioxidants modulate acute solar ultraviolet radiation-induced NF-kappa-B activation in a human keratinocyte cell line. Free Radic Biol Med 26:174–183, 1999.
8. Packer L, Yodoi J. Redox Regulation of Cell Signaling and Its Clinical Application. New York: Marcel Dekker, 1999.
9. Smith JA. Neutrophils, host defense, and inflammation: a double-edged sword. J Leukoc Biol 56:672–686, 1994.
10. De Groote MA, Ochsner UA, Shiloh MU, Nathan C, McCord JM, Dinauer MC, Libby SJ, Vazquez-Torres A, Xu Y, Fang FC. Periplasmic superoxide dismutase protects Salmonella from products of phagocyte NADPH-oxidase and nitric oxide synthase. Proc Natl Acad Sci USA 94:13997–14001, 1997.
11. Babior BM. NADPH oxidase: an update. Blood 93:1464–1476, 1999.
12. Kelly FJ. Use of antioxidants in the prevention and treatment of disease. J Int Fed Clin Chem 10:21–23, 1998.
13. Fuchs J, Kern H. Modulation of UV-light-induced skin inflammation by D-alpha-tocopherol and L-ascorbic acid: a clinical study using solar simulated radiation. Free Radic Biol Med 25:1006–1012, 1998.

14. Jesberger JA, Richardson JS. Oxygen free radicals and brain dysfunction. Int J Neurosci 57:1–17, 1991.
15. Lee AY, Chung SS. Contributions of polyol pathway to oxidative stress in diabetic cataract. FASEB J 13:23–30, 1990.
16. Maitra I, Serbinova E, Trischler H, Packer L. Alpha-lipoic acid prevents buthionine sulfoximine-induced cataract formation in newborn rats. Free Radic Biol Med 18: 823–829, 1995.
17. Awasthi S, Srivastava SK, Piper JT, Singhal SS, Chaubey M, Awasthi YC. Curcumin protects against 4-hydroxy-2-trans-nonenal-induced cataract formation in rat lenses. Am J Clin Nutr 64:761–766, 1996.
18. Reilly CA, Aust SD. Iron loading into ferritin by an intracellular ferroxidase. Arch Biochem Biophys 359:69–76, 1998.
19. Cadenas E, Packer L, eds. Handbook of Antioxidants. New York: Marcel Dekker, 1996.
20. Packer JE, Slater TF, Willson RL. Direct observation of a free radical interaction between vitamin E and vitamin C. Nature 278:737–738, 1979.
21. Packer L. Vitamin E. Sci Am Sci Med 1:54–63, 1994.
22. Packer L. Prevention of free radical damage in the brain: protection by α-lipoic acid. In: Packer L, Hiramatsu M, Yoshikawa T, eds. Free Radicals in Brain Physiology and Disorders. New York: Academic Press, 1996.
23. Kagan VE, Serbinova EA, Forte T, Scita G, Packer L. Recycling of vitamin E in human low density lipoproteins. J Lipid Res 33:385–397, 1992.
24. Thomas PR, Earl R, eds. Opportunities in the Nutrition and Food Sciences, Research Challenges and the Next Generation of Investigators. Washington, DC: National Academy Press, 1994.
25. Garcia DJ. Omega-3 long chain PUFA nutraceuticals. Food Technol 52:44, 1998.
26. DeFelice SL. Nutraceuticals. New York: Marcel Dekker, 1997.
27. Packer L, Fuchs J, eds. Vitamin E in Health and Disease. New York: Marcel Dekker, 1993.
28. Packer L, Hiramatsu M, Yoshikawa T, eds. Antioxidant Food Supplementation in Human Health. New York: Academic Press, 1999.
29. Gey KF, Puska P, Jordan P, Moser UK. Inverse correlation between plasma vitamin E and mortality from ischemic heart disease in cross-cultural epidemiology. Am J Clin Nutr 53:326S–334S, 1991.
30. Stampfer MJ, Hennekens CH, Manson JE, Colditz GA, Rosner B, Willett WC. Vitamin E consumption and the risk of coronary disease in women [see comments]. N Engl J Med 328:1444–1449, 1993.
31. Rimm EB, Stampfer MJ, Ascherio A, Giovannucci E, Colditz GA, Willett WC. Vitamin E consumption and the risk of coronary heart disease in men [comment] [see comments]. N Engl J Med 328:1450–1456, 1993.
32. Stephens NG, Parsons A, Schofield PM, Kelly F, Cheeseman K, Mitchinson MJ. Randomised controlled trial of vitamin E in patients with coronary disease: Cambridge Heart Antioxidant Study (CHAOS). Lancet 347:781–786, 1996.
33. Sano M, Ernesto C, Thomas RG, Klauber MR, Schafer K, Grundman M, Woodbury P, Growdon J, Cotman CW, Pfeiffer E, Schneider LS, Thal LJ. A controlled trial of selegiline, alpha-tocopherol, or both as treatment for Alzheimer's disease. The

Alzheimer's Disease Cooperative Study [see comments]. N Engl J Med 336:1216–1222, 1997.
34. Knekt P. Vitamin E and cancer prevention: methodological aspects of human studies. In: Ohigshi H, Osawa T, Terao J, Watanabe S, Yoshikawa T, eds. Food Factors for Cancer Prevention. New York: Springer, 1997.
35. Regnström J, Nilsson J, Moldeus P, Ström K, Båvenholm P, Tornvall P, Hamsten A. Inverse relation between the concentration of low-density-lipoprotein vitamin E and severity of coronary artery disease. Am J Clin Nutr 63:377–385, 1996.
36. Esterbauer H, Jürgens G, Quehenberger O. Modification of human low density lipoprotein by lipid peroxidation. Basic Life Sci 49:369–373, 1988.
37. Traber MG, Serbinova EA, Packer L. Biological activities of tocotrienols and tocopherols. In: Packer L, Hiramatsu M, Yoshikawa T, eds. Antioxidant Food Supplements in Human Health. New York: Academic Press, 1999.
38. Serbinova E, Kagan V, Han D, Packer L. Free radical recycling and intramembrane mobility in the antioxidant properties of alpha-tocopherol and alpha-tocotrienol. Free Radic Biol Med 10:263–275, 1991.
39. Suzuki YJ, Tsuchiya M, Wassall SR, Choo YM, Govil G, Kagan VE, Packer L. Structural and dynamic membrane properties of alpha-tocopherol and alpha-tocotrienol: implication to the molecular mechanism of their antioxidant potency. Biochemistry 32:10692–10699, 1993.
40. O'Byrne D, Grundy S, Packer L, Devaraj S, Baldenius K, Hoppe P, Kramer K, Jialal I, Traber M. Studies of LDL oxidation following α-, γ-, or δ-tocotrienyl acetate supplementation of hypercholesterolemic humans. Free Rad Biol Med 29, 2000.
41. Suzuki YJ, Packer L. Inhibition of NF-kappa B DNA binding activity by alpha-tocopheryl succinate. Biochem Mol Biol Int 31:693–700, 1993.
42. Stäuble B, Boscoboinik D, Tasinato A, Azzi A. Modulation of activator protein-1 (AP-1) transcription factor and protein kinase C by hydrogen peroxide and D-alpha-tocopherol in vascular smooth muscle cells. Eur J Biochem 226:393–402, 1994.
43. Traber MG, Packer L. Vitamin E: beyond antioxidant function. Am J Clin Nutr 62: 1501S–1509S, 1995.
44. Boscoboinik D, Szewczyk A, Hensey C, Azzi A. Inhibition of cell proliferation by alpha-tocopherol. Role of protein kinase C. J Biol Chem 266:6188–6194, 1991.
44a. Sen CK, Khanna S, Roy S, Packer L. Molecular basis of vitamin E action: tocotrienol potently inhibits glutamate-induced pp60c-src kinase activation and death of HT-4 neuronal cells. J Biol Chem 275:13049–13055, 2000.
45. Weber SU. Oxidants in skin pathophysiology. In: Sen CK, Packer L, Hanninen O, eds. Exercise and Oxygen Toxicity. 2d ed. Amsterdam: Elsevier Science, 1999.
46. Shindo Y, Witt E, Han D, Epstein W, Packer L. Enzymic and non-enzymic antioxidants in epidermis and dermis of human skin. J Invest Dermatol 102:122–124, 1994.
47. Weber SU, Jothi S, Thiele JJ. High pressure liquid chromatography analysis of ozone-induced depletion of hydrophilic and lipophilic antioxidants in murine skin. Methods Enzymol, in press.
48. Thiele JJ, Packer L. Noninvasive measurement of α-tocopherol gradients in human stratum corneum by high-performance liquid chromatography analysis of sequential tape strippings. In: Methods in Enzymology. New York: Academic Press, 1999: 413–419.

49. Thiele JJ, Traber MG, Packer L. Depletion of human stratum corneum vitamin E: an early and sensitive in vivo marker of UV induced photo-oxidation. J Invest Dermatol 110:756–761, 1998.
50. Weber SU, Thiele JJ, Packer L. Ozone depletes vitamin C, urate and glutathione in murine stratum corneum. Free Radic Biol Med 25:100, 1998.
51. Thiele JJ, Traber MG, Polefka TG, Cross CE, Packer L. Ozone-exposure depletes vitamin E and induces lipid peroxidation in murine stratum corneum. J Invest Dermatol 108:753–757, 1997.
52. Thiele JJ, Traber MG, Re R, Espuno N, Yan LJ, Cross CE, Packer L. Macromolecular carbonyls in human stratum corneum: a biomarker for environmental oxidant exposure? FEBS Lett 422:403–406, 1998.
53. Podda M, Weber C, Traber MG, Packer L. Simultaneous determination of tissue tocopherols, tocotrienols, ubiquinols, and ubiquinones. J Lipid Res 37:893–901, 1996.
54. Weber C, Podda M, Rallis M, Thiele JJ, Traber MG, Packer L. Efficacy of topically applied tocopherols and tocotrienols in protection of murine skin from oxidative damage induced by UV-irradiation. Free Radic Biol Med 22:761–769, 1997.
55. Thiele JJ, Traber MG, Podda M, Tsang K, Cross CE, Packer L. Ozone depletes tocopherols and tocotrienols topically applied to murine skin. FEBS Lett 401:167–170, 1997.
56. Lopez-Torres M, Thiele JJ, Shindo Y, Han D, Packer L. Topical application of alpha-tocopherol modulates the antioxidant network and diminishes ultraviolet-induced oxidative damage in murine skin. Br J Dermatol 138:207–215, 1998.
57. McVean M, Liebler DC. Inhibition of UVB induced DNA photodamage in mouse epidermis by topically applied alpha-tocopherol. Carcinogenesis 18:1617–1622, 1997.
58. Eberlein-Konig B, Placzek M, Przybilla B. Protective effect against sunburn of combined systemic ascorbic acid (vitamin C) and d-alpha-tocopherol (vitamin E). J Am Acad Dermatol 38:45–48, 1998.
59. Yuen KS, Halliday GM. Alpha-tocopherol, an inhibitor of epidermal lipid peroxidation, prevents ultraviolet radiation from suppressing the skin immune system. Photochem Photobiol 65:587–592, 1997.
60. Halliday GM, Bestak R, Yuen KS, Cavanagh LL, Barnetson RS. UVA-induced immunosuppression. Mutat Res 422:139–145, 1998.
61. Kramer-Stickland K, Liebler DC. Effect of UVB on hydrolysis of alpha-tocopherol acetate to alpha-tocopherol in mouse skin. J Invest Dermatol 111:302–307, 1998.
62. Weber SU, Luu C, Traber MG, Packer L. Tocotrienol acetate penetrates into murine skin and is hydrolyzed in vivo. Oxygen Club of California, Book of Abstracts, 1999.
63. Jeune B, Kannisto V. Emergence of centenarians and super-centenarians. In: Robine JM, Vaupel JW, Jeune B, Allard M, eds. Longevity: To the Limits and Beyond. Heidelberg: Springer, 1997.

3

S-Adenosylmethionine (SAMe): Preclinical and Clinical Studies in Depression

Teodoro Bottiglieri
Baylor Institute of Metabolic Disease, Dallas, Texas

I. INTRODUCTION

S-Adenosylmethionine (SAMe), first discovered in 1952 (1), is formed from the essential amino acid methionine and adenosine triphosphate (ATP). SAMe is found in every living cell, where it functions as a donor of methyl groups in over 100 different reactions catalyzed by methlytransferase enzymes, which act on substrates such as DNA, proteins, phospholipids, monoamine neurotransmitters, and many other low molecular weight compounds (2,3). In its native form SAMe is labile and degrades rapidly. However, several patents on SAMe stable salts have been granted. Among them, SAMe-1,4-butanedisulfonate has been chosen for pharmaceutical development because of its high stability and tolerability, allowing preclinical and clinical studies to be performed. Numerous studies over the last two decades have shown SAMe to be effective in the treatment of depression (4–6), osteoarthritis (7,8), and liver disease (9–11). Moreover, SAMe has a very low side effect profile, comparable to that of placebo, affording considerable advantages as an alternative to standard antidepressant and anti-inflammatory prescription medications that have unwanted and, in many cases, intolerable side effects.

Since March 1999 SAMe has been introduced to the American market under the Dietary Supplement and Health Education Act (DSHEA) as an over-the-counter dietary supplement. Although SAMe is a relatively new product in the

United States, it has been available by prescription in Italy since 1979, Spain since 1985, and Germany since 1989. The numerous clinical trials and frequent daily use in the European population has provided considerable evidence to confirm its therapeutic effects and high safety profile. In addition, since its discovery, SAMe has been intensely studied by the scientific community in many diverse fields of biochemistry because of the pivotal role it plays in cellular metabolism. This research has provided some understanding of the mechanisms involved in the health-promoting and therapeutic effects of SAMe.

II. METABOLIC ROLE OF SAMe

SAMe serves an important biological function as the sole methyl donor in a multitude of cellular methylation reactions (2,3). Most cells contain numerous SAMe-dependent methyltransferases that can transfer the methyl group (CH_3) to the oxygen, nitrogen, or sulfur atoms of both small and large molecules. The synthesis of creatine from guanidinoacetate, sarcosine from glycine, phosphatidylcholine from phosphatidylethanolamine, epinephrine from norepinephrine, methylation of carboxyl residues of various proteins, and cytosine residues of DNA all use SAMe as the methyl donor. The product of all SAMe-dependent methylation reactions is S-adenosylhomocysteine (SAH) (Fig. 1). SAH is rapidly

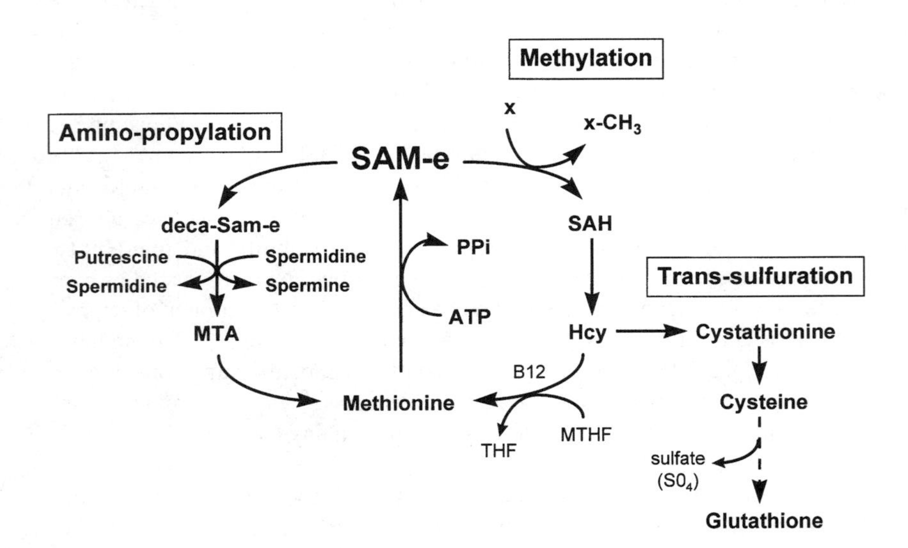

Figure 1 Metabolism of SAMe through methylation, aminopropylation, and transsulfuration pathways.

metabolized to homocysteine and then enters into the trans-sulfuration pathway, ultimately leading to the synthesis of glutathione, a major cellular antioxidant. Alternatively, homocysteine may be remethylated to methionine, with the methyl group originating from methyltetrahydrofolate (MTHF), by a vitamin B_{12}–dependent enzyme reaction. The daily amount of SAMe that is required by the body is dependent on the availability of methionine that is produced by de novo synthesis, involving MTHF and vitamin B_{12} and also methionine obtained from the diet, mainly from the breakdown of proteins ingested.

Another important metabolic role of SAMe is in the synthesis of polyamines through a pathway known as aminopropylation. SAMe may be metabolized to decarboxylated SAMe, and the aminopropyl group is transferred to putrescine and then on to form the polyamines spermidine and spermine (Fig. 1). In this process methylthioadenosine is produced, which is then converted back to methionine. The polyamines spermidine and spermine are involved in the control of cell growth (12) and have also been shown to have analgesic and anti-inflammatory properties (13).

III. PHARMACOKINETICS OF SAMe

The pharmacokinetics of SAMe has been studied by measuring the decay of the compound in plasma after i.v. administration of 100 mg (1.49 ± 0.08 mg/kg) and 500 mg (7.45 ± 0.4 mg/kg) to six healthy volunteers (14). A biexponential decay was observed with a terminal disposition phase starting about 60 minutes after the administration. The apparent volumes of distribution after the low and high doses were 407 ± 27 and 443 ± 36 mL/kg (mean $\pm$ SEM), respectively. Total urinary excretion of the SAMe was 30 ± 3 and 34 ± 8 mg at 8 and 24 hours after the administration of 100 mg dose. At the same times after a 500 mg dose the excretion rate was 189 ± 11 and 201 ± 10 mg, respectively. The disposition and renal excretion were almost complete within 24 hours, and the ratio between renal and total clearances indicate that at both doses more than half of the SAMe administered was metabolized. This suggests that body accumulation of SAMe is unlikely at least up to the doses studied.

Experimental studies have shown that SAMe is able to cross the intestinal wall and increase plasma levels. Early studies in rats revealed that absorption of the SAMe is much better after intraduodenal administration compared to oral administration (15). In a phase I study the administration of enteric-coated capsules of SAMe in varying doses of 400, 600, and 1000 mg to four male subjects increased plasma concentrations, in a dose-dependent manner, between 30 to 50 times basal values (16) (Fig. 2). Despite substantial increases above physiological concentrations, the systemic bioavailability after oral SAMe administration appears to be low. However, oral administration of [methyl-^{14}C]SAMe (200 mg;

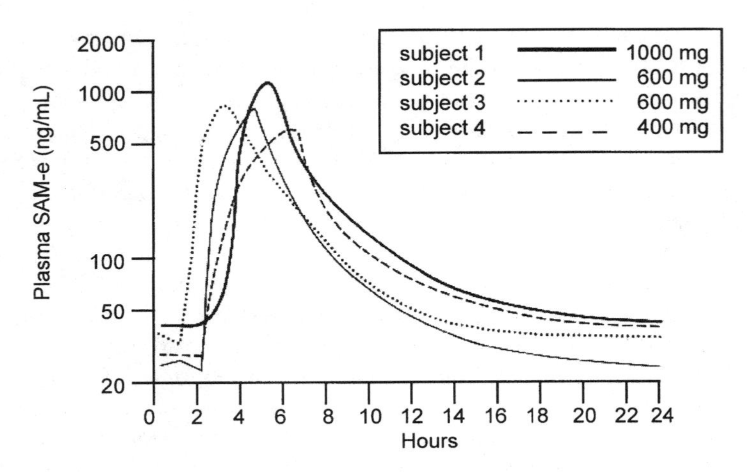

Figure 2 Absorption of oral SAMe in healthy volunteers. (From Ref. 16.)

0.02 μCi/μmol) to three adult volunteers showed that urinary excretion of radioactivity during the first 48 hours was 15.5 ± 1.5% and feces contained 23.5 ± 3.5% of the radioactivity up to 72 hours (17). These findings indicate that approximately 60% of the radioactivity is incorporated into stable pools. A comparison of the rapid metabolism of SAMe after an intravenous or oral dose of [methyl-^{14}C]SAMe (50 mg; 0.4 mCi/mmol) has been performed in six male volunteers (15). Plasma radioactivity rapidly decreased after intravenous administration corresponding to the decay of the unmodified product. In contrast, after oral administration plasma radioactivity increased with time reaching a peak between 8 and 24 hours after treatment. The higher radioactivity found after oral administration compared to intravenous administration at the later time intervals suggests that SAMe given orally is actively metabolized, with the methyl group being incorporated into stable pools such as proteins and phospholipids. These observations are supported by a recent study showing that after oral administration of a single 100 mg dose of double labeled [methyl-^{3}H:^{35}S]SAMe, 62% of [^{3}H] and 43.7% of [^{35}S] radioactivity still remained in the body after 5 days (17). Plasma concentrations of radioactivity were much higher than those of the unmodified compound, suggesting a strong presystemic metabolism of absorbed SAMe.

In relation to the neuro-pharmacological action of SAMe, it is essential to demonstrate that SAMe can pass across the blood-brain barrier. Several studies indicate that parenteral and oral administration of SAMe can increase CSF concentrations. In dogs an intravenous injection of 8 mg/kg of SAMe followed by an intravenous infusion of 12 mg/kg of SAMe for 6 hours was associated with a steady hourly increase in CSF SAMe levels, with a 20- to 40-fold increase over basal values after 6 hours (15). CSF SAMe levels have also been studied in a placebo-controlled trial after the parenteral administration of 200 mg SAMe daily for 14 days to depressed patients (18). At 2 and 24 hours after the last injection, CSF SAMe levels were significantly increased by 65% and 12%, respectively, compared to baseline values, indicating that compound can cross the blood-brain barrier. Similarly, administration of oral SAMe (400 mg t.d.s. for 4–8 months) to four patients with Alzheimer's dementia significantly increased both plasma and CSF SAMe levels (18). There is also additional evidence that SAMe crosses the blood-brain barrier intact. In a recent study the parenteral administration of 800 mg SAMe-1,4-butanedisulfonate daily for 14 days to 7 HIV-infected patients was associated with a marked increase in CSF SAMe (19).

In relation to the efficacy of SAMe in the treatment of osteoarthritis, it is important to know if SAMe is able to increase levels in the synovial fluid of the joint. In one study four patients with osteoarthritis received SAMe (400 mg orally) at 8-hour intervals for 7 days (15). SAMe levels were determined in synovial fluid taken from the patients before treatment and 4 hours after the last dose. In each patient there was a significant increase in SAMe content in the synovial fluid indicating that the compound is able to reach the disease ''site.''

IV. DISTRIBUTION OF SAMe IN TISSUES AND BIOLOGICAL FLUIDS

A. Animal Studies

The distribution of SAMe throughout various organs of the body has been studied in several animal species. In the most frequently studied species, the laboratory rat, the highest concentration is found in the liver followed by adrenal, heart, spleen, kidney, lung, and brain tissue (20). SAMe levels in both liver and brain tissue are much higher in newborn rats and decrease toward a stable level with maturation (21,22). SAMe levels have been shown to be decreased throughout various tissues (liver 35%, adrenal 22%, lung 20%, muscle 7%, brain 13%, and blood 16%) in aged (30-month-old) rats compared to young (3-month-old) rats (20). The decrease in SAMe levels in tissues of aged rats parallels the decrease in activity of methyltransferase enzymes involved with phospholipid metabolism (23).

B. Human Studies

Studies of SAMe levels in various human disease states have relied mainly on blood or CSF determinations. In a few studies SAMe levels have been studied in either brain postmortem or liver biopsy samples. In humans, SAMe concentrations are high in both blood (24) and CSF (25) at birth and rapidly decline during

Table 1 Studies of SAMe in Human Biological Fluids and Tissues

Disorder	Fluid or tissue	SAMe level	Ref.
Disease			
Depression	CSF	Decreased	18
Alzheimer's disease	CSF/Brain	Decreased	18, 36
Parkinson's disease	Whole blood	Decreased	35
	CSF	Decreased	34
Liver disease (cirrhosis)	Liver	Decreased	38
Heart disease	Whole blood	Decreased	27
Acute lymphoblastic leukemia	CSF	Decreased	31
HIV infection	CSF	Decreased	19,28,29
	Erythrocytes	Normal	19
	Plasma	Increased	19
Genetic deficiency			
MAT I/III deficiency	CSF	Decreased	42
	Plasma	Decreased	41
MTHFR deficiency	CSF	Decreased	42
Cobalamine G, C, D defect	CSF	Decreased	42
Nutritional deficiency			
Folate deficiency	CSF	Decreased	26
Vitamin B_{12} deficiency	CSF	Decreased	26

the first 24 months. Table 1 lists the major disorders in which a SAMe deficiency has been found.

Folate or vitamin B_{12} deficiency, either drug induced, genetically acquired, or as a result of dietary insufficiency, has a direct effect on SAMe metabolism. Both vitamins are required as cofactors in the synthesis of methionine, upon which formation of SAMe is dependent (Fig. 1). A defect in some methylation pathways due to SAMe deficiency is believed to be the biochemical lesion responsible for the neurological and psychiatric complications often associated with both folate and vitamin B_{12} deficiency (26). In one study involving depressed patients, CSF SAMe was significantly lower in patients with low red cell folate levels and high serum homocysteine levels (26). In another study, decreased concentrations of SAMe in blood was reported in patients with heart disease who have low red cell folate and high serum homocysteine levels (27). Folate deficiency can therefore impair the remethylation of homocysteine to methionine and synthesis of SAMe. Decreased SAMe levels have been found in CSF from patients with HIV infection (19,28,29). Although folate and vitamin B_{12} deficiency is common in HIV-infected patients due to intestinal malabsorption, patients with low CSF SAM levels were not deficient in these vitamins. The exact cause of

SAMe deficiency in HIV infection is not yet known, but it may play a role in the etiology of the neurological disorders that are common in the later stages of this disease.

Drugs that affect folate metabolism, such as the anticancer agent methotrexate (MTX), may also cause depletion of SAMe. Patients with acute lymphoblastic leukemia treated with MTX have been shown to have increased homocysteine (30) and decreased SAMe levels in CSF (31). These changes are postulated to be involved in the neurotoxicity associated with high-dose MTX therapy.

Levodopa is the mainstay treatment for Parkinson's disease. A metabolic consequence of levodopa treatment is a marked deficiency of SAMe. Animal studies have shown that levodopa decreases both liver and brain SAMe concentrations (32,33). Similar observations in humans treated with levodopa have shown reduced blood and CSF SAMe concentrations (34,35). Low SAMe levels in Parkinson's disease may be a contributing factor to the underlying depression that frequently occurs in Parkinson's disease.

SAMe levels have been shown to be reduced in Alzheimer's disease where a 40% decrease has been reported in CSF (18) and a similar decrease in postmortem brain tissue (36). The cause of brain SAMe deficiency in Alzheimer's disease is not known. Folate and vitamin B_{12} deficiency, which can result in decreased SAMe levels, are common in the elderly, and elevated blood homocysteine levels have been reported to be a risk factor for Alzheimer's disease (37).

The hepatic concentration of SAMe is decreased in patients with cirrhosis of the liver (38). In cirrhotic patients methionine metabolism is decreased and the activities of methionine adenosyltransferase (MAT) and phospholipid methyltransferase are reduced (39). Supplemental use of SAMe is a rational and effective mode of overcoming this metabolic block.

SAMe deficiency may also occur as a result of congenital genetic defects affecting enzymes related to methionine and SAMe metabolism. The cloning and characterization of the transcription unit of the human methionine adenosyltransferase (MAT*1A*) gene was completed in 1995 (40). The MAT*1A* gene is expressed solely in nonfetal liver to form two isoenzymes called MAT I and MAT III. To date 16 mutations in the MAT*1A* gene have been identified in 43 individuals (41). Most of the mutations have been expressed and shown to severely decrease MAT I/III activity in mammalian and/or bacterial systems. Most patients are clinically normal, but only 20 are known and many are still young. Three cases (2 girls, both aged 11 years, and a boy aged 4.2 years) have been shown by MRI examination to have brain demyelination. In one case treatment with oral SAMe for 12 months led to a complete reversal of the MRI changes with normal myelination (42). Other genetic enzyme defects that lead to SAMe deficiency include those involved with the synthesis of methionine, such as 5,10-methylene-tetrahydrofolate reductase deficiency and cobalamin C, D, and G defects (42). In all these cases demyelination is a clinical feature indicating that a deficiency of SAMe in the brain is likely to be involved in the etiology of this disorder.

V. SAMe IN DEPRESSION

A. Preclinical Studies

The neuropharmacology of SAMe was the subject of three extensive reviews in 1986 (43), 1987 (44), and 1994 (45). Preclinical studies indicate that SAMe has stimulatory effects on monoamine metabolism and/or turnover. Thus, SAMe treatment has been reported to increase rat brain concentrations of norepinephrine (NE) (46,47) and serotonin (5HT) (47,49). The stimulatory effect of SAMe on central monoaminergic neurotansmitters has been postulated to be the mechanism of its antidepressant effect. Recent in vivo microdialysis studies in the rat indicate that SAMe increase dopaminergic tone. In one study chronic but not acute SAMe (200 mg/kg daily i.p. for 7 days) inhibited the apomorphine-induced decrease in striatal dopamine (50). Another study reported that chronic administration of SAMe (200 mg/kg daily i.p. for 7 days) increased striatal dopamine and the accumulation of L-dopa after inhibition of aromatic amino acid decarboxylase (AADC) with NSD 1015 (51). The accumulation of L-dopa is indicative of an increase in tyrosine hydroxylase activity.

SAMe has been studied in several animal models that are predictive of possible antidepressant activity (52). SAMe dose-dependently (12.5, 25, 50, 100, and 200 mg/kg s.c.) decreased immobility time in the forced swimming test in mice and rats, an effect that was antagonized by haloperidol. The reduction of the immobility time evoked by antidepressants is regarded as a result of activation of the dopamine system. In addition, D-amphetamine–induced locomotor hyperactivity in rats was significantly increased by chronic SAMe (50 mg/kg s.c. twice daily for 14 days). SAMe dose-dependently (12.5, 25, and 50 mg/kg s.c.) reduced hypothermia induced by apomorphine in mice, although it did not affect hypothermia induced by clonidine or reserpine. Apomorphine hypothermia is potentially antagonized by antidepressants (mainly tricylics), as well as by amphetamine-like compounds and β-adrenergic agonists. The effect of SAMe on apomorphine-induced hypothermia is consistent with its effect on inhibition of apomorphine-induced decrease in striatal dopamine measured by in vivo microdialysis (51).

Several studies have shown that administration of SAMe can affect various receptor systems associated with neurotransmitter function. Chronic treatment with SAMe increases the density of β-receptors in rat cerebral membranes (53). In 30-month-old rats the binding of the β-adrenergic agonist [^{3}H]dihydroalprenolol to rat brain membranes is decreased compared to young rats (3 months old). Chronic treatment of old rats with SAMe was shown to reverse this effect and also decrease the membrane microviscosity (54). Dopamine-sensitive adenylate cyclase activity, which was reduced in aged rats, was also restored to normal (54). These effects of SAMe on β-adrenergic receptors are consistent with earlier findings that an increase in erythrocyte phospholipid methylation increases β-adrenoreceptor–adenylate cyclase coupling. The number of muscarinic receptors in the striatum and hippocampus of aged rats is significantly lower than the number in young animals. Treatment of aged rats with 50 mg/kg of SAMe for 30 days restored the number of muscarinic receptors to levels found in the striatum and hippocampus of young animals (55). In this study the in vitro addition of SAMe to hippocampal membranes from aged rats resulted in a significant increase in the number of muscarinic binding sites, an effect antagonized by S-adenosylhomocysteine (SAH), a methyltransferase inhibitor. The reduction in muscarinic receptor density was postulated to be related to a decrease in neuronal membrane fluidity induced by aging. SAMe treatment by virtue of its ability to act as a methyl donor may increase the fluidity of cell membranes by stimulating phospholipid methylation. Other investigators have shown that treatment with 10 mg/kg of SAMe for 30 days significantly increased the number of M1 muscarinic receptors in young rat forebrain. No changes were reported for the M3 and M4 muscarinic subtypes (56).

The effect of SAMe on receptor systems is of particular interest as recent evidence suggests that age changes in the plasma environment, especially those resulting in increased viscosity, may be responsible for G protein–receptor coupling/uncoupling dysfunction (57). The beneficial effects of SAMe treatment suggest a possible strategy for various systems that exhibit G protein-receptor coupling/uncoupling dysfunction.

B. Clinical Studies

Review articles on the efficacy of SAMe in the treatment of depressive disorders were published in 1988 (4), 1989 (5), and in 1994 (6). The later and most comprehensive review performed a meta-analysis of clinical trials with SAMe between 1973 and 1992. Overall, there were 13 uncontrolled trials enrolling 377 patients, 11 controlled trials with SAMe versus placebo enrolling 402 patients, and 14 controlled trials with SAMe versus other tricylic antidepressants enrolling 389 patients. The results of the meta-analysis showed a greater response rate with SAMe when compared to placebo with a global effect size of 38% for partial to full responders (decrease in Hamilton score >25%) and 17% for full responders (decrease in Hamilton score >50%), with an average effect size of 27.5%. Meta-analysis of trials comparing SAMe versus other antidepressants gave among partial to full responders a global response of 92% for SAMe and 85% for tricylic antidepressants (global effect size of 7%) and a global response among full responders of 61% for SAMe and 59% for tricyclic antidepressants (global effect size of 1%). These results indicate that the efficacy of SAMe in treating depressive disorders is superior to that of placebo and comparable to that of standard tricylic antidepressants. Furthermore, relatively few side effects were reported in the various trials after administration of SAMe.

The efficacy of SAMe in treating depressive disorders has been confirmed in several other studies since the meta-analysis report by Bressa (6). In a multicenter open-label study involving 195 outpatients, the administration of SAMe (400 mg daily i.m.) was accompanied by a relatively fast symptomatic improvement (58). In this study mean Hamilton scores (HAM-D) were significantly reduced by 28.9% and 48.7% after 7 and 15 days of treatment, respectively, compared to the baseline value (mean ± SD; 22.8 ± 5.3). In another double-blind study in which 40 patients received either 200 mg per day i.m. of SAMe or placebo in addition to oral imipramine (IMI), the onset of clinical response occurred earlier in the SAMe-IMI group than in those receiving the placebo-IMI combination (59). The SAMe-IMI combination is suggested to accelerate neurochemical changes associated with antidepressant effects, thereby shortening the therapeutic latency. It is relevant to note that both acute and chronic administration of imipramine significantly reduce rat brain SAMe concentrations by 57% (60).

VI. OTHER HEALTH BENEFITS OF SAMe

SAMe has been shown to be effective in the treatment of osteoarthritis. Clinical studies comparing SAMe to placebo or a nonsteroidal anti-inflammatory drug (NSAID) (8) indicates that it is effective in controlling the symptoms of osteoarthritis by improving joint mobility and relieving joint pain. Controlled clinical trials have shown that SAMe improved both subjective and objective symptoms of osteoarthritis significantly more than placebo and to the same extent as the comparison NSAIDs. Furthermore, there is evidence both in experimental models (61) and in patients with finger osteoarthritis that SAMe can promote cartilage growth (62).

Clinical trials in patients with various types of chronic liver disease, including biliary or alcohol cirrhosis, hepatitis, or drug-induced cholestasis, have confirmed the effect of SAMe (given intravenously or orally) relative to placebo in normalizing measures of liver function (63). In addition, SAMe has been shown to protect against hepatic dysfunction caused by other drugs, including steroids (64), various psychoactive drugs (65), paracetamol (66), and alcohol (67). A recent study has investigated the effect of long-term treatment with SAMe on human alcohlic liver cirrhosis (11). In this randomized double-blind trial involving 123 patients, the overall mortality/liver transplantation at the end of the trial decreased from 30% in the placebo group to 16% in the SAMe group, although the difference was not statistically significant. When patients with Child C class

(8 severely affected patients) were excluded from the analysis, the overall mortality/liver transplantation was significantly greater in the placebo group than in the SAMe group (29% vs. 12%, $p = 0.025$), and differences between the two groups in the 2-year survival curves (defined as the time to death or liver transplantation) were also statistically significant ($p = 0.046$). The results indicate that long-term treatment with SAMe may improve survival or delay liver transplantation in patients with alcoholic liver cirrhosis, especially in those with less advanced liver disease.

Primary fibromyalgia is a chronic nonarticular rheumatism associated with pain and stiffness in multiple areas and commonly associated with depression, hypochondriasis, and paranoia. The efficacy of SAMe in primary fibromyalgia has been evaluated in three double-blind placebo-contolled trials. Two studies reported significant improvement in tender point score, pain, fatigue, morning stiffness, and mood in the SAMe-treated group compared to placebo (68,69). Another study reported no significant difference in improvement in the primary outcome: tender point change between the two treatment groups (70). However, there was a tendency toward statistical significance in favor of SAMe on subjective perception of pain at rest ($p = 0.08$), pain on movement ($p = 0.11$), and overall well-being ($p = 0.17$) and slight improvement only on fatigue, quality of sleep, morning stiffness, and on the Fibromyalgia Impact Questionnaire for pain. Further clinical trials are warranted to fully assess the efficacy of SAMe in primary fibromyalgia.

VII. CONCLUSIONS

SAMe is a biological compound that is involved in many diverse and important cellular reactions. Methyl group deficiency, as a result of reduced SAMe levels, is associated with neurological and psychiatric complications. This emphasizes the role SAMe plays in maintaining normal brain function. Parenteral and oral forms of SAMe have been tested in clinical trials involving severely depressed patients. In several European countries SAMe is available in doses ranging from 100 to 500 mg in intravenous, intramuscular, and oral preparations only by prescription from a physician. In the United States SAMe is available as a dietary supplement only in the oral form (100, 200, and 400 mg tablets). Clinical severe depression is a serious health-threatening condition that requires proper medical attention. In such cases, self-treatment is not an option, and it is recommended that SAMe should be used under the supervision of a physician. For many people that experience mild to moderate depression, the use of SAMe as a dietary supplement is potentially useful. SAMe may be used in combination with other antidepressants to speed the onset of action or to reduce the dose and associated side effects of prescription antidepressants and in a prophylactic manner. There are no reports of any drug or supplement interactions with SAMe. Other health benefits from taking SAMe include relief of pain due to osteoarthritis, improved liver function, and relief from the symptoms of fibromyalgia. Depression and osteoarthritis are frequently found to exist co-morbidly in the elderly population, who generally do not tolerate well the side effects of standard prescription antidepressants and NSAIDs. SAMe may prove to be a better choice of treatment as a natural, nontoxic, and safe alternative, especially in the elderly, as well as in the remaining general population.

REFERENCES

1. Cantoni GL. The nature of the active methyl donor formed enzymatically from L-methionine and adenosine triphosphate. J Am Chem Soc 74:2942–2943, 1952.
2. Cheng X, Blumenthal RM. S-Adenosylmethionine-Dependent Methyltransferases: Structures and Functions. Singapore: World Scientific Pub Co., 1999.
3. Chiang PK, Gordon RK, Tal J, Zeng GC, Doctor BP, Pardhasaradhi K, McCann PP. S-Adenosylmethionine and methylation. FASEB J 10(4):471–480, 1996.
4. Janicak PG, Lipinski JD, Comaty JE, Waternaux C, Cohen B, Altman E, Sharma RP. S-Adenosylmethionine—a literature review and preliminary report. Alabama J Med Sci 25:306–313, 1988.
5. Friedel HA, Goa KL, Benfield P. S-Adenosyl-L-methionine: A review of its therapeutic potential in liver dysfunction and affective disorders in relation to its physiological role in cell metabolism. Drugs 38(3):389–416, 1989.
6. Bressa GM. S-Adenosyl-L-methionine (SAMe) as antidepressant: meta-analysis of clinical studies. Acta Neurol Scand 154(suppl):7–14, 1994.
7. Bradley JD, Flusser D, Katz BP, Schumacher HR Jr, Brandt KD, Chambers MA, Zonay LJD. A randomized, double blind, placebo controlled trial of intravenous loading with S-adenosylmethionine (SAM) followed by oral SAM therapy in patients with knee osteoarthritis. J Rheumatol 21(5):905–911, 1994.
8. Padova C. S-Adenosylmethionine in the treatment of osteoarthritis: review of the clinical studies. Am J Med 83(5A):60–65, 1987.
9. Lieber CS. Role of S-adenosyl-L-methionine in the treatment of liver diseases. J Hepatol 30(6):1155–1159, 1999.
10. Liber CS, Willams R. Recent advances in the treatment of liver diseases. Drugs 40(suppl 3):1–138, 1990.
11. Mato JM, Camara J, Fernandez de Paz J, Caballeria L, Coll S, Caballero A, Garcia-Buey L, Beltran J, Benita V, Caballeria J, Sola R, Moreno-Otero R, Barrao F, Martin-Duce A, Correa JA, Pares A, Barrao E, Garcia-Magaz I, Puerta JL, Moreno J, Boissard G, Ortiz P, Rodes J. S-Adenosylmethionine in alcoholic liver cirrhosis: a randomized, placebo-controlled, double-blind, multicenter clinical trial. J Hepatol 30(6):1081–1089, 1999.
12. Herby O. Role of polyamines in the control of cell proliferation and differentiation. Differentiation 19:1–20, 1981.
13. Oyanagui Y. Anti-inflammatory effects of polyamines in serotonin and carrageenan

paw edemata—possible mechanism to increase vascular permeability inhibitory protein level which is regulated by glucocorticoids and superoxide radical. Agents Actions 14(2):228–237, 1984.
14. Giulidori P, Cortellaro M, Moreo G, Stramentinoli G. Pharmacokinetics of S-adenosyl-L-methionine in healthy volunteers. Eur J Clin Pharmacol 227:119–121, 1984.
15. Stramentinoli G. Ademethionine as a drug. Am J Med 83(suppl 5A):35–42, 1987.
16. Bottiglieri T, Chary TKN, Laundy M, Carney MWP, Godfrey P, Toone BK, Reynolds EH. Transmethylation and depression. Alabama J Med Sci 25:296–300, 1988.
17. Giulidori P, Fellin M, Di Padova C. Metabolism of exogenous S-adenosylmethionine in humans and its significance in the therapeutic use of the drug. Proceedings of a IV Workshop on Methionine Metabolism, Sierra Nevada, Spain, 1998, pp 159–163.
18. Bottiglieri T, Chary TKN, Carney MWP, Godfrey P, Toone BK, Reynolds EH. Cerebrospinal fluid S-adenosylmethionine in depression and dementia: the effect of parenteral and oral treatment. J Neurol Neurosurg Psychiatr 53:1096–1098, 1990.
19. Castagna A, Le Grazie C, Giulidori P, Bottiglieri T, Lazzarin A. Deficiency of CSF S-adenosylmethionine (SAMe) and glutathione in HIV infected patients: the effect of parenteral treatment with SAMe. Neurology 45:1678–1683, 1995.
20. Stramentinoli G, Gualano M, Catto E, Algeri S. Tissue levels of S-adenosylmethionine in aging rats. J Gerontol 32(4):392–394, 1977.
21. Shivapurkar N, Poirier LA. Levels of S-adenosylmethionine and S-adenosylethionine in four different tissues of male weanling rats during subchronic feeding of DL-ethionine. Biochem Pharmacol 34(3):373–375, 1985.
22. Finkelstein JD, Kyle WE, Harris BJ, Martin JJ. Methionine metabolism in mammals: concentration of metabolites in rat tissues. J Nutr 112(5):1011–1018, 1982.
23. Sarda N, Reynaud D, Gharib A. S-adenosylmethionine, S-adenosylhomocysteine and adenosine system. Age-dependent availability in rat brain. Dev Pharmacol Ther 13(2–4):104–112, 1989.
24. Bohuon C, Callard L. S-adenosylmethionine in human blood. Clin Chim Acta 33: 256–257, 1971.
25. Surtees R, Hyland K. Cerebrospinal fluid concentrations of S-adenosylmethionine, methionine, and 5-methyltetrahydrofolate in a reference population: cerebrospinal fluid S-adenosylmethionine declines with age in humans. Biochem Med Metab Biol 44(2):192–199, 1990.
26. Bottiglieri T. Folate, vitamin B12, and neuropsychiatric disorders. Nutr Rev 54(12): 382–390, 1996.
27. Loehrer FM, Angst CP, Haefeli WE, Jordan PP, Ritz R, Fowler B. Low whole-blood S-adenosylmethionine and correlation between 5-methyltetrahydrofolate and homocysteine in coronary artery disease. Arterioscler Thromb Vasc Biol 16(6):727–733, 1996.
28. Surtees R, Hyland K, Smith I. Central-nervous-system methyl-group metabolism in children with neurological complications of HIV infection. Lancet 335:619–621, 1990.
29. Keating JN, Trimble KC, Mulcahy F, Scott JM, Weir DG. Evidence of brain methyltransferase inhibition and early involvement in HIV positive patients. Lancet 337: 935–939, 1991.
30. Quinn CT, Griener JC, Bottiglieri T, Hyland K, Farrow A, Kamen BA. Elevation

of homocysteine and excitatory amino acid neurotransmitters in the CSF of children who receive methotrexate for the treatment of cancer. J Clin Oncol 15(8):2800–2806, 1997.
31. Surtees R, Clelland J, Hann I. Demyelination and single-carbon transfer pathway metabolites during the treatment of acute lymphoblastic leukemia: CSF studies. J Clin Oncol 16(4):1505–1511, 1998.
32. Wurtman RJ. Effect of L-DOPA on S-adenosylmethionine levels and norepinephrine metabolism in rat brain. Adv Biochem Psychopharmacol 6:241–246, 1972.
33. Miller JW, Shukitt-Hale B, Villalobos-Molina R, Nadeau MR, Selhub J, Joseph JA. Effect of L-Dopa and the catechol-O-methyltransferase inhibitor Ro 41-0960 on sulfur amino acid metabolites in rats. L-dopa—human CSF SAMe. Clin Neuropharmacol 20(1):55–66, 1977.
34. Pall HS, Surtees R, Sturman SG. S-adenosylmethionine in cerebrospinal fluid in Parkinson's disease (abstr.) Neurology 42:283, 1992.
35. Cheng H, Gomes-Trolin C, Aquilonius SM, Steinberg A, Lofberg C, Ekblom J, Oreland L. Levels of L-methionine S-adenosyltransferase activity in erythrocytes and concentrations of S-adenosylmethionine and S-adenosylhomocysteine in whole blood of patients with Parkinson's disease. Exp Neurol 145:580–585, 1997.
36. Morrison LD, Smith DD, Kish SJ. Brain S-adenosylmethionine levels are severely decreased in Alzheimer's disease. J Neurochem 67(3):1328–1331, 1996.
37. Clarke R, Smith AD, Jobst KA, Refsum H, Sutton L, Ueland PM. Folate, vitamin B12, and serum total homocysteine levels in confirmed Alzheimer disease. Arch Neurol 55(11):1449–55, 1998.
38. Mato JM, Corrales F, Martin-Duce A, Ortiz P, Pajares MA, Cabrero C. Mechanisms and consequences of the impaired trans-sulphuration pathway in liver disease: Part I. Biochemical implications. Drugs 40 3(suppl):58–64, 1990.
39. Duce AM, Ortiz P, Cabrero C, Mato JM. S-Adenosyl-L-methionine synthetase and phospholipid methyltransferase are inhibited in human cirrhosis. Hepatology 8(1): 65–68, 1988.
40. Ubagai T, Lei K-J, Huand S, Mudd SH, Levy HL, Chou JY. Molecular mechaniss of an inborn error of methionine pathway: methionine adenosyltransferase deficiency. J Clin Invest 96:1943–1947, 1995.
41. Mudd SH, Chamberlin ME, Yang-Chou J. Isolated persistent hypermethioninemia: genetic metabolic and clinical aspects. Proceedings of a IV Workshop on Methionine Metabolism, Sierra Nevada, Spain, 1998, pp 3–13.
42. Surtees R, Leonard J, Austin S. Association of demyelination with deficiency of cerebrospinal fluid S-adenosylmethionine in inborn errors of methyl-transferase pathway. Lancet 338:1550–1554, 1991.
43. Carney MWP. Neuropharmacology of S-adenosylmethionine. Clin Neuropharmacol 9:235–243, 1986.
44. Baldessarini RJ. Neuropharmacology of S-adenosyl-L-methionine. Am J Med 83(suppl 5A):95–103, 1987.
45. Bottiglieri T, Hyland K, Reynolds EH. The clinical potential of ademethionine (S-adenosylmethionine) in neurological disorders. Drugs 48:1137–1152, 1994.
46. Algeri S, Catto E, Curcio M, Ponzio F, Stramentinoli G. Changes in rat brain noradrenaline and serotonin after administration of S-adenosylmethionine. In: Zappia

V, Usdin E, Salvatore S, eds. Biochemical and Pharmacological Roles of Adenosylmethionine and the Central Nervous System. New York: Pergamon Press, 1979: 81–87.

47. Otero-Losado ME, Rubio MC. Acute effects of S-adenosyl-L-methionine on catecholaminergic central function. Eur J Pharmacol 163:353–356, 1989.
48. Otero-Losado ME, Rubio MC. Acute changes in 5HT metabolism after S-adenosylmethionine administration. Gen Pharmacol 20:403–406, 1989.
49. Curcio M, Catto E, Stramentinoli G, Algeri S. Effect of SAMe on 5HT metabolism in rat brain. Prog Neuropsychopharmacol 2:65–71, 1978.
50. Mishima K, Higuchi H, Kamata M, Yoshimoto M, Hishikawa Y. Effect of acute and chronic S-adenosylmethionine (SAM) administration on dopaminergic function in rat striatum (abstr). Proc 15 JSBP: 714, 1994.
51. Bottiglieri T, Hyland K. Effect of S-adenosylmethionine on dopamine metabolism in the rat striatum: an in-vivo microdialysis study (abstr). Soc Neurosci Abstr 2(2): 834, 1996.
52. Czyrak A, Rogoz Z, Skuza G, Zajaczkowski W Maj J. Antidepressant activity of S-adenosylmethionine in mice and rats. J Basic Clin Physiol Pharmacol 3:1–17, 1992.
53. Cohen B, Stramentinoli G, Sosa AL, Babb SM, Olgiati V. Effects of the novel antidepressant S-adensosylmethionine on α1 and β-adrenoreceptors in rat brain. Eur J Pharmacol 170:201–207, 1989.
54. Cimino M, Vantini G, Algeri S, Curala G, Pezzoli C, Stramentinoli G. Age-related modification of dopaminergic and beta-adrenergic receptor systems: restoration to normal activity by modifying membrane fluidity with S-adenosylmethionine. Life Sci 34:2029–2039, 1984.
55. Muccioli G, Scordamaglia A, Bertacco S, Di Carlo R. Effect of S-adenosyl-L-methionine on brain muscarinic receptors. Eur J Pharmacol 227:293–299, 1992.
56. Sanchez de la Cuesta F, Martos F, Marquex F, Gonzalez J, Martinez G, Garcia A, Ruis F, Pavia J. Effect of S-adenosylmethionine on brain muscarinic subtypes of young rats (abstr). First European Congress of Pharmacology, Milan, 1995: 287.
57. Kowatch MA Roth GS. Effect of specific membrane perturbations on alpha-adrenergic and muscarinic-cholinergic signal transduction in rat parotid cell aggregates. Life Sci 55:2003–2010, 1994.
58. Fava M, Giannelli A, Rapisarda V, Petralia A, Guaraldi GP. Rapidity of onset of the antidepressant effect of parenteral S-adenosylmethionine. Psychiatry Res 56: 295–297, 1995.
59. Berlanga C, Ortega-Soto HA, Ontiveros M, Senties H. Efficacy of S-adenosyl-L-Methionine in speeding the onset of action of imipramine. Psychiatry Res 44:257–262, 1992.
60. Taylor KM, Randall PK. Depletion of S-adenosylmethionine in mouse brain by antidepressive drugs. J Pharmacol Exp Ther 194:303–310, 1995.
61. Barcelo HA, Wiemeyer JCM, Sagasta CL, Macia M, Barreira JC. Effect of S-adenosylmethionine on experimental osteoarthritis in rabbits. Am J Med 83(suppl 5A): 55–59, 1987.
62. Konig H, Stahl H, Sieper J, Wolf KJ. Magnetic resonance tomography of finger

polyarthritis: morphology and cartilage signals after ademetionine therapy (in German). Aktuelle Radiol 5(1):36–40, 1995.

63. Friedal HA, Karen LG, Benfield P. S-adenosylmethionine: a review of its pharmacological properties and therapeutic potential in liver dysfunction and affective disorders in relation to its physiological role in cell metabolism. Drugs 38:389–416, 1989.
64. Piccinino F, Sagnelli E, Pasquale G, Giusti G. S-adenosylmethionine in patients with chronic active hepatitis treated with steroids. Ital J Gastroenterol 14:186–188, 1982.
65. Torta R, Zanalda E, Rocca P, Ravizza L. Inhibitory activity of S-adenosylmethionine on serum gamma-glutamyl-transpeptidase increase induced by psychodrugs and anticonvulsants. Curr Ther Res 44:144–159, 1988.
66. Vendemiale G, Altomare E, Trizio T, Le Grazie C, Di Padova C, Salerno MT, Carrieri V, Albano O. Effects of oral S-adenosyl-L-methionine on hepatic glutathione in patients with liver disease. Scand J Gastroenterol 24(4):407–15, 1989.
67. Cibin M, Gentile N, Ferri M, Canton G, Gallimberti L. S-Adenosylmethionine (SAMe) is effective in reducing ethanol abuse in an outpatient program for alcoholics. In: Kuriyama et al., eds. Biomedical and Social Aspects of Alcohol and Alcoholism. Amsterdam: Elsevier Science Publishers B.V., 1988, pp 357–360.
68. Jacobsen S, Danneskiold-Samsoe B, Andersen RB. Oral S-adenosylmethionine in primary fibromyalgia. Double-blind clinical evaluation. Scand J Rheumatol 20(4): 294–302, 1991.
69. Tavoni A, Vitali C, Bombardieri S, Pasero G. Evaluation of S-adenosylmethionine in primary fibromyalgia. A double-blind crossover study. Am J Med (suppl 5A) 83: 107–110, 1987.
70. Volkmann H, Norregaard J, Jacobsen S, Danneskiold-Samsoe B, Knoke G, Nehrdich D. Double-blind, placebo-controlled cross-over study of intravenous S-adenosyl-L-methionine in patients with fibromyalgia. Scand J Rheumatol 26(3):206–211, 1997.

4

S-Adenosyl-L-Methionine: The Healthy Joint Product

Giorgio Stramentinoli
Crosspharma S.A., Milan, Italy

I. INTRODUCTION

S-Adenosyl-L-methionine (SAMe) is a naturally occurring molecule present in all living organisms and present in the food chain (Table 1). SAMe is synthesized from methionine and ATP by S-adenosylmethionine synthetase (ATP-L-methionine-S-adenosyltransferase, EC 2.5.1.6) (1) and takes part in several biological reactions, either as a group donor or as an enzymatic inducer. SAMe is probably second only to ATP in the variety of reactions for which it serves as a cofactor (2). The involvement of SAMe in three important biochemical pathways—transmethylation, transsulfuration, and aminopropylation (Fig. 1)—depends on its particular structure with a positive charge on the sulfur atom, which favors the cleavage of sulfur-carbon bonds. The denomination ''active methyl'' for SAMe indicates the important role of this metabolite in transmethylation processes (3).

In higher organisms more than 40 either anabolic or catabolic reactions involve the transfer of the methyl group of SAMe to various substrates, such as nucleic acids, proteins, and lipids (4) (Table 2). On the other hand, the release of the methyl group from the molecule is the starting point for the ''transsulfuration'' pathway, which gives rise to all endogenous sulfur compounds (5).

Polyamine synthesis is another important metabolic pathway in which SAMe takes part (6). After being transformed into a decarboxylated analog (DecaSAMe) by SAMe decarboxylase (EC 4.1.1.50), the aminopropyl group is transferred to putrescine to form polyamines, whereas the remaining portion of the molecule gives rise to methylthioadenosine (MTA).

Table 1 SAMe Content in Selected Foods

Food	SAMe content (μg/100 g)
Fruit	
Pear	47
Apple	36
Banana	365
Grape	329
Orange	139
Grapefruit	183
Peach	164
Vegetables	
Lettuce	540
Spinach	478
Carrot	6
Tomato	737
Meat-fish-egg-milk	
Beef liver	74
Beef steak	587
Pig muscle	423
Chicken breast	643
Sea bream (orata)	503
Trout	278
Egg	6
Milk (fresh, whole)	10
Miscellaneous	
Flour (dry)	3
Baker's yeast	552
Bread (inner)	180

Samples taken as early as possible in the production-to-consumption chain.

The importance of adequate SAMe concentrations in the conservation of cell homeostasis has been assessed for membrane fluidity, through methylation of membrane phospholipids, and for the generation of sulfurated compounds like proteoglycans, one of the major components of cartilage.

Several studies have been carried out in order to prove the utilization and the metabolism of SAMe administered exogenously both in animals (7) and in humans (8).

In a recent study performed in six male healthy volunteers, 100 mg of [methyl-^{3}H, ^{35}S] SAMe 1,4-butanedisulfonate was given by oral route: blood sam-

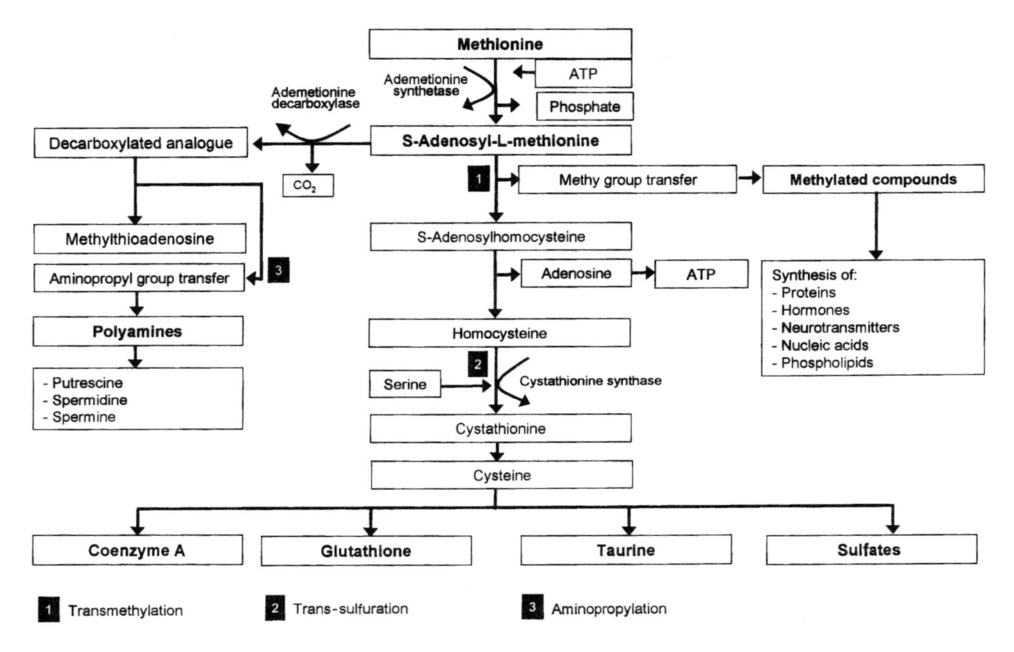

Figure 1 SAMe metabolic pathways.

ples were taken and urine and feces collected. The time courses of plasma concentrations of unmodified SAMe and of total ^{3}H and ^{35}S radioactivity (SAMe + metabolites) are shown in Figure 2. Both ^{3}H and ^{35}S radioactivity were higher than those of unmodified compounds, suggesting that circulating radioactivity is associated with metabolites rather than with the unmodified drug. After sharp initial increases of plasma concentrations, relatively late peaks were observed, most likely due to the redistribution of metabolite species present in plasma at various times after the administration.

The cumulative urinary excretion values over the 0- to 120-hour observation period accounted for 42 ± 13% and 19 ± 5% (mean ± SD) of the applied ^{35}S and ^{3}H radioactive doses, respectively. The analysis of metabolites in urine allowed the characterization and quantification of SAMe and main ^{35}S metabolites: the profile of main urinary metabolites in a representative subject is shown in Figure 3. The main metabolite in urine was sulfate, which in the 5 days following administration accounted for 65% of the total radioactive ^{35}S excreted.

The metabolism of applied SAMe, as reflected in the urinary metabolic profile, goes through transmethylation (SAH) and transsulfuration (taurine and

Table 2 Principal Transmethylation Reactions

O-Methylation		
Catecholamines	→	3-O-methylcatecholamines
Catechol estrogens	→	2-methyl-catechol estrogens
N-Acetyl serotonin	→	melatonin
Proteins		
N-Methylation		
Noradrenaline	→	adrenaline
Ethanolamine	→	choline
Histamine	→	methylhistamine
Cephaline	→	lecithin
Guanido acetic acid	→	creatine
Serotonin	→	methylserotonin
Proteins		
Nucleic acids		
C-Methylation		
Nucleic acids		
S-Methylation		
Exogenous compounds with sulfhydryl group		

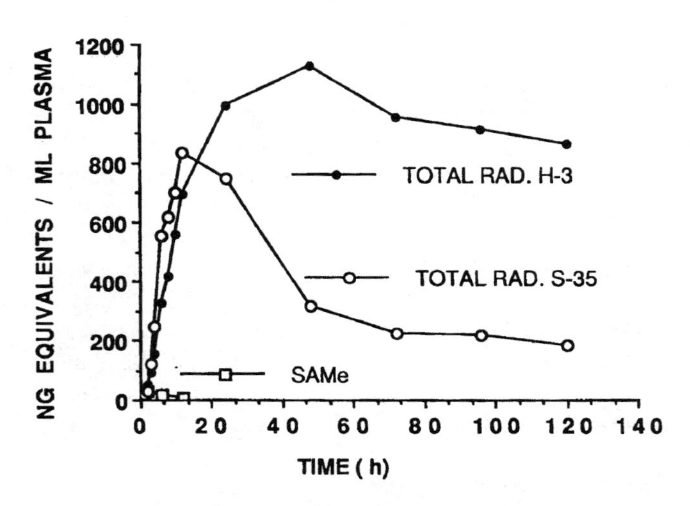

Figure 2 Mean concentrations of SAMe and of ^{3}H and ^{35}S radioactivity in the plasma of healthy volunteers ($n = 6$) receiving 100 mg of [methyl-^{3}H] and [^{35}S]SAMe by oral route.

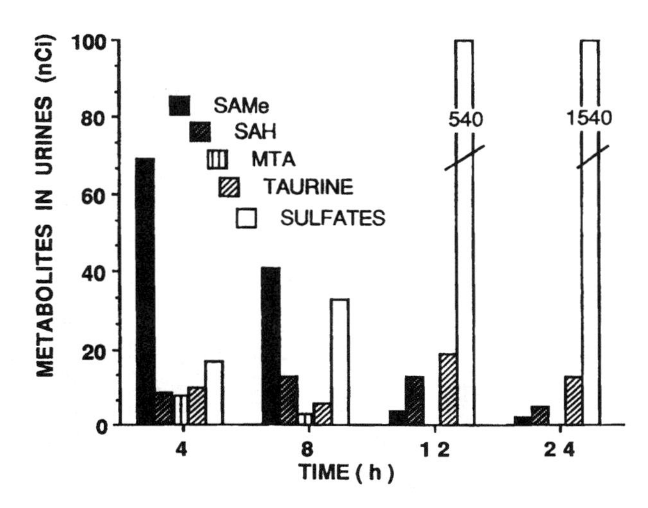

Figure 3 ^{35}S SAMe and main metabolites in urine from a healthy volunteer.

sulfates). Sulfates, an ultimate metabolite of cysteine formed by transsulfuration, are the main form of urinary excretion of ^{35}S SAMe metabolites, and its excretion greatly exceeds those of other metabolites and of unmodified SAMe.

The presystemic metabolism of SAMe, besides reducing the systemic availability of the unmodified drug, does not prevent, more likely promotes, the utilization of SAMe for the formation of sulfates. The finding that SAMe is actively metabolized to sulfate correlates very well with the effect of SAMe in maintaining the correct sulfuration status of the proteoglycans, a major component of cartilage. Cartilage is a connective tissue composed of two elements: cartilage cells (chondrocytes) and the acellular matrix, which surrounds the chondrocytes and constitutes about 90% of the articular cartilage. The matrix is formed by collagen fibers and a ground substance in which the collagen fibers are embedded; this ground substance is composed of glycosaminoglycans (GAGs). These polysaccharide molecules have attached numerous carboxyl and sulfate groups, which are negatively charged at physiological pH and therefore give an overall negative charge to the glycosaminoglycan chain. Because of their negative charge, the polysaccharide chains strongly repel each other and are highly hydrophilic. These physical characteristics of the GAGs are the basis for the resilient and flexible nature of cartilage.

The ability of SAMe to reach the disease ''site'' after oral administration was studied in patients with osteoarthritis to determine SAMe levels in synovial

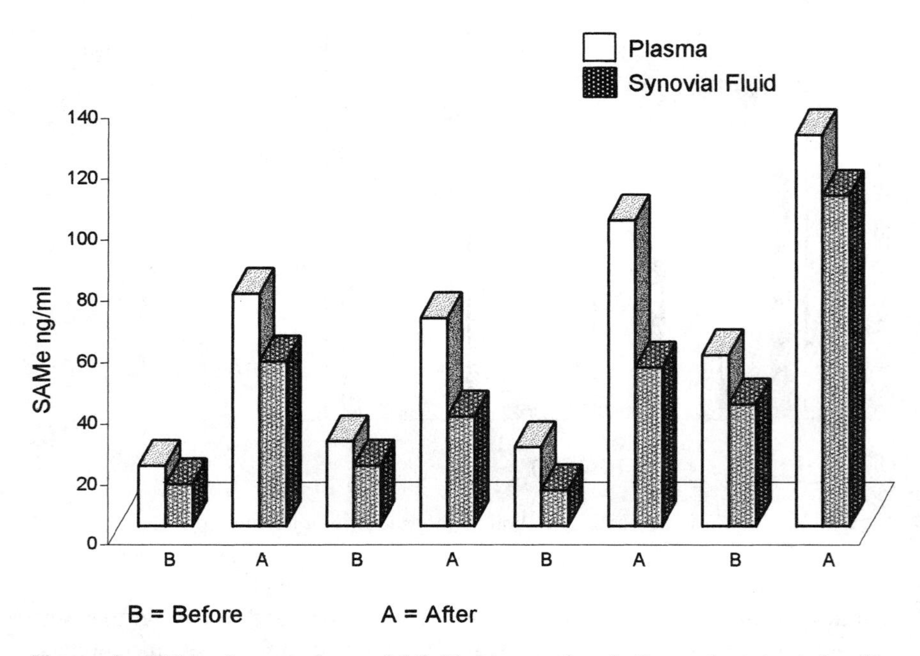

Figure 4 SAMe plasma and synovial fluid concentrations in four patients treated orally for 7 days with 400 mg twice a day. Samples were withdrawn before the first drug administration and on day 7, 4 hours after the last treatment.

fluid. The drug (400 mg as two enteric-coated tablets) was given daily to four patients at 8-hour intervals for 7 days. Before treatment and 4 hours after the last dose, samples of plasma and synovial fluid were collected and the SAMe concentration was determined. Plasma levels increased after treatment as expected, and a parallel increase was observed in the synovial fluid of all patients (Fig. 4).

II. SAMe IN OSTEOARTHRITIS: PRECLINICAL AND CLINICAL RESULTS

Osteoarthritis is characterized by a loss of joint cartilage and by hypertrophy of the adjacent bone. The American Arthritis Foundation estimates that about 43 million people in the United States have radiological evidence of osteoarthritis, including 85% of persons over the age of 70.

The exact mechanisms for cartilage damage in osteoarthritis have not been defined, but the loss of compressibility of cartilage secondary to proteoglycan malfunction seems to be a central feature in the development of the disease (9,10). In degenerative lesions of joint cartilage, the size of proteglycan molecules is reduced, because of either degradation or altered synthesis. In addition, the content of proteases and other hydrolases is increased in degenerative lesions. These observations, along with the findings of accelerated metabolic activity and increased chondrocyte division, indicate that increased degradation and increased synthesis of cartilage matrix occur concurrently.

Extensive research has clearly shown that SAMe plays a significant role in cellular physiology, such as the methylation of phospholipids, which is important in the transduction of biological response mediated by receptors located in the cell membrane, as well as in transsulfuration processes, which are relevant for the synthesis of proteoglycans. Harmand et al. (11) showed that SAMe appears to enhance native proteoglycan synthesis and secretion in human chondrocyte cultures arising from the cartilage of patients with osteoarthritis. This experiment showed that SAMe prevalently increased the synthesis of native proteoglycans, which are important for cartilage repair (Fig. 5).

Additional experiments in vivo have shown that SAMe also prevents surgically induced experimental osteoarthritis in rabbits. In particular, SAMe antagonized degenerative joint lesions following partial meniscectomy performed according to the method of Moskowitz et al. (12). In SAMe-treated animals, significantly greater cartilage thickness as well as higher chondrocyte counts compared to placebo-treated rabbits have been reported (13) (Fig. 6). Moreover, the proteoglycan content of cartilage assessed by histochemistry (14) appeared greater in SAMe-treated animals than in control animals, indirectly confirming the previous in vitro data by Harmand et al. (11) that SAMe stimulates proteoglycan biosynthesis.

From a clinical point of view, SAMe has been evaluated extensively in different studies (15–30). More than 22,000 patients have been enrolled in these trials. The period of treatment ranged between 3 weeks and 2 years. The dosage of SAMe varied between 400 and 1200 mg per day orally. The controlled clinical trials have shown that SAMe improved both subjective and objective symptoms of osteoarthritis more than placebo and to the same extent as nonsteroidal anti-inflammatory drugs. SAMe was very well tolerated, so that it was possible to administer the compound for long periods (up to 24 months). Based on these findings we can state that SAMe is an ideal product to be utilized as a nutraceutical because it is a physiological compound and it is extremely safe; it is also a good example of how the biochemistry correlates very well with the clinical expected activity.

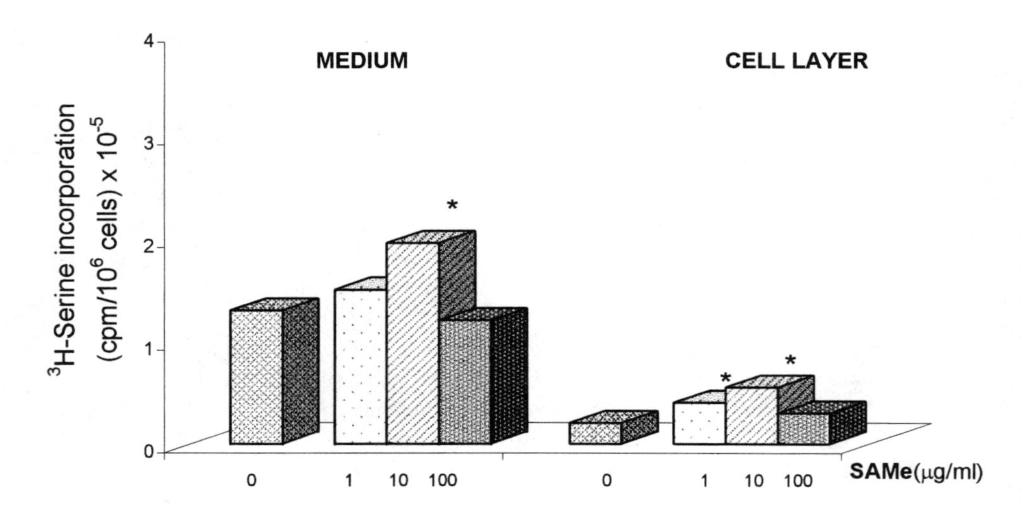

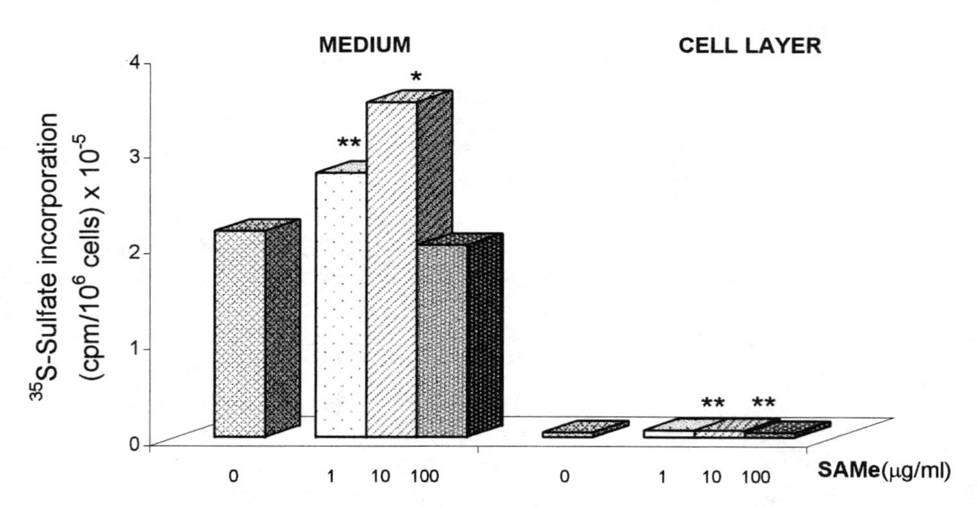

Figure 5 Effect of SAMe on ^{3}H-serine incorporation (top) and ^{35}S-sulfate incorporation (bottom) obtained in fractions from media and cell layers of osteoarthritis cultures. $*p < 0.001$; $**p < 0.01$.

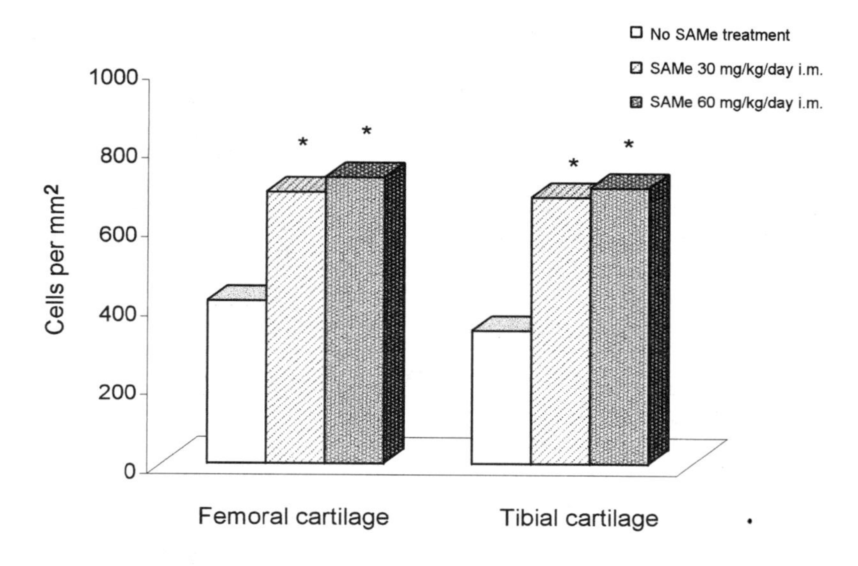

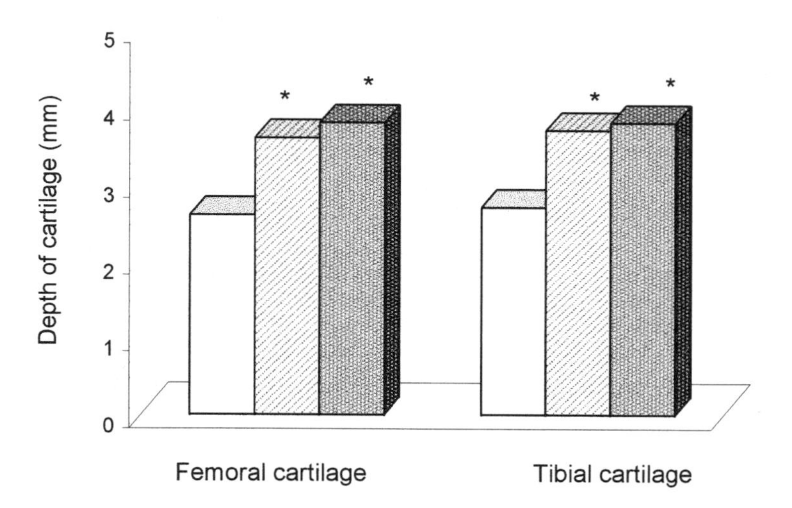

Figure 6 Cell numbers (top) and depth of articular cartilage (bottom) in rabbits with experimental osteoarthritis 12 weeks after surgery. $*p < 0.001$.

REFERENCES

1. Cantoni GL. The nature of the active methyl donor formed enzymatically from L-methionine and adenosine triphosphate. J Am Chem Soc 74:2942–2943, 1952.
2. Salvatore F, Borek E, Zappia V, et al. The Biochemistry of Adenosylmethionine. New York: Columbia University Press, 1977.
3. Greenberg GM. Biological methylation. Adv Enzymol 25:395–431, 1963.
4. Mudd SH, Cantoni GL. Biological transmethylation, methyl groups neogenesis and other ''one carbon'' metabolic reactions dependent upon tetrahydrofolic acid. In: Comprehensive Biochemistry. Amsterdam: Elsevier, 1964.
5. Finkelstein JD. Control of sulfur metabolism in mammals. In: OH Muth, Oldfield JE, eds. Sulfur in Nutrition. Westport, CT: AVI Publishing Co., 1970:46–60.
6. Williams-Ashman HG, Pegg AE. Aminopropyl group transfers in polyamine biosynthesis. In: Morris DR, Marton LJ, eds. Polyamines in Biology and Medicine. New York: Marcel Dekker, 1981:43–68.
7. Giulidori P, Stramentinoli G, et al. Transmethylation, transsulfuration and aminopropylation reactions of S-adenosyl-L-methionine in vivo. J Biol Chem 259(7):4205–4211, 1984.
8. Giulidori P, Fellin M, Di Padova C. Metabolism of exogenous S-adenosylmethionine in humans and its significance in the therapeutic use of the drug. In: IV Workshop on Methionine Metabolism: Molecular Mechanisms and Clinical Implications. Sierra Nevada, Granada: JM Mato, A Caballero, 1998:157–163.
9. Brandt KD. Photogenesis of osteoarthritis. In: Kelley WN, et al. Textbook of Rheumatology. Philadelphia: WB Saunders Co., 1985:1417–1431.
10. Dieppe P, et al. Osteoarthritis: progressive or controllable? A review of new research developments and their clinical significance. Morristown, NJ: Pharmalibri, 1986.
11. Harmand MF, et al. Effects of S-adenosylmethionine on human articular chondrocyte differentiation: an in vitro study. Am J Med 83(suppl 5A):48–54, 1987.
12. Moskowitz RW, et al. Experimentally induced degenerative joint lesions following partial meniscectomy in the rabbit. Arthritis Rheum 16:397–405, 1973.
13. Barcelò HA, et al. Effect of S-Adenosylmethionine on experimental osteoarthritis in rabbits. Am J Med 83(suppl 5A):55–59, 1987.
14. Barcelò HA, et al. Morphologische Untersuchungen zur Struktur degenerative Gelenklasionen beim Kaninchen ohne und mit Behandlung mit GAG-Peptid-komplex (GAG-Pep). Akt Rheumatol 9:113–121, 1984.
15. Ballabio CB, et al. Le traitement medical de la coxarthrose. J Med Strasbourg (Eur Med) 9(7):313–319, 1978.
16. Capretto C, et al. A double-blind controlled study of S-adenosylmethionine (SAMe) v. ibuprofen in gonarthrosis, coxarthrosis and spondylarthrosis. Clin Trials J 22:15–24, 1985.
17. Glorioso S, et al. Double-blind multicentre study of the activity of S-adenosylmethionine in hip and knee osteoarthritis. Int J Clin Pharm Res 1:39–49, 1985.
18. Marcolongo R, et al. Double-blind multicentre study of the activity of S-adenosylmethionine in hip and knee osteoarthritis. Curr Ther Res 37(1):82–94, 1985.
19. Caruso I, et al. Double-blind study of S-adenosyl-methionine versus placebo in hip

and knee arthrosis. Biological Methylation and Drug Design—Experimental and Clinical Roles of S-Adenosylmethionine.'' Totowa, NJ: Humana Press, 1986:363.
20. Harmand MF, et al. Effects of S-adenosylmethionine on human articular chondrocyte differentiation. Am J Med 83(suppl 5A):48–54, 1987.
21. Di Padova C, et al. S-Adenosylmethionine in the treatment of osteoarthritis. Review of the clinical studies. Am J Med 83(suppl 5A):60–65, 1987.
22. Maccagno A, et al. Double-blind controlled clinical trial of oral S-adenosylmethionine versus piroxicam in knee osteoarthritis. Am J Med 83(suppl 5A):72–77, 1987.
23. Vetter G. Double-blind comparative clinical trial with S-adenosylmethionine and indomethacin in the treatment of osteoarthritis. Am J Med 83(suppl 5A):78–80, 1987.
24. Müller-Fassbender H. Double-blind clinical trial of S-adenosylmethionine versus ibuprofen in the treatment of osteoarthritis. Am J Med 83(suppl 5A):81–83, 1987.
25. Berger R, et al. A new medical approach to the treatment of osteoarthritis. Report of an open phase IV study with ademetionine (Gumbaral). Am J Med 83(suppl 5A): 84–88, 1987.
26. Konig B. A long-term (two years) clinical trial with S-adenosylmethionine for the treatment of osteoarthritis. Am J Med 83(suppl 5A):89–94, 1987.
27. Delrieu F, et al. Etude preliminaire de la L-methionine dans le traitement de la polyarthrite rhumatoide. Rev Rhumat 55(12):995–997, 1988.
28. Domljan Z, et al. A double-blind trial of ademethionine vs naproxen in activated gonarthrosis. Intal J Clin Pharmacol Ther Toxicol 27(7):329–333, 1989.
29. Kalbhen DA, et al. Pharmakologische Untersuchungen zur antidegenerativen Wirkung von Ademetonin bei der tierexperimentellen Arthrose. Arzneir-Forsch Drug Res 40(11), 9:1017–1021, 1990.
30. Konig H, et al. Magnetresonanztomographie der Fingerpolyarthrose: Morphologie und Knorpelsignalverhalten unter Ademetonintherapie. Akt Radiol 5:36–40, 1995.

5

Methyltetrahydrofolate: The Superior Alternative to Folic Acid

John Scott
Trinity College, Dublin, Ireland

I. FOLATE COFACTORS IN NATURE

The folates are the collective name for the 10 or so different forms of this vitamin that occur in nature (1). They all consist of a pteridine ring, which is attached to *p*-aminobenzoic acid, which in turn is attached to the amino acid glutamate (Fig. 1). In all of the naturally occurring forms of the vitamin, the pteridine ring is in the reduced state, as tetrahydrofolate, either on its own or with different so-called carbon one units attached to it, i.e., formyl (—CHO), methylene ($—CH_2—$), methenyl (—CH=), or methyl ($—CH_3$). The sole exception is dihydrofolate, formed as a result of the action of the enzyme thymidylate synthase, which, as discussed later, is involved in the conversion of the uracil-type base found in RNA to the thymine-type base found in DNA. In all cells not one but several glutamates are attached to the folates. These are linked to each other through the γ-carboxyl group. During intestinal absorption this polyglutamate chain is removed by an enzyme present in the brush border of the duodenal mucosal cells called folate polyglutamate conjugase. This enzyme converts all of the naturally occurring folate polyglutamates into monoglutamates.

II. FOLATE ABSORPTION FROM THE INTESTINE

A mixture of various folate monoglutamates, e.g., tetrahydrofolate, 10-formyltetrahydrofolate, and 5-methyltetrahydrofolate, cross the intestinal mucosal cells. During this transit, all of these different forms are converted to a single form,

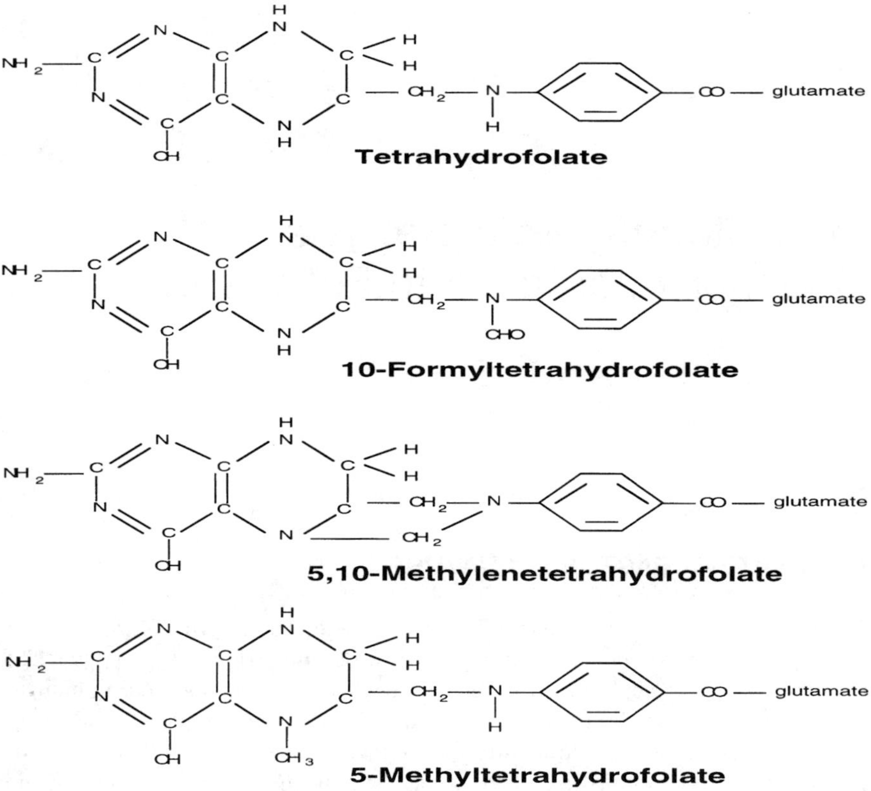

Tetrahydrofolate

10-Formyltetrahydrofolate

5,10-Methylenetetrahydrofolate

5-Methyltetrahydrofolate

Figure 1 Structures of some common naturally occurring folates, including 5-methyltetrahydrofolate.

5-methyltetrahydrofolate, if they are not in that form already (2). Thus, under normal circumstances only a single form of folate crosses into the human circulation. However, the capacity of this system to convert everything into 5-methyltetrahydrofolate is limited (see later).

III. FOLATE UPTAKE BY CELLS FROM THE CIRCULATION

For the reasons stated above, in the human circulation there is usually only one form of folate, namely, 5-methyltetrahydrofolate monoglutamate. This is thus the only form normally presented to human cells. It appears that cells take up this cofactor by passive or facilitated diffusion. It is, however, clear that this 5-methyltetrahydrofolate monoglutamate can pass back out of cells.

The system of uptake or, more importantly, the retention of the circulating 5-methyltetrahydrofolate monoglutamate occurs as follows: after uptake, the vitamin can and will pass back out of the cells unless it is converted into a polyglutamate and thus retained. In the cell there is only one enzyme that uses 5-methyltetrahydrofolate as a substrate—the vitamin B_{12}–dependent enzyme methionine synthase. This enzyme is part of the methylation cycle (Fig. 2). Its role is to remethylate homocysteine back to methionine. This methionine is then activated by ATP to produce s-adenosylmethionine (SAM). This form of methionine, sometimes called ''active methionine,'' is the methyl donor for dozens of methyltransferases that exist in all cells. These methyltransferases methylate a wide

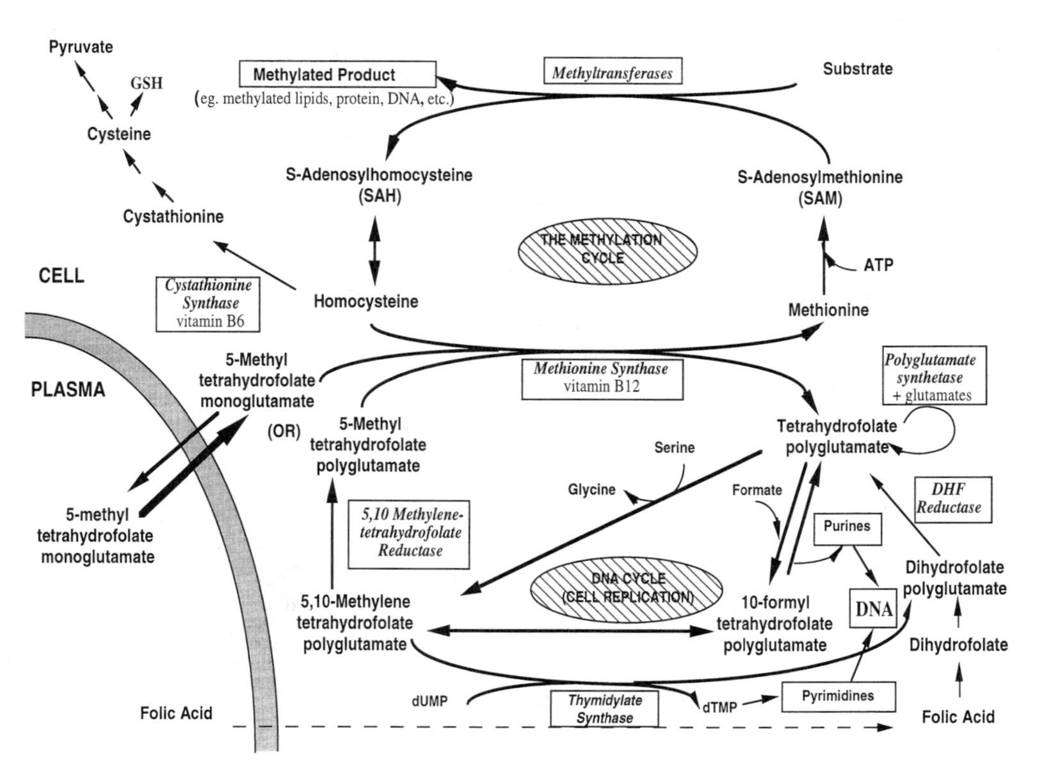

Figure 2 Metabolic pathways in which folate cofactors are involved showing difference in cellular uptake and retention of 5-methyltetrahydrofolate monoglutamate compared to folic acid.

range of substrates as diverse as hormones such as dopamine, lipids such as phosphatidylethanolamine, and proteins such as myelin basic protein. Thus, 5-methyltetrahydrofolate effectively continuously supplies the methylation cycle with methyl groups.

The cell has adapted to use this methionine synthase reaction as the method to control the retention of 5-methyltetrahydrofolate (3). It does this as follows: 5-methyltetrahydrofolate is a very poor substrate for polyglutamate synthase. However, after it is acted upon by this enzyme as part of the methylation cycle, it is converted into tetrahydrofolate. This cofactor, as well as other reduced carbon one–substituted folates, such as 10-formyltetrahydrofolate, are very good substrates for polyglutamation (3). Thus, once 5-methyltetrahydrofolate is metabolized to tetrahydrofolate monoglutamate, it will be converted into a polyglutamate and retained. The deciding factor for methionine synthase to use newly taken-up 5-methyltetrahydrofolate monoglutamate is its concentration relative to the concentration of 5-methyltetrahydrofolate polyglutamate already present in the cell. Both the monoglutamate and the polyglutamate form of 5-methyltetrahydrofolate can be used by methionine synthase, but under normal circumstances in folate-replete cells the concentration of the polyglutamate is high and that of the monoglutamate is low. Thus, very little of the latter is converted to tetrahydrofolate and retained. It will therefore diffuse back out of the cell. However, if the cells become folate deficient, then the relative concentration of cellular folate polyglutamates to monoglutamates begins to decrease. Then, more and more of the 5-methyltetrahydrofolate monoglutamate will be used by methionine synthase and converted into tetrahydrofolate monoglutamate and 10-formyltetrahydrofolate monoglutamate. These are good substrates for polyglutamate synthetase and are thus converted into polyglutamates and retained within cells. As more and more of these latter cofactors are polyglutamated and retained, they are recycled back to 5-methyltetrahydrofolate polyglutamates, which progressively compete with the newly taken-up 5-methyltetrahydrofolate monoglutamates for methionine synthase. Thus, as the cells become folate replete they will retain less and less of recently taken-up 5-methyltetrahydrofolate. Apart from where cells need to take up and retain more folate because they are folate deficient, when cells divide the daughter cells will initially have half of the original concentration of folate that existed in the parent cells. This will result in a lower than optimal concentration of 5-methyltetrahydrofolate polyglutamate being available to methionine synthase. Methionine synthase will thus use 5-methyltetrahydrofolate monoglutamate taken up from the circulating plasma. As this is converted into tetrahydrofolate and retained, the folate concentration of the cell begins to build up. The concentration of 5-methyltetrahydrofolate will also build up. Thus less and less of the monoglutamate is used by methionine synthase and retained. Another factor that will influence the ultimate concentration retained by cells is the concentration of 5-methyltetrahydrofolate monoglutamates in the plasma. The higher this is, the higher will be the monoglutamate intracellular concentration and the higher the chances that it will be used by methionine synthase and thus retained.

IV. FOLIC ACID UPTAKE BY CELLS

Folic acid is the synthetic form of the vitamin (Fig. 3). It differs from the naturally occurring folates in that the pterdine ring is not reduced. Folic acid does not occur naturally since all of the cellular forms of the vitamin are either in the tetrahydro or dihydro state of reduction (Fig. 1). A very small amount of folic acid can be isolated from cells. In fact it was the form of the vitamin originally isolated from spinach and named folic acid after *folium*, the Latin word for leaf (4). It is now recognized that folic acid occurs through the in vitro oxidation of some natural tetrahydrofolates. Synthetic folic acid, whether taken as a supplement or in fortified food, can be converted like the other folate monoglutamates to 5-methyltetrahydrofolate during its passage through the intestinal mucosal cells. However, the capacity of the intestinal cells to do this is limited. It has been shown that at supplement levels greater than 300 μg, one begins to see unaltered folic acid in the plasma (5). This synthetic form of the vitamin is rapidly excreted by the kidney. However, during the period when it is in the plasma, it is presented to cells via the circulation. In common with 5-methyltetrahydrofolate it diffuses into cells. One might expect that, since it does not occur in nature, folic acid would be inactive in cells. However, it transpires that it is acted upon by the enzyme dihydrofolate reductase. This enzyme's function is normally to convert dihydrofolates that arise during the action of the enzyme thymidylate synthetase back to tetrahydrofolates. Thymidylate synthetase converts deoxyuridine monophosphate to deoxythymidine monophosphate during pyrimidine biosynthesis (Fig. 2). The carbon one–substituted cofactor used by the enzyme, namely 5,10-

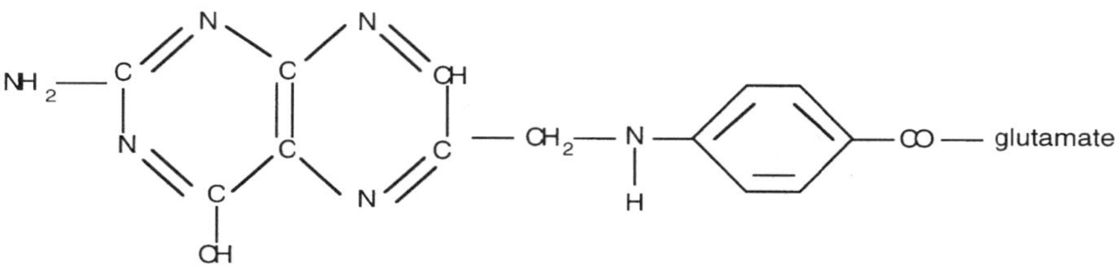

Folic acid

Figure 3 Structure of folic acid, the synthetic form of the vitamin.

methylenetetrahydrofolate, is unique in folate-dependent carbon one donations in that the product is not tetrahydrofolate but dihydrofolate. This must constantly be recycled back to tetrahydrofolate for the cell to keep folate metabolism going. This is achieved by the enzyme dihydrofolate reductase. After converting folic acid to dihydrofolate, the same enzyme then converts it to tetrahydrofolate. Once folic acid is converted to dihydrofolate or tetrahydrofolate, it will be made into a polyglutamate and retained by the cells. Thus, folic acid is really an inactive provitamin that happens to be acted upon by a folate-dependent enzyme whose natural function is to carry out a different reaction. In any event, by the above means the non–naturally occurring provitamin folic acid gains access to the cell's metabolic pathway and, because it is converted into a polyglutamate, it is retained by cells.

This entry and retention of folic acid by human cells is fundamentally different from that which applies to 5-methyltetrahydrofolate monoglutamate, the sole circulating natural form of the vitamin. As discussed above, this cofactor must be demethylated to tetrahydrofolate before it will be made into a polyglutamate and retained by the cells. In fact, as described, increasing or decreasing use of 5-methyltetrahydrofolate monoglutamate instead of 5-methyltetrahydrofolate polyglutamate is the way that cells increase or decrease retention of circulating folates. Thus, increased retention will occur in deficient cells or where cell division has reduced the intracellular 5-methyltetrahydrofolate polyglutamate content relative to its corresponding monoglutamate content. In addition, raising the circulating level of 5-methyltetrahydrofolate will have some effect on raising intracellular levels, thus leading to somewhat more 5-methyltetrahydrofolate monoglutamate being used by methionine synthase and retained as a polyglutamate. Thus, the system is designed to regulate retention of new folates commensurate with the needs of the cell but will be somewhat influenced by the plasma level. By contrast, the uptake of folic acid has no such constraint for retention. Once cells express the enzyme dihydrofolate reductase, a feature common to all dividing cells, they will metabolize and retain folic acid. The higher the plasma level and consequently the intracellular level, the greater this uptake and retention will be. Thus, folic acid is not subject to the usual control of cellular uptake to which 5-methyltetrahydrofolate in the circulation is subjected.

V. THE ROLE OF VITAMIN B_{12} IN CELLULAR RETENTION OF CIRCULATING 5-METHYLTETRAHYDROFOLATE AND FOLIC ACID

As mentioned above, the enzyme methionine synthase is vitamin B_{12} dependent (Fig. 2). It is well known that deficiency of vitamin B_{12} such as occurs in the autoimmune disease pernicious anemia (PA) has two distinct clinical consequences, anemia and neuropathy. It is now recognized that neuropathy is due to interruption of the methylation cycle (6), which for reasons now beginning to emerge produces destruction of the myelin sheath (7,8). In PA there is also anemia, which is identical to that seen in folate deficiency (9). It thus seems probable that interruption of the activity of methionine synthase in some way disrupts normal folate function. The explanation that seems most likely to fit with most of the experimental and clinical evidence is called the ''methyl-trap hypothesis.'' It suggests that in vitamin B_{12}—deficient cells, cellular folate becomes trapped as 5-methyltetrahydrofolate polyglutamates. Thereafter, progressively more and more of the cellular folates in PA will find their way into this form and will be trapped and incapable of further metabolism. This progressive trapping would consequently deplete the cells of the other forms of folate necessary for purine (10-formyltetrahydrofolate) and pyrimidine (5,10-methylenetetrahydrofolate) biosynthesis. Thus, cells would undergo a sort of pseudo folate deficiency. They would have folate, but it would be in a form that could not be used for purine and pyrimidine biosynthesis. Consequently, DNA biosynthesis and cell division would stop, just as if the cells were folate deficient. When this would happen in the bone marrow, the resultant anemia would be identical to that seen in folate deficiency. It might at first seem hard to believe that cells would respond to vitamin B_{12} deficiency in such an inappropriate way. However, it appears that the cell has evolved to expect not to become vitamin B_{12} deficient and interprets what happens in vitamin B_{12} deficiency in an inappropriate way. During vitamin B_{12} deficiency, as the level of methionine synthase diminishes, the recycling of homocysteine back to methionine also diminishes. This in turn causes the level SAM to start to decrease. Because SAM is vital as a methyl donor for some dozens of methyltransferases in all mammalian cells, the vitamin B_{12}–deficient cells set about reestablishing the level of SAM. The way they do this is to encourage more methionine synthesis and with it SAM synthesis. To make more methionine the cells need to increase the cellular concentration of the two substrates for vitamin B_{12}–dependent methionine synthase—homocysteine and 5-methyltetrahydrofolate. It increases the level of the former by reducing its SAM-dependent inhibition of the enzyme 5,10-methylenetetrahydrofolate (MTHF) reductase. This inhibition is achieved by the enzyme having an allosteric binding site for SAM. When SAM is bound to the enzyme, its activity is decreased, which indicates to the cell that there are adequate concentrations of the constituents of the methylation cycle. What is more important from the point of view of the methyl trap hypothesis is that the reductase enzyme that makes 5-methyltetrahydrofolate is also influenced by low levels of SAM. As the level of SAM begins to decrease, the activity of the reductase progressively increases, thus converting more and more of the folate cofactors into 5-methyltetrahydrofolate. The methyl trap hypothesis also requires that the action of the MTHF reductase is irreversible. This does in fact appear to be the case. For the reductase to be reversed requires the presence of a very strong electron acceptor. While this can and is achievable in vitro using an artificial electron acceptor such as menadione, it appears that no such acceptor exists in cells. In addition the methyl trap hypothesis requires that the only enzyme that can metabolize 5-methyltetrahydrofolate is the vitamin B_{12}–dependent enzyme methionine synthase. This appears to be correct in that no other enzyme has ever been identified. Thus in vitamin B_{12}–deficient bone marrow, once formed, 5-methyltetrahydrofolate is metabolically trapped and cannot be used for folate-dependent DNA biosynthesis. This in turn prevents cell division and produces an identical anemia to that seen in folate deficiency.

Treatment of the anemia in folate deficiency with folate or folic acid will replenish cellular folates and thus restart purine and pyrimidine biosynthesis and with it DNA biosynthesis and cell division. Treatment with vitamin B_{12} will do nothing since methionine synthase is already in a fully active state.

Treatment of the identical anemia found in conditions of vitamin B_{12} deficiency such as PA with vitamin B_{12} will reactivate methionine synthase and release the trapped methyltetrahydrofolate to make tetrahydrofolate and the other folate cofactors. This quickly leads to purine and pyrimidine biosynthesis and the synthesis of DNA and cell division, i.e., to the treatment of the anemia. Treatment of vitamin B_{12} deficiency with the folate cofactor 5-methyltetrahydrofolate would not be expected to do anything. It would just become added to the already trapped folate of the same form. Just like the endogenous folate of the same form, it would not be able to pass through the enzyme methionine synthase now inactive because of inadequate vitamin B_{12}. In fact, one would expect that it would not even be retained in such vitamin B_{12}–deficient cells, because since it is not a substrate for polyglutamate synthethase it would just exit the cell. There is in fact ample evidence that this happens naturally in the case of circulating 5-methyltetrahydrofolate. A feature of vitamin B_{12} deficiency is that cellular folate levels are markedly reduced even in the face of normal or even elevated plasma 5-methyltetrahydrofolate.

However, if such vitamin B_{12}–deficient bone marrow is treated with folic acid, a different pattern emerges. As described above, when folic acid enters cells, such as bone marrow cells, that are dividing and contain the enzyme dihydrofolate reductase, it is converted to dihydrofolate. This in turn is converted to tetrahydrofolate and the formyl and methylene derivatives that participate respectively in purine and pyrimidine biosynthesis. The latter forms are also converted into polyglutamates, thus ensuring that the folic acid so taken up by cells and metabolized will be retained. This process happens in normal cells, but it will also happen in vitamin B_{12}–deficient cells. This is because the activity of methionine synthase is not involved in the above process. Thus in normal cells and vitamin B_{12}–deficient cells, folic acid will quickly and directly permit the synthesis of the folate cofactors needed for purine and pyrimidine biosynthesis. Thus folic acid will initiate DNA biosynthesis and cell division. Eventually these folate derivatives will be channeled toward MTHF reductase, now very active because of low cellular SAM levels. They will eventually be trapped. However, they will have permitted some cell division and thus a bone marrow response. If the folic acid is given continuously to a person with vitamin B_{12} deficiency, the bone marrow will continue to respond and the anemia that was present will be treated. It might be felt that this would be appropriate. However, this so-called masking of the anemia is dangerous and inappropriate. This is because most people with PA are diagnosed by the presence of the anemia. The neuropathy, which is also a feature of PA, is much more difficult to recognize clinically. Thus, by masking the anemia, PA may not be diagnosed at the appropriate time. While the anemia is being treated the neuropathy will progress. This is because folic acid itself, or even when it is metabolized to dihydro, tetrahydro, or to the corresponding formyl and methylene forms, cannot restart the methylation cycle. It is the absence of the methylation cycle that is the cause of the neuropathy. Likewise, the eventual conversion of folic acid, after metabolism, to 5-methyltetrahydrofolate will also not restart the methylation cycle because it will remain interrupted due to the inactivity of methionine synthase, which is essential for the cycle. Thus, folic acid treatment will prevent the diagnosis of PA by masking the presence of the anemia, but it will not treat the neuropathy. There is even some support for the possibility that treatment with folic acid will exacerbate the neuropathy, causing it to progress at a faster rate, all the time becoming more and more irreversible (10). When the diagnosis is eventually made and proper treatment with intramuscular vitamin B_{12} is instituted, much of this nerve damage will remain.

VI. THE NECESSITY TO IMPROVE FOLATE STATUS IN MOST INDIVIDUALS AND POPULATIONS

Traditionally, it was believed that anybody who consumed three or four meals per day of a mixed diet would obtain enough of every nutrient to ensure optimal health. There is now very good evidence that this is not true for folate status. It is now agreed that the diet as currently eaten and constituted, even in the most developed countries of Europe and North America, will not produce optimal status to prevent certain conditions. Thus it has been shown that in the majority of women, the risk of having a baby affected by spina bifida can be reduced dramatically if folate/folic acid is taken periconceptionally (11). There is now very strong (and some would say almost conclusive) evidence that any elevation of plasma homocysteine causes an increased risk of heart disease (12) and stroke (13). Homocysteine is an amino acid that occurs naturally in plasma. It arises from the breakdown of the dietary amino acid methionine, which is found in about 60% excess over the body needs in most diets. This excess is broken down and used for energy via a metabolic pathway that involves the syntheses and subsequent breakdown of homocysteine (Fig 2). The level of homocysteine is rigorously controlled, both in cells and in plasma, either by its degradation or by its reconversion back to methionine, the latter being used to maintain the level of SAM and to ensure adequate provision of methyl groups for the methylation cycle. This is achieved by three enzymes. Two of these enzymes require folate cofactors for their activity. It is clear that in the majority of populations and in almost all of the elderly, insufficient folate is provided by the diet to allow these enzymes to function optimally (14). Thus, most apparently normal people have homocysteine levels that can be lowered by ingestion of small physiological levels of folic acid (15). The overall result is that most diets, without having their folic acid/folate level enhanced, carry with them an increased but preventable risk of heart disease and stroke (16).

Several lines of evidence have suggested that increased intake of folic acid/folate in the diet will reduce the risk of colorectal cancer (17). A recent study has added greatly to this evidence by showing in a large group of apparently normal women followed for decades that the long-term ingestion of a vitamin supplement that contains folic acid very significantly lowered the prevalence of colorectal cancer (18). What was particularly impressive about this study was that this protective effect was not found in those who had only recently taken supplements. There was increased protection as one extended the taking of supplements from years to decades, as one would expect on biological grounds.

VII. COMPARISON OF FOLIC ACID AND 5-METHYLTETRAHYDROFOLATE TO IMPROVE FOLATE STATUS

If one accepts the case that folate status must be improved in most individuals and populations, there are three ways in which this might be achieved:

1. Changing dietary intake patterns toward foods that are high in naturally occurring folates
2. Taking supplements
3. Fortifying the diet with vitamins

Option 1 is in practice not easily achieved. It has proven notoriously difficult to get the average person to change their usual diet and to maintain a new dietary pattern of intake. This is exacerbated by the fact that, while folate is widely distributed in nature, it is not really abundant in any particular food. The sole exception would be liver, which forms a very insignificant part of most diets. Thus, improving intake has mostly been addressed through either taking supplements or taking foods fortified with the vitamin. In both instances the form of the vitamin used to date has been the synthetic form, folic acid. This form, as mentioned above, does not occur in nature and is really a provitamin. It is certainly well suited to the task of changing folate status. It is chemically extremely stable and probably totally absorbed. However, in the final analysis it is a synthetic derivative that human cells were not designed to encounter. As discussed above, this is reflected in the way in which folic acid can gain access to cells. It is not limited by the system that regulates the uptake and cellular retention of the naturally occurring form in plasma, namely 5-methyltetrahydrofolate. It could be argued that since folic acid is converted into this natural form during its passage across the intestinal mucosal cells, giving folic acid is the equivalent of giving the natural form. However, as mentioned earlier the capacity of the intestinal mucosa to do this is extremely limited and consequently even a single supplement of 300 μg of folic acid results in the synthetic provitamin appearing in the circulation. If, in all circumstances one could be sure that less than this amount, say 200 μg, was going to be taken by an individual person, then clearly the provitamin would always be converted to the natural form and this would be the only form presented to cells other than those of the intestinal mucosa. However, virtually all supplements contain 400 μg per tablet, and it seems very probable that this will continue. This is because the current thinking is to revise the recommendation for daily intakes upward.

The most recent revision of the Recommended Dietary Allowances (RDA) just completed in the United States changed the RDA for adults to up to 400 μg of dietary folate equivalent per day (19). This is equivalent to 200 μg of pure folic acid. If one seeks to increase intake using fortified food, there is an even bigger potential for unaltered folic acid to appear in the plasma. This is because the food to which folic acid would be added, be it flour or breakfast cereal, will have a range of intake, unlike supplements, which will be usually taken at a fixed amount. To be effective there will have to be a minimum concentration of the vitamin added to such foods. This will inevitably result in higher exposures in others in the population who happen to eat quite a lot of this particular fortified food. Thus, unless one restricts fortification to an extremely low level it is almost inevitable that certain members of the population will succeed in taking levels of the fortified food that will contain enough folic acid to exceed the capacity of the intestinal mucosa to convert it into the usual circulatory form of 5-methyltetrahydrofolate. It will be discussed later whether such unaltered folic acid prevents any potential problems for individuals or for populations as a whole. However, one clear way to avoid this happening is for the supplements or the fortified food to contain, instead of folic acid, the natural form of the vitamin, namely, 5-methyltetrahydrofolate.

VIII. 5-METHYLTETRAHYDROFOLATE AS A SUPPLEMENT OR IN FORTIFIED FOOD

This option certainly exists and has the advantage of not introducing a provitamin into the circulation with its known and possible unknown consequences. However, for this to happen two technical problems must be overcome: chemically producing the natural isomer and stabilizing the natural isomer.

A. Producing the Natural Isomer

The reduction of the pteridine ring of folic acid to the tetrahydro form produces an asymmetrical molecule. Thus, the conventional chemical synthesis gives equal amounts of both C-6 epimers, namely the biologically active (6S) diastereoisomer and the biologically inactive (6R) diastereoisomer (20). The starting material for the 5-methyltetrahydrofolate available commercially and used in supplements is thus this mixture. The corresponding enzymatic reduction of folic acid to dihydrofolate and tetrahydrofolate produces only the active (6S) diastereoisomer. When folates are synthesized in plants and bacteria, only the active (6S) diastereoisomer is produced, so all naturally occurring reduced folates will be in this form. Only this active form is biologically active. It is the form recognized by all folate transport systems and used by all folate-dependent reactions. The (6R) isomer, being the mirror image of the active form, is not bound to any of the biologically active folate binders or transport systems. Likewise, it does not fit into the active site of any folate-dependent enzyme. Thus, while its chemical and physical properties will be identical to the active (6S) isomer, e.g., stability, diffusion, and solubility, as far as is known it will be completely devoid of any biological function. As such, it might be considered to be just a passive and inactive bystander if taken in by humans. Thus, on chemical and biological grounds one would expect it to be absorbed passively across the intestinal mucosa at the same rate as the active isomer. It would equally diffuse into cells, but it would not be acted upon by the enzyme methionine synthase. Thus, unlike the active form it would not be converted in the tetrahydro form, made into a polyglutamate, and retained by cells. It would eventually clear from the cells and from the body without exercising any biological function. Both on biological and chemical grounds there is no reason to believe that the (6R) diastereoisomer would have any biological function. The mixture of the two isomers has been given to humans in certain research studies and also therapeutically without any apparent ill effects. It is, however, impossible to say that it definitely would not interact with any biological system. It should be remembered that the antifolate drug methotrexate, which is a synthetic analog of folic acid, binds to its target enzyme dihydrofolate reductase in an inverse position to folic acid. Thus, while there is no direct evidence of any problem of using the racemic mixture, it would clearly be better to use only the biologically active (6S) diastereoisomer.

B. Stabilizing the Natural Isomer

Folic acid is extremely stable chemically (21). At room temperature either in solution or as a solid, it undergoes virtually no degradation over periods of weeks or even months. However, when the pteridine ring is reduced to the dihydro or tetrahydro forms, the chemistry of the molecule changes dramatically. Dihydrofolate or tetrahydrofolate are both extremely susceptible to oxidative cleavage of the molecule at C9-N10 bond producing two degradation products, a pteridine and *p*-aminobezoylglutamate (22). Both of these molecules are inactive in themselves and cannot be biologically converted back to any active folate. The introduction of a group onto the N-5 nitrogen has a stabilizing effect on this oxidative cleavage process. Thus 5-methyltetrahydrofolate does not cleave like tetrahydrofolate. However, it is susceptible to a different type of oxidative attack. This chemical process initially produces 5-methyldihydrofolate. This form can be reduced back to 5-methyltetrahydrofolate by the enzyme MTHF reductase (Fig. 2). While the usual initial substrate for this enzyme is 5,10-methylenetetrahydrofolate, it seems very probable that 5-methyldihydrofolate is an intermediate form in the active site on its way to the product of this enzyme reaction 5-methyltetrahydrofolate. However, once the partly oxidized form of the 5-methyldihydrofolate is formed it becomes susceptible to further chemical oxidation. This involves the rearrangement of the ring to produce a new derivative. This was initially ascribed a structure of a 4a-hydroxy 5-methyldihydrofolate (22) but has since been shown to have a different chemical structure (23). In any event, this structure is completely inactive biologically. In addition it cannot either chemically or enzymatically be converted back to an active folate. There are two distinct considerations when one considers the stability of 5-methyltetrahydrofolate. First, there is the question of its stability in a preparation that might be used either in supplements or added to food for the purpose of fortification. Technically, Knoll achieved a product that appears to be sufficiently stable for these purposes. Second, there is the question of the stability of 5-methyltetrahydrofolate during its various phases of ingestion and absorption, merging eventually with the concept of its overall bioavailability. This requires information on its likely stability in the acid environment of the stomach, followed by its survival in the intestine. Some guidance as to the probable stability under these circumstances is available. It would appear very probable that it is stable enough to remain active during these stages. However, it is difficult to simulate the conditions of oxidation and chemical exposure that are likely to be encountered during this complex process. To resolve this a full comparative bioavailability study between folic acid and 5-methyltetrahydrofolate needs to be undertaken.

IX. POSSIBLE ADVANTAGES OF 5-METHYLTETRAHYDROFOLATE OVER FOLIC ACID IN SUPPLEMENTS OR FORTIFIED FOOD

A. The Natural Vitamin as Opposed to a Provitamin

There is the obvious general advantage that given equal bioavailability, etc., one would prefer to treat humans with the form of the vitamin that has evolved in nature. One would assume that evolution would have ensured a safety and tolerance for it.

B. Pernicious Anemia

There is no doubt that the biggest advantage would be that 5-methyltetrahydrofolate would be less likely to mask the anemia in PA, thus preventing its timely diagnosis. Any 5-methyltetrahydrofolate presented to vitamin B_{12}–deficient bone marrow cells would be predicted to be poorly metabolized and poorly retained. This is because the only way that its metabolism can occur is through the vitamin B_{12}–dependent enzyme methionine. As discussed earlier, it is the reduced or absent activity of this enzyme that gives rise to the trapping of the cellular folate as 5-methyltetrahydrofolate. Thus, it seems clear that the intracellular polyglutamates of this form are not effectively utilized. It would seem equally likely that the 5-methyltetrahydrofolate monoglutamate would not be utilized or retained by such vitamin B_{12}–deficient cells. It would thus not cause the bone marrow to make DNA and in turn prevent the masking of the anemia.

Experimental evidence of two types exist showing that 5-methyltetrahydrofolate will not cause vitamin B_{12}–deficient bone marrow to respond. First, three separate investigations have shown that marrow taken from vitamin B_{12}–deficient subjects does not respond to 5-methyltetrahydrofolate, while it does to folic acid, with respect to DNA biosynthesis (24–26). These studies looked at the response of recently collected bone marrow cells in vitro by measuring their increase in de novo pyrimidine biosynthesis comparing the addition of the two different forms of the vitamin (27). There is also an in vivo study on a single vitamin B_{12}–deficient subject. This subject showed no hematological response as measured by his reticulocyte count when given 5-methyltetrahydrofolate at 100 μg per day for 10 days. Neither did he respond to 100 μg given intravenously. Treatment with intravenous B_{12} caused a steady increase in reticulocyte count.

C. Reduction in Plasma Homocysteine

As discussed earlier, 5-methyltetrahydrofolate is involved in the metabolism of homocysteine. It would thus seem very probable that this form of the vitamin would be as effective as folic acid in lowering elevated plasma homocysteine concentrations, which many lines of investigation have shown is an independent risk factor for heart disease and stroke (28).

D. Endothelial Function

Verhaar et al. (29) reported that 5-methyltetrahydrofolate, but not folic acid, restores in vivo endothelial cell function in patients with familial hypercholesterolemia. It is suggested that this happens by stimulation of the regeneration of endogenous tetrahydrobiopterin, which in turn could restore nitric oxide activity.

E. Recovery from Psychiatric Illness

Godfrey et al. (30) claim to have shown a significant improvement in a placebo-controlled trial using 15 mg of 5-methyltetrahydrofolate daily for 6 months compared to placebo in 123 patients with acute psychiatric disorders.

REFERENCES

1. McPartlin J, Weir DG, Scott JM. Folic acid—physiology, dietary sources and requirements. In: MJ Sadler, B Caballero, JJ Strain, eds. Encyclopaedia of Human Nutrition. London: Academic Press, 1998:803–811.
2. Scott JM, Weir DG. Folate/Vitamin B_{12} interrelationships. In: KF Tipton, ed. Essays in Biochemistry. Vol 28: London: Portland Press, 1994:63–72.
3. Shane B. Folate Chemistry and Metabolism. In: L Bailey, ed. Folate in Health and Disease. New York: Marcel Dekker, 1995:1–22.
4. Mitchell HK, Snell EE, Williams RJ. The concentration of "folic acid." J Am Chem Soc 63:2284, 1941.
5. Kelly P, McPartlin J, Goggins M, Weir DG, Scott JM. Unmetabolized folic acid in serum: acute studies in subjects consuming fortified food and supplements. Am J Clin Nutrition 65:1790–1795, 1997.
6. Scott JM, Weir DG. The methyl folate trap. Lancet ii:337–340, 1981.
7. Bergmann S, Vladimir S, Ratter F, Schiemann S, Schulze-Osthoff K, Lehman V. Adenosine and homocysteine together enhance TNF-mediated cytotoxicity but do not alter activation of nuclear factor-κB in L929 cells. J Immunol 153:1736–1743, 1994.
8. Buccellato FR, Miloso M, Braga M, Nicolini G, Moralito A, Pravettoni G, Tredici G, Scalabrino G, Myelinolytic lesions in spinal cord of cobalamin-deficient rats are TNF-alpha-mediated. FASEB J 13:297–304, 1999.
9. Chanarin I. The Megaloblastic Anaemias. 2nd ed. Oxford: Blackwell Scientific Publications, 1979:198–229.
10. Savage DG, Lindenbaum J. Neurological complications of acquired cobalamin deficiency: clinical aspects. In: SM Wickramasinghe, ed. Balliére's Clinical Haematology. Megaloblastic Anaemia. London: Balliére Tindall, 1995:657–678.
11. Scott JM, Weir DG, Kirke P. Folate and neural tube defects. In: LB Bailey, ed. Folate in Health and Disease. New York: Marcel Dekker, 1994:329–360.
12. Wald NJ, Watt HC, Law MR, Weir DG, McPartlin J, Scott JM. Homocysteine and ischaemic heart disease: results of a prospective study with implications on prevention. Arch Intern Med 158:862–867, 1998.
13. Perry IJ, Refsum H, Morrise RW, Ebrahim SB, Ueland PM, Shaper AC. Prospective study of serum total homocysteine concentrations and risk of stroke in middle aged British men. Lancet 346:1395–1398, 1995.
14. Selhub J, Jacques PF, Wilson PWF, Rush D, Rosenberg IH. Vitamin status and intake as primary determinants of homocysteinemia in an elderly population. JAMA 270:2693–2698, 1993.

15. Ward M, McNulty H, McPartlin J, Strain JJ, Weir DG, Scott JM. Plasma homocysteine, a risk factor for cardiovascular disease can be effectively reduced by physiological amounts of folic acid. Q J Med 90:519–524, 1997.
16. Scott JM, Weir DG. Homocysteine and cardiovascular disease. Q J Med 89:561–563, 1996.
17. Mason JB. Folate status: effects on casrcinogenesis. In: L Bailey, ed. Folate in Health and Disease. New York: Marcel Dekker, 1995:361–378.
18. Giovannucci E, Stampfer MJ, Colditz GA, Hunter DJ, Fuchs C, Rosner BA, Speizer FE, Willett WC. Multivitamin use, folate and colon cancer in women in the Nurses' Health Study. Ann Intern Med 129:517–524, 1998.
19. Dietary Reference Intakes: Thiamin, Riboflavin, Niacin, Vitamin B_6, Folate, Vitamin B_{12}, Pantothenic Acid, Biotin and Choline. Institute of Medicine. Washington, DC: National Academy Press, 1998:1–68.
20. Bailey SW, Ayling JE. Total chemical synthesis of chirally pure (6S)-tetrahydrofolic acid. In: DB McCormick, JW Suttie, C Wagner, eds. Methods in Enzymology. New York: Academic Press, 1997:3–16.
21. Blakley RL. In: RL Blakley, ed. The Biochemistry of Folic Acid and Related Compounds, Amsterdam: North-Holland Publishing Company, 1969:76–96.
22. Gapski GR, Whiteley JM, Hennekens FM. Hydroxylated derivatives of 5-methyl-5,6,7,8-tetrahydrofolate. Biochemistry 10:2930–2934, 1971.
23. Mager HIX, Berends W. Activation and transfer of oxygen VIII. Autooxidative ring contraction of blocked dihydroalloxiazines and tetrahydropteridines in the presence of H_2, ^{18}O and $^{18}O_2$. Tetrahedron Lett 41:4051–4052, 1973.
24. Metz J, Kelly A, Swett VC, Waxman S, Herbert V. Deranged DNA synthesis by bonemarrow from vitamin B_{12}-deficient humans. Br Med J iii:403–406, 1967.
25. Ganeshagura K, Hoffbrand AV. The effect of deoxyuridine, vitamin B_{12}, folate and alcohol on the uptake of thymine and on the deoxynucleoside triphosphate concentrations in normal and megaloblastic cells. Br J Haematol 40:29–41, 1978.
26. Zittoun J, Marquet J, Zittoun R. Effect of folate and cobalamin compounds on the deoxyuridine suppression test in vitamin B_{12} and folate deficiency. Blood 51:119–128, 1978.
27. Gutstein S, Bernstein LH, Levy L, Wagner G. Failure of response to N^5-methyltetrahydrofolate in combined folate and vitamin B_{12} deficiency. Evidence in support of the ''folate trap'' hypothesis. Digest Dis 18:142–146, 1973.
28. Weir DG, Scott JM. Homocysteine as a risk factor for cardiovascular and related disease: nutritional implications. Nutr Res Rev 11:311–338, 1998.
29. Verhaar MC, Wever RM, Kastelein JJ, van Dam T, Koomans HA, Rabelink TJ. 5-Methyltetrahydrofolate, the active form of folic acid, restores endothelial function in familiar hypercholesterolemia. Circulation 97:237–241, 1998.
30. Godfrey PSA, Toone BK, Carney MWP, Flynn TG, Bottiglieri T, Laundy M, Chanarin I, Reynolds EH. Enhancement of recovery from psychiatric illness by methylfolate. Lancet 336:329–395, 1990.

6

Lycopene and Lutein: The Next Steps to the Mixed Carotenoids

Robert M. Russell
Schools of Medicine and Nutrition, Tufts University, Boston, Massachusetts

There is public health interest in the potential of lycopene and lutein for the prevention of particular chronic diseases: cancer (prostate) and age-related macular degeneration, respectively. This chapter reviews what is known about lycopene and lutein from a metabolic point of view and their possible roles in the prevention of chronic disease. The chapter also focuses on what is *not* known about these compounds and what needs to be accomplished before health professionals can embrace them as part of a disease-prevention strategy.

Different populations in the world have vastly different carotenoid profiles in their blood. For example, a large percentage of total carotenoids is made up by lycopene in the American population as compared to a very small percentage in the Korean and Chinese populations. On the other hand, the Korean population has more than 50% of total circulating carotenoids made up by cryptoxanthin, and in the Chinese population 50% total carotenoids is made up by lutein (unpublished observations). These blood carotenoid profiles reflect different dietary patterns and food choices in the various populations. Other factors besides diet that can modulate serum levels of carotenoids are age and body composition (1,2). For example, aging has been correlated with the decline of serum lycopene in the American population, which could reflect the decreased popularity of pizza in this older age group (1,2). Greater body mass index has been inversely correlated with lower levels of all carotenoids (3,4).

I. LYCOPENE

Lycopene is found in a limited number of foods, not in the diverse array of foods that β-carotene, for example, is found in. The primary sources of lycopene in the diet are tomatoes and tomato products, although other foods such as apricots, pink grapefruit, watermelon, guava, and papaya are also dietary sources. Despite tomatoes being the prime source of dietary lycopene, various strains of tomatoes contain vastly different amounts of lycopene. We assayed the lycopene content of various tomatoes taken during the summer from a market near Boston. The lycopene content varied from 0 in the yellow varieties to 24 μg/g wet weight in the red varieties. In the 1998 U.S. Department of Agriculture (USDA)–National Cancer Institute (NCI) Carotenoid Data Base, the average lycopene content of red, ripe, raw tomatoes is given as 30 μg/g wet weight (5). This points out a problem in coming up with standardized reliable tables for use in various epidemiological studies. It remains very difficult to translate food intake into exact quantities of lycopene consumption due to variation in the lycopene content of the many varieties of tomatoes grown around the world.

Lycopene appears to be a very stable compound during food processing; however, the bioavailability of carotenoids, and lycopene in particular, appears to be increased by heating the food substance (6,7). Heating dissociates protein-carotenoid complexes and disrupts carotenoid crystals. Dietary fat is needed for optimal carotenoid absorption, in particular for the nonpolar carotenoids such as lycopene and β-carotene. In addition, bile salts and pancreatic enzymes are needed for absorption of these compounds. Most lycopene and other nonpolar carotenoids are transported in low-density lipoproteins. This is in contrast to polar carotenoids such as lutein and zeaxanthin, which are more equally distributed between low-density lipoproteins and high-density lipoproteins (8). A study by Gärtner et al. illustrates how food processing, particularly in which cell walls are broken down, can increase the bioavailability of lycopene (6). Five subjects underwent two studies 2 weeks apart. In a first study, 400 g of tomatoes with 15 g of corn oil were fed, and in a second study, 40 g of tomato paste with 15 g of corn oil were fed. Each feeding contained 23 mg of lycopene. Lycopene appearing in the chylomicron fraction over a 12-hour period was markedly higher in those fed tomato paste as compared to those fed the fresh tomatoes. Chylomicron carotenoid levels, rather than plasma responses, are more appropriate for studying intestinal absorption kinetics of carotenoids than are simple concentrations in plasma, since plasma concentrations represent not only newly absorbed carotenoids, but also a rate of tissue uptake and resecretion.

As an example of a longer-term feeding study, we recently reported plasma lycopene responses and other carotenoid responses in blood after changing from a self-selected diet to a diet that included 10 servings of fruits and vegetables per day (9). Thirty-six subjects were studied on a 3-day rotating plan. The amount of lycopene contained in the diet was approximately 3.3 mg/day, and the total carotenoid content of the diet was 16 mg/day. The macronutrient content of the diet was made up of 26% of calories from fat. Although older studies had suggested that the ingestion of purified lycopene would be needed to achieve major increases in plasma concentrations, this study clearly indicated that lycopene and, indeed, most carotenoids, were increased in only 5 days in both young and old men and women. We also studied a group of 25 males who were placed on a low-carotenoid diet containing approximately 0.05 mg total carotenoids per day while residing in a metabolic ward. In these 25 subjects over a 2-week period, levels of all carotenoids dropped, including lycopene (unpublished data). From this and other studies, the half-life for plasma depletion of lycopene is estimated to be in the range of 12–30 days (10).

The tissue distribution of lycopene, from various reports, varies quite substantially. For example, lycopene is highly concentrated in testes, adrenal gland, and liver tissue (11–14). Lower concentrations are found in such organs as the kidney, lung, and stomach. In tissue, the *cis* form of lycopene makes up approximately 50% of the isomeric profile, and in prostate 80% of lycopene has been reported to be in the *cis* form (9,14). This is in stark contrast to the isomeric form found in vegetables, which is predominantly all-*trans*. In looking for appropriate animal models to be used for the study of lycopene, the ferret appears to be suitable. Zhao et al. have shown that the rat will accumulate lycopene when fed in extremely high doses (15).

It does not appear that there are significant interactions between lycopene and other carotenoids. Although some studies have shown β-carotene supplementation to reduce serum lycopene levels over time, other studies have shown just the opposite. At this point in time, very little is known about the in vivo metabolism of lycopene. Although Khachik demonstrated a few metabolites in human plasma or tissues such as 5,6-dihydroxy-5,6-dihydro lycopene (thought to be an in vivo oxidation product), nothing is known of the possible biological activity of such compounds (16).

Major interest in lycopene was sparked by a series of reports showing that high dietary intakes of lycopene were associated with a lower risk of developing prostate cancer. One of these studies was reported in 1989 in a cohort of 14,000 Seventh Day Adventists (17). This study showed a nonsignificant inverse association between tomato intake and risk of prostate cancer. A subsequent study by Hsing and colleagues in 1990 showed that high plasma lycopene levels were associated with a reduced risk of prostate cancer, with a relative risk of 0.5 between the highest and lowest quartiles (18). The study was very small, and this relative risk reduction did not reach statistical significance. A report by Giovannucci and colleagues from the Health Professionals Study examined the relationship between tomato intake as assessed by food frequency questionnaire and subsequent prostate cancer development (19). The study began in 1986 and was completed in 1992, a 6-year period. In this study, the only carotenoid for which intake was clearly related to lower risk for developing subsequent prostate cancer was lycopene, with a relative risk of 0.79 in the highest quintile of intake as compared to the lowest quintile of intake. Similarly, of the fruits and vegetables that were assessed, four were significantly associated with lower prostate cancer risk: pizza, tomato sauce, tomatoes, and strawberries, three of which are important sources of lycopene.

However, the association between high lycopene intake and lower prostate cancer risk has not been universally found. For example, in a recent case-control study reported from England by Key et al., high lycopene intake was not associated with reduced risk (20). Also, the effect may not be unique to lycopene: from the Finnish ATBC study, long-term supplementation of vitamin E was shown to substantially reduce prostate cancer incidence and mortality in male smokers (a 32% decrease) (21). In contrast to the findings in the ATBC study, a recent abstract from the Physician's Health Study showed that men in the lowest quartile of β-carotene intake benefited from β-carotene supplementation due to an apparent reduction in the risk of prostate cancer (22). Nevertheless, the question of whether lycopene or the consumption of tomato products reduces prostate cancer risk certainly warrants further study, including mechanistic studies.

Interest also has been sparked in lycopene as a possible preventive agent for skin damage by ultraviolet irradiation. For example, we showed that when skin is subjected to ultraviolet light stress, far more skin lycopene is destroyed as compared to β-carotene, suggesting a role of lycopene in mitigating oxidative damage in this tissue (23). Also in the multicenter case-control EURAMIC study, adipose tissue levels of lycopene, independently of other carotenoids, was associated with protection against myocardial infarction (24). That is, lycopene showed a protective effect with an *inverse* odds ratio with increasing adipose tissue concentrations. These areas of research also appear to be worth exploring more fully.

II. LUTEIN

As with lycopene, the carotenoid values for spinach also vary with source and with season. In the USDA-NCI 1998 Carotenoid Tables, the average lutein plus zeaxanthin content in spinach is listed as 11.9 mg/100 g of spinach (5). However, as with lycopene in tomatoes, the different lutein and zeaxanthin values in spinach according to source and season make interpretation of epidemiological studies difficult.

As for bioavailability of lutein, the mode of presentation of lutein makes a difference. We studied the bioavailability of lutein from spinach as compared to lutein extract in a pill. Twenty healthy adult men were studied after being on a low-carotenoid diet for 2 weeks. Subjects consumed either spinach or the lutein with a standard meal, which contained 21 g of fat but no other carotenoids or retinoids. The study involved the oral ingestion of 48 mg of purified lutein or 48 mg of lutein contained in cooked, chopped spinach. Each subject consumed the purified lutein or spinach with the liquid diet after the first blood sample was obtained. We found that there was little difference in the plasma response curves from taking either purified lutein or the chopped spinach. Thus, the bioavailability of a more polar carotenoid such as lutein in spinach, in contrast to the bioavailability of a nonpolar carotenoid such as β-carotene, appears to be equal that of the purified lutein in a gelatin capsule. Similar to lycopene, the bioavailability of lutein is increased with food processing, particularly when the cell walls are broken (e.g., by pureeing).

With regard to lutein interactions with other carotenoids, several studies are worth noting. In one study a mixed carotenoid source (betatene) was given, consisting of 0.5% lutein, 0.7% zeaxanthin, 3.6% α-carotene, 70.3% all-*trans* β-carotene, 22% *cis* β-carotene, and 2.1% unidentified carotenoids and no lycopene (25). Betatene was given as a single dose together with 500 mL of 2.5% fat content milk, and blood was drawn at 0 and at 3, 6, 9, and 10 hours after the betatene ingestion. Lutein, α-carotene, and zeaxanthin all showed rises in blood after the mixed carotenoid ingestion, with a peak maximum at 9 hours. Of interest in this study was that the carotenoid pattern in the chylomicron fraction did not match the pattern of the mixed carotenoid source with a 14-fold higher level of lutein and a 4-fold higher level of zeaxanthin compared to their relative contents in the carotenoid mixture. Although the absolute amount of all-*trans* β-carotene in serum showed a marked rise, the rise was actually relatively low compared to the all *trans* β-carotene content of the betatene. This may reflect a higher bioavailability of lutein as opposed to β-carotene when given together. In a second paper by Kostic et al., single equimolar doses of lutein β-carotene or lutein plus β-carotene together were fed in a random mixed order (26). Each of the three phases of the schedule lasted for 5 weeks. Blood was drawn just before dosing and at various time points after dosing for up to 840 hours. When given in combined equal molar dose, lutein and β-carotene interacted with each other such that β-carotene reduced the mean area under the curve for lutein to 54–61% of its value when given alone. Seven of eight subjects showed this effect. However, lutein affected the area under the curve for β-carotene to a lesser extent. Van der berg and van Vliet have shown that lutein affects β-carotene absorption when given simultaneously, but that lutein has little effect on β-carotene cleavage to vitamin A (27). It should be realized that in the context of the entire diet, however, these observations on bioavailability after giving pure compounds together in the same meal might have little relevance. This is borne out by long-term intervention studies using β-carotene in which β-carotene administration did not have an effect on other carotenoid levels over time (28).

As with lycopene, little is known about the intermediate metabolism of lutein or zeaxanthin in the body. Khachik et al. have identified several metabolites of lutein and zeaxanthin resulting from oxidation and/or enzymatic dehydration in both blood and the eye (29,30). Once again the biological activity of these metabolites is uncertain. Bone and Landrum et al. showed that concentrations of the nondietary mesozeaxanthin are extremely high in the central fovea, whereas concentrations of lutein become higher at a further radial distance from the fovea (31). The authors speculate that lutein can be converted to mesozeaxanthin in the eye.

The major interest in lutein and zeaxanthin as chemopreventive agents originated in a report by Seddon et al., which analyzed dietary carotenoids as related to the prevalence of age-related macular degeneration (32). This was a case-control study involving 356 cases of advanced-stage age-related macular degeneration and 520 control subjects. It was found that after adjusting for other risk factors for macular degeneration, lutein and zeaxanthin intakes were most strongly associated with reduced risk of macular degeneration; thus those in the highest quintile of lutein and zeaxanthin intake had a multivariate odds ratio of 0.43 as opposed to those in the lowest quintile. In addition, a higher dietary intake of spinach was related to a significantly lower risk of macular degeneration with a p value of 0.001.

However, a subsequent case-control study by Mares-Perlman et al. showed that high levels of serum lycopene but not lutein and zeaxanthin were related to a lower incidence of macular degeneration (33). Further, the Eye Disease Case-Control Study Group reported that, although blood levels of carotenoids in the medium and highest tertiles had reduced risk of age-related macular degeneration as compared to the lowest tertile, the risk reduction was the same whether all carotenoids, β-carotene alone, or lutein and zeaxanthin alone were considered (34). Finally, in the Baltimore Longitudinal Study of Aging, high levels of α-tocopherol appeared to be protective against macular degeneration, although other studies evaluating vitamin E effects on macular degeneration have been equivocal (35).

We wished to see whether or not a moderate dietary intervention could influence blood carotenoid levels and macular pigment density of the fovea. In this study we were particularly interested in the question of whether feeding additional spinach and corn with only one meal a day could raise blood and macula lutein and zeaxanthin levels over a period of several weeks (36). Twelve subjects, 6 males and 6 females, ate additional chopped spinach and corn with one meal a day. They were instructed to eat the spinach and corn with a meal that contained at least some fat. The cooked spinach and corn supplements were supplied to the volunteers. The spinach weighed 60 g and contained 10.8 g of lutein and 0.3 mg of zeaxanthin, whereas the corn weighed 105 g and contained 0.4 mg of zeaxanthin. We found that one meal a day containing some spinach and corn caused initial significant rises in serum lutein and zeaxanthin levels. Whereas the blood lutein levels remained high throughout the study and declined only after stopping the spinach supplement, zeaxanthin levels tended to drift back to normal after the initial rise even though the spinach and corn supplements continued. In this study, only 1 out of 12 individuals on this spinach and corn supplement did not show a 20% or greater rise in blood lutein, whereas 4 of 12 did not show a rise in blood zeaxanthin. For the overall group the increase in dietary intake of lutein by feeding additional spinach and corn was sufficient to raise the mean serum concentration of lutein by 33%. At this point, there is no explanation for the few individuals who can be classified as blood nonresponders to the diet, although such cases of nonresponsiveness have been seen with other carotenoids as well.

Mean macular pigment density and serum concentrations of lutein were also examined during the intervention. Three different types of responses were seen in response to this simple dietary modification. There were seven retinal responders: these individuals showed rises both in macular pigment density and serum lutein. Two individuals responded with high blood lutein levels, but no macular pigment response was noted. Data from one person whose serum lutein did not change also showed that his macular pigment did not increase. From further studies (unpublished), it appears that the explanation for retinal and blood nonresponders, in part, has to do with how much body fat an individual has. At least in females, the greater the amount of body fat, the less the responsiveness of the retina to lutein/zeaxanthin supplementation.

III. LESSONS FROM THE β-CAROTENE EXPERIENCE

What can be learned from the β-carotene intervention trial experiences? Although epidemiological data are consistent that high dietary and blood levels of β-carotene predict a low prevalence of certain cancers, particularly lung cancer, the findings of two intervention trials using high-dose β-carotene in smokers or asbestos-exposed workers showed that high-dose β-carotene supplements actually resulted in a greater number of lung cancers as compared to the non–β-carotene-treated groups (37,38). We wanted to see if similar results could be reproduced in an animal model (39). Thus, we turned to the ferret model and divided ferrets into two groups, either β-carotene exposed or non–beta-carotene exposed. The dose of β-carotene used was equivalent to 30 mg/day in the human intervention trials. Each of the β-carotene- and non–β-carotene-treated groups were further divided into smoke-exposed and non–smoke-exposed groups. The animals were exposed to cigarette smoke twice in the morning and twice in the afternoon for 30 minutes each time, giving these animals an exposure equivalent to smoking 1½ packs of cigarettes per day in the human. A smoking machine would expel smoke into a chamber into which ferrets were placed. After the period of exposure was over, the ferrets were removed from the chamber. The animals tolerated this exposure well and did not have any decrease in appetite or weight, and they did not behave differently than the non–smoke-exposed animals. Animals were treated for a 6-month period of time and then killed.

Large increases in the concentration of β-carotene were seen in the plasma of ferrets supplemented with β-carotene. However, plasma β-carotene levels were significantly lower in the β-carotene–supplemented animals exposed to smoke than in the β-carotene–supplemented animals not exposed to cigarette smoke. Similarly, lung tissue levels of β-carotene were significantly lower in the smoke-exposed ferrets than in the non–smoke-exposed ferrets in both the β-carotene–supplemented and nonsupplemented animals. It should also be noted that the concentrations of retinoic acid in lung tissue were also significantly lower in all three treatment groups as compared to the control group. We showed that the dramatic decreases in lung and blood β-carotene levels due to smoke were the result of enhanced breakdown of β-carotene into excentric cleavage oxidation products. This enhanced breakdown was shown by in vitro incubations of β-carotene with the postnuclear fractions of lung tissue in smoke-exposed animals as compared to non–smoke-exposed ferrets. When we examined the lung sections of the four groups of ferrets, we found that smoke exposure caused mild aggregation and proliferation of macrophages. However, localized proliferation of alveolar cells and alveolar macrophages and keratinized squamous epithelial cells were observed in the ferrets in the two high-dose beta-carotene–supplemented groups. The most severe proliferation of alveolar cell squamous metaplasia and destruction of alveolar cells were observed in the smoke-exposed ferrets that were given high-dose β-carotene as compared to any other group. Keratinized squamous metaplasia was confirmed in the lung sections of all ferrets exposed to either high-dose β-carotene without smoke or high-dose β-carotene with smoke by immunohistochemical staining with anti-keratin antibody.

To assess a potential increase in cell proliferation in whole lung, we analyzed proliferating-cell nuclear antigen (PCNA) expression from the right upper lobes of ferrets from all four groups. PCNA expression was increased in both the lungs of the β-carotene–supplemented ferrets exposed to smoke as well as of the β-carotene–supplemented ferrets not exposed to smoke. Because retinoic acid levels were lower in the smoke-exposed ferrets than in non–smoke-exposed ferrets due to increased oxidative breakdown, we wished to see if there was diminished retinoid signaling, since retinoic acid is a ligand for two classes of nuclear receptors: the retinoic acid receptors (RAR) and the retinoid x receptors (RXR). We found that the expression of RAR-β was downregulated in the three treatment groups as compared with the control group. RAR-β is known to play an important role in normal lung development, and primary lung tumors and lung cell cancer lines lack RAR-β expression (40,41). Thus, a role for RAR-β as a tumor suppressor gene has been proposed. RAR-α expression was not affected. Since lung carcinogenesis is also associated with an alteration in retinoid signaling involving the activator protein AP1 complex, we looked at AP1 transcriptional activities in our ferrets. C fos and C jun make up the AP1 complex, and both were upregulated three- to fourfold in the smoke-exposed β-carotene–supplemented ferrets as compared with control animals. Moreover, expression of AP1 was positively correlated with squamous metaplasia and with increased PCNA expression and inversely with the expression of RAR-β in these animals.

Thus, we feel that high doses of β-carotene in highly oxidative conditions result in a number of excentric cleavage oxidative breakdown products, which have biological activity of their own. One possibility is that these products interfere with retinoic acid binding to retinoid receptors. Another possibility is that these metabolites induce local enzymes in the lung, such as P450 enzymes, which cause an increased catabolism of retinoic acid and thus diminish retinoic acid signaling. A local deficiency of retinoic acid then results in squamous metaplasia. We are now carrying out dose-response experiments under similar conditions.

IV. THE NEXT STEPS

What then needs to be done next with regard to lycopene and lutein before they can gain legitimacy and acceptance by the medical and regulatory communities? I have already alluded in my comments to many of the missing pieces of knowledge that need to be determined before these compounds can be accepted as safe and effective for prevention of certain chronic diseases. First of all, additional prospective and observational data are necessary in order to understand the strength and consistency of the disease relationships—in the case of lycopene for cancer (and possibly cardiovascular disease) and in the case of lutein for macular degeneration.

Second, the metabolism of both compounds must be better understood. Carotenoids can be metabolized by hydroxylation, enzymatic and chemical oxidation, cleavage, reduction, and isomerization. The identification of major metabolites and the testing of them for possible biological activities and toxicities needs to be carried out using both in vitro studies and appropriate animal models. Using animal models, the timing of an intervention in a disease process can also be ascertained. Is, for example, lutein effective in preventing macular degeneration, or is it effective in slowing the disease process down once it has begun, or both? We don't know how lutein interacts with rods and cones in retinal pigment epithelium. Indeed, we do not know how it moves from one cell to the other, let alone knowing whether lutein is converted to mesozeaxanthin in the eye, as has been proposed.

Third, long-term intervention studies should be carried out using appropriate animal models, as should long-term intervention studies in a limited number of humans, with careful monitoring for toxicity as well as for possible interactions with other nutrients, such as other carotenoids, vitamin D, or vitamin E. No long-term studies with lycopene or lutein have been carried out, and it has not been proven that the psychophysiological measures of macular pigment density truly reflect tissue macular pigment density in a clinic population.

Fourth, dose-response studies need to be carried out. Do serum and tissue levels in the human plateau on a given dose of the carotenoid, or do they continue to build up? Serum adipose tissue and buccal mucosal cells can be intermittently assayed along with blood. If a desirable level of macular pigment density could be defined, lutein doses could be individualized to achieve that desirable level.

We have begun to work on some of these problems, for example, by using deuterated lycopene in humans. It will take a concerted effort to answer these questions before convincing any government agency here or abroad to support costly, long-term, large intervention trials in a human population, particularly after the β-carotene experience. Lycopene and lutein are promising compounds, but we do not want to have a repeat of the β-carotene story, where we were blind-sided due to a lack of basic knowledge about how these compounds are handled and metabolized in vivo under oxidative stress conditions.

REFERENCES

1. Brady WE, Mares-Perlman JA, Bowen P, Stacewicz-Sapuntzakis M. Human serum carotenoid concentrations are related to physiologic and lifestyle factors. J Nutr 1996; 1126:129–137.
2. Peng YM, Peng YS, Lin Y, et al. Concentrations and plasma-tissue-diet relationships of carotenoids, retinoids, and tocopherols in humans. Nutr Cancer 1995; 23:233–246.
3. Zhu YI, Hsieh W, Parker RS, et al. Evidence of a role for fat-free body mass in modulation of plasma carotenoid concentrations in older men: studies with hydrodensitometry. J Nutr 1997; 127:321–326.
4. Yeum KJ, Booth SL, Rounenoff R, Russell RM. Plasma carotenoid concentrations are inversely correlated with fat mass in older women. J Nutr Health Aging 1998; 2:79–83.
5. USDA-NCC Carotenoid Database for U.S. Foods, 1998. Nutrient Data Laboratory Home Page, http://www.nal.usda.gov/fnil/foodcomp.
6. Gärtner C, Stahl W, Sies H. Lycopene is more bioavailable from tomato paste than from fresh tomatoes. Am J Clin Nutr 1997; 66:116–122.
7. Zhou JR, Gugger ET, Erdman Jr JW. The crystalline form of carotenes and the food matrix in carrot root decrease the relative bioavailability of β- and α-carotene in the ferret model. J Am Coll Nutr 1996; 15:84–91.
8. Krinsky NI, Cornwell DG, Oncley JL. The transport of vitamin A and carotenoids in human plasma. Arch Biochem Biophys 1958; 73:233–246.
9. Yeum KJ, Booth SL, Sadowski JA, et al. Human plasma carotenoid response to the ingestion of controlled diets high in fruits and vegetables. Am J Clin Nutr 1996; 64:594–602.

10. Rock CL, Swendseid ME, Jacob RA, McKee RW. Plasma carotenoid levels in human subjects fed a low carotenoid diet. J Nutr 1992; 122(1):96–100.
11. Stahl W, Schwartz W, Sundquist AR, Sies H. *Cis-trans* isomers of lycopene and β-carotene in human serum and tissues. Arch Biochem Biophys 1992; 294:173–177.
12. Kaplan LA, Lau JM, Stein EA. Carotenoid composition, concentrations, and relationships in various human organs. Clin Physiol Biochem 1990; 8:1–10.
13. Schmitz HH, Poor CL, Wellman RB, Erdman Jr JW. Concentrations of selected carotenoids and vitamin A in human liver, kidney and lung tissue. J Nutr 1991; 121: 1613–1621.
14. Clinton SK, Emenhiser C, Schwartz SJ, et al. *Cis-trans* lycopene isomers, carotenoids, and retinol in the human prostate. Cancer Epidemiol Biomarkers Prev 1996; 823–833.
15. Zhao Z, Khachik F, Richie JP Jr, Cohen LA. Lycopene uptake and tissue disposition in male and female rats. Proc Soc Exp Biol Med 1998; 218(2):109–114.
16. Khachik F, Spangler CJ, Smith JC Jr, et al. Identification, quantification, and relative concentrations of carotenoids and their metabolites in human milk and serum. Anal Chem 1997; 69:1873–1881.
17. Mills PK, Beeson WL, Phillips RL, Fraser GE. Cohort study of diet, lifestyle, and prostate cancer in Adventist men. Cancer 1989; 64:598–604.
18. Hsing AW, Comstock GW, Abbey H, Polk BR. Serologic precursors of cancer: retinol, carotenoids, and tocopherol and risk of prostate cancer. J Natl Cancer Inst 19990; 82:941–946.
19. Giovannucci EL, Ascherio A. Rimm EB, et al. Intake of carotenoids and retinol in relationship to risk of prostate cancer. J Natl Cancer Inst 1995; 87:1767–1776.
20. Key TJA, Silicocks PH, Davey GK, Appleby PN, Bishop DT. A case-control study of diet and prostate cancer. Br J Canc 1997; 76:(5)678–687.
21. Heinonen OP, Albanes D, Virtamo J, Taylor PR, Huttunen JK, Hartman AM, et al. Prostate cancer and supplementation with alpha-tocopherol and beta-carotene: incidence and mortality in a controlled trial. J Natl Cancer Inst 1989; 90:440–446.
22. Stampfer MJ, Cook NR, Hennekens CH. Effects of beta-carotene supplementation on total and prostate cancer incidence among randomized participants with low baseline plasma levels: The Physician's Health Study. American Society of Clinical Oncology, 1997 (abstr).
23. Ribaya-Mercado JD, Garmyn M, Gilchrest BA, Russell RM. Lycopene in human skin is preferentially consumed, compared to β-carotene, during ultraviolet irradiation. J Nutr 1995; 125:1854–1859.
24. Kohlmeier L, Kark JD, Gomez-Garcia E, Martin BC, Steck SE, Kardinaal AFM et al. Lycopene and myocardial infarction risk in the EURAMIC Study. Am J Epidemiol 1997; 146:618–626.
25. Gärtner C, Stahl W, Sies H. Preferential increase in chylomicron levels of the xanthophylls lutein and zeaxanthin compared to β-carotene in the human. Int J Vit Nutr Res 1996; 66:1–7.
26. Kostic C, White WS, Olson JA. Intestinal absorption, serum clearance, and interactions between lutein and β-carotene when administered to human adults in separate or combined oral doses. Am J Clin Nutr 1995; 62:604–610.

27. Van den Berg H, van Vliet T. Effect of simultaneous, single oral doses of β-carotene with lutein or lycopene on the β-carotene and retinyl ester responses in the triacylglycerol-rich lipoprotein fraction of men. Am J Clin Nutr 1998; 68:(1)82–89.
28. Mayne ST, Carmel B, Silva F, Chi SK, Fallon BG, Briskin K et al. Effect of supplemental β-carotene on plasma concentrations of carotenoids, retinol, and α-tocopherol in humans. Am J Clin Nutr 1998; 68:642–647.
29. Khachik F, Bernstein PS, Garland DL. Identification of lutein and zeaxanthin oxidation products in human and monkey retinas. Invest Ophthalmol Vis Sci 1997; 38: 1802–1811.
30. Khachik F, Beecher GR, Smith JC Jr. Lutein, lycopene, and their oxidative metabolites in chemoprevention of cancer. J Cell Biochem 1995; 22(suppl):236–246.
31. Bone RA, Landrum JT, Friedes LM, Gomez CM, Kilburn MD, Menendez E, Vidal I, Wang W. Distribution of zeaxanthin stereoisomers in the human retina. Exp Eye Res 1997; 64:211–218.
32. Seddon JM, Ajani UA, Sperduto RD, Hiller R, Blain N, Burton TC et al. Dietary carotenoids, vitamins A, C, and E and advanced age-related macular degeneration. JAMA 1994; 272:1413–1420.
33. Mares-Perlman JA, Brady WE, Klein R, Klein BE, Bowen P, et al. Serum antioxidants and age-related macular degeneration in a population-based case-control study. Arch Ophthalmol 1995; 113:1518–1523.
34. Eye Disease Case-Control Study Group. Antioxidant status and neovascular age-related macular degeneration. Arch Ophthalmol 1993; 111:104–109.
35. West S, Vitale S, Hallfrisch J, et al. Are antioxidants or supplements protective for age-related macular degeneration? Arch Ophthalmol 1994; 112:222–227.
36. Hammond BR, Johnson EJ, Russell RM, Krinsky NI, Yeum KJ, Edwards RB, Snodderly DM. Dietary modification of macular pigment density. Invest Ophthalmol Vis Sci 1997; 88:1795–1801.
37. The Alpha-Tocopherol, Beta-Carotene Cancer Prevention Study Group. The effect of vitamin E and beta carotene on the incidence of lung cancer and other cancers in male smokers. N Engl J Med 1994; 330:1029–1035.
38. Omenn GS, Goodman GE, Thornquist MD, Balmes J, Cullen MR et al. Effects of a combination of beta-carotene and vitamin A on lung cancer and cardiovascular disease. N Engl J Med 1996; 334:1150–1155.
39. Wang XD, Liu C, Bronson RT, Smith DE, Krinsky NI, Russell RM. Alteration of retinoid signaling and AP1 expression by B-carotene supplements in smoke exposed ferrets. J Natl Cancer Inst 1999; 91:60–66.
40. Gebert JF, Moghal N, Frangioni JV, Sugarbaker DJ, Neel BG. High frequency of retinoic acid receptor β abnormalities in human lung cancer [published erratum appears in Oncogene 1992; 7:821]. Oncogene 1991; 6:1859–1868.
41. Lotan R. Retinoids in cancer chemoprevention. FASEB J 1996; 10:1031–1039.

7

n-3 Polyunsaturated Fatty Acids from Fish: Effects on Coronary Artery Disease

Erik Berg Schmidt
Hjørring/Brønderslev Hospital, Copenhagen, Denmark

Jørn Dyerberg
Nova Medical Medi-Lab, Copenhagen, Denmark

Coronary artery disease (CAD) is caused by atherosclerosis in the coronary arteries. Serious complications of CAD, notably acute myocardial infarction (AMI), is nearly always caused by a thrombus formed on top of a ruptured or eroded atherosclerotic plaque (1,2). The risk of plaque rupture is related to the extent of atherosclerosis. However, the composition of the plaques may be even more important, because plaques with a high content of lipid and macrophages and a thin overlying fibrous cap are particularly prone to rupture (1,2).

In this chapter we will focus on the effects of marine n-3 polyunsaturated fatty acids (PUFA) in atherogenesis and thrombogenesis and discuss the clinical effects of these n-3 PUFA on the risk of CAD.

I. INTRODUCTION

The n-3 polyunsaturated fatty acids (n-3 PUFA) are essential fatty acids characterized by having their first double bond at carbon atom number 3 (opposed to the more common n-6 PUFA, having their first double bond at carbon atom number 6) counted from the methyl end of the carbon chain that constitutes the backbone of fatty acids (3,4).

There are two subgroups of n-3 PUFA: γ-linolenic acid derived from plant oils (canola oil, rapeseed oil, and linseed oil), composed of 18 carbon atoms and 3 double bonds (nomenclature 18:3) and especially present in a Mediterranean-type diet, and a group of n-3 PUFA derived from seafood; the major marine n-3 PUFA are eicosapentaenoic acid (EPA; 20:5) and docosahexaenoic acid (DHA; 22:6). Because of a larger number of carbon atoms (20 and 22, respectively), these are also called long-chain n-3 PUFA. γ-Linolenic acid can to a limited extent be converted in the human body to the long-chained n-3 PUFA; otherwise they are acquired from eating seafood or taking fish oil supplements (cod liver oil/fish oil capsules).

The content of n-3 PUFA varies between fish species (5), being high in fatty fish like salmon, herring, and mackerel (2–5 g/100 g edible fish) and low in lean fish like flounder and cod (0.2 g/100 g edible fish).

The intake of long-chained n-3 PUFA varies considerably between populations, being very high in traditionally living Eskimos (10–14 g/day), low in western populations (<0.3 g/day), and intermediate in countries like Japan, Iceland, and Norway.

The content of n-3 PUFA in cod liver oil is about 20%, but it can be up to 90% in fish oil concentrates. Most studies investigating the effects of fish oil supplements have used daily doses of n-3 PUFA between 2 and 6 g. The difference in dosage between different studies should be kept in mind, because the effects of n-3 PUFA are dose-dependent.

In this chapter we focus on the effect of the marine long-chain n-3 PUFA and will not further discuss the possible effects of γ-linolenic acid.

II. MARINE n-3 PUFA AND ATHEROSCLEROSIS

There is some evidence from epidemiological studies that ingestion of marine n-3 PUFA reduces the risk of CAD. This has been most clearly shown in Greenland Eskimos (6), a population with a very high intake of n-3 PUFA. A recently published autopsy study found that the extent of atherosclerosis was very low in Greenland Eskimos living on a traditional diet rich in long-chain n-3 PUFA (7). Interestingly, advanced atherosclerosis at necropsy was also less prevalent in Alaskan Eskimos than in Alaskan nonnatives eating less seafood (8). Pulse wave velocity of the aorta was slower (indicating less atherosclerosis) in subjects living in Japanese fishing villages compared to people from farming villages elsewhere in Japan (9). In western countries the results of studies of the effect of fish consumption on CAD have not been consistent, but studies from the Netherlands, Italy, and the United States have reported an inverse correlation between CAD and fish intake (3,10–12).

n-3 PUFA are readily incorporated into human atherosclerotic plaques (13), and, considering the importance of plaque structure on future clinical events (1,2), the effect of dietary n-3 PUFA on plaque composition and characteristics is an area of great interest. It has, however, been studied to a rather small extent. Interestingly, it was recently reported that adipose tissue levels of DHA inversely correlated to the extent of coronary atherosclerosis at autopsy (14).

A beneficial effect of marine n-3 PUFA on atherosclerosis is also supported from the majority of animal studies showing that fish oil feeding may decrease atherosclerosis (15).

III. n-3 PUFA AND THROMBOSIS

Dietary n-3 PUFA modestly reduce platelet reactivity in part because of an inhibition of thromboxane production (3,4). Coagulability and fibrinolysis do not seem to be affected by n-3 PUFA to any major extent, although some data suggest that fibrinolysis may be impaired by n-3 PUFA due to an increase in plasma levels of plasminogen activator inhibitor-1 (3,4).

In a series of studies, Hornstra has shown an antithrombotic effect of n-3 PUFA in rats, but only when n-3 PUFA were given in combination with a diet low in saturated fat (16). Cod liver oil reduced platelet deposition to carotid arteries subjected to deep intimal injury by balloon angioplasty in pigs and reduced injury-related vasoconstriction (17). Also, when blood from cod liver oil–treated pigs perfused normal aortas, ex vivo platelet deposition to the aortas was lower than when blood from control pigs was used. These results indicate a beneficial effect of n-3 PUFA on the platelet-vessel wall interaction.

In a comprehensive study in baboons, a very high daily dose of fish oil (1 g/kg/day) was administered for 22 weeks (18). Femoral arteriovenous Dacron shunts were surgically implanted, and thrombotic responses of blood to segments of the grafts were determined. Later, endarterectomies were performed on carotid arteries. Vascular thrombus formation and lesions were inhibited by n-3 PUFA. The authors concluded that n-3 PUFA modestly reduced thrombotic responses of blood to thrombogenic surfaces and largely eliminated both the thrombotic and proliferative responses of endarterectomized carotid arteries. These results corroborate a reduction in microthrombi over atherosclerotic lesions found in hyperlipidemic swine fed fish oil (19).

IV. n-3 PUFA AND EXPERIMENTAL ACUTE MYOCARDIAL ISCHEMIA

There are several lines of evidence indicating that dietary n-3 PUFA reduce neutrophil reactivity. Thus it has been shown that neutrophil adhesion to endothelium, chemotaxis, chemiluminescence, and production of proinflammatory leukotriene B_4 are reduced by n-3 PUFA (20–22). This is of interest because there is growing evidence of an important role for neutrophils in acute myocardial ischemia (AMI) (23). Activated neutrophils may liberate proteases, leukotrienes, free oxygen radicals, and enzymes and by these and other mechanisms increase tissue injury during ischemia and reperfusion (23). Recently, Nakamura et al. (24) showed that intravenous infusion of docosahexaenoic acid into rabbits approximately halved the formation of leukotriene B_4 from stimulated neutrophils 6 hours after infusion. This method of administration of n-3 PUFA is ultimately proved to be safe and effective in humans and calls for studies in patients with unstable angina and AMI.

Furthermore, n-3 PUFA have been reported to reduce myocardial infarct size and infiltration of neutrophils into the myocardium (4). Improvement of blood rheology (25) and changes in vasoactive responses in direction of vasodilation and reduced platelet aggregability (3,26) by n-3 PUFA may also counteract acute myocardial ischemia and its consequences.

V. n-3 PUFA AND ARRHYTHMIAS IN EXPERIMENTAL MODELS

In a series of studies in rats and monkeys, McLennan et al. have convincingly shown that dietary n-3 PUFA reduce the incidence and severity of malignant ventricular tachyarrhythmias after coronary artery ligation and during reperfusion (27,28). n-6 PUFA also possess antiarrhythmic properties compared to saturated fat, but they are less effective than n-3 PUFA in ameliorating arrhythmias, while diets rich in monounsaturated fatty acids are neutral in this respect (28). The mechanisms by which n-3 PUFA inhibit ventricular tachyarrhythmias remain to be established but may be related to changes in eicosanoid formation (27) or may be caused by a modulation of calcium flux across cell membranes (29), but they are likely to include other mechanisms as well (30).

VI. CLINICAL STUDIES IN PATIENTS WITH CAD

A. Angina Pectoris

Saynor et al. in 1984 reported an astonishing symptomatic effect of dietary n-3 PUFA supplementation on anginal attacks in patients with stable angina pectoris in an open, uncontrolled trial (31). We were, however, unable to confirm this in a larger controlled trial (32), and other studies on small groups of patients have also been negative (4).

No studies have been published on the effect of n-3 PUFA in patients with unstable angina pectoris.

B. Secondary Prevention After AMI

Burr et al. (33) randomized more than 2000 men with recent AMI to various dietary changes, including an increased intake of n-3 PUFA (eating fatty fish twice weekly or, alternatively, fish oil capsules) for 2 years. There was a significant (29%) reduction in total mortality and deaths from CAD in those given fish advice (increasing their dietary intake of n-3 PUFA to approximately 1 g/day), whereas the other dietary changes (low fat, high fiber) had no effects. The number of nonfatal AMI increased, but not significantly, in the group given fish advice. This makes the underlying mechanism of protection in the fish group unlikely to be of antithrombotic nature, and the authors suggested an antiarrhythmic effect of n-3 PUFA as an explanation for their findings. However, in 18 men recovering from AMI, dietary supplementation with 6 g of n-3 PUFA/day for 6 weeks had no effect on the prevalence of ventricular extrasystoles or other arrhythmias (34). We found a nonsignificant decrease in ventricular extrasystoles after fish oil supplementation to patients with previously documented ventricular tachyarrhythmias (35). In another study, mainly including healthy subjects, supplementation with fish oil capsules reduced the number of ventricular extrasystoles in subjects with a high baseline number of extrasystoles (36).

C. Restenosis After PTCA

A rather high number of patients treated with percutaneous transluminal coronary angioplasty (PTCA) develops restenosis. The effect of dietary supplementation with n-3 PUFA in the prevention of restenosis has been evaluated in several trials. The results were initially promising, with significant beneficial effects reported in five of eight randomized controlled trials, an effect that was significant in a meta-analysis (37). However, recent larger trials set up to finally prove a beneficial effect of n-3 PUFA in these patients failed to show any effect of n-3 PUFA at all (38,39).

Today approximately two-thirds of patients are treated with stents during PTCA, which has considerably reduced the risk of restenosis. The studies with n-3 PUFA in the prevention of restenosis were all performed in the prestent era, and studies investigating the possible effect of n-3 PUFA in stented patients after PTCA should be undertaken.

D. Coronary Bypass Surgery

It has been reported that the incidence of late vein graft occlusion after coronary artery bypass surgery did not differ between patients randomized to fish oil or to aspirin (40).

In a recently published study from Norway, 610 patients undergoing coronary bypass surgery were supplemented with approximately 3.5 g of n-3 fatty acids daily as fish oil capsules or with placebo capsules for one year. Graft patency for venous but not for arterial (mammary) grafts was significantly better after 1 year of follow-up in those randomized to fish oil (41).

E. Cardiac Transplant Patients

It is not known if n-3 PUFA affect graft survival, development of coronary atherosclerosis, or prognosis in cardiac transplant recipients. However, n-3 PUFA improved endothelium-dependent coronary vasodilation (42), reduced plasma triglycerides (43), and reduced cyclosporine-induced hypertension in cardiac transplant patients (44,45).

F. Sudden Cardiac Death

The content of long-chain n-3 PUFA in coronary arteries was lower in subjects dying from sudden cardiac death than controls dying of other causes (46), and intake of n-3 fatty acids was associated with a reduced risk of cardiac arrest in previously healthy subjects (47). Furthermore, in the Physician's Health Study it was recently reported that the risk of sudden cardiac death was reduced by fish consumption (48). This is in line with the animal data mentioned above and a reduction in ventricular extrasystoles in humans eating n-3 PUFA (35,36). However, a better indicator for the risk of sudden cardiac death than the number of ventricular extrasystoles is heart rate variability (49). We therefore believe it is of major interest that in several studies on different patient groups our group has found that intake of n-3 PUFA improves heart rate variability (50–52). Thus, our studies suggest that the major cause of death from CAD, sudden cardiac death, may be reduced by intake of n-3 PUFA.

VII. MARINE n-3 PUFA AND RISK FACTORS FOR CAD

Dietary n-3 PUFA in practical doses have no effect on low-density lipoprotein (LDL) cholesterol levels, may slightly increase high-density lipoprotein (HDL) cholesterol levels (in particular antiatherogenic HDL2 cholesterol), but substantially decrease plasma triglycerides (53,54). n-3 PUFA may also slightly decrease blood pressure (55), while most studies have indicated no effect of n-3 fatty acids on the coronary risk factors fibrinogen and coagulant factor VII levels (4,56). There is little doubt that n-3 PUFA reduce platelet reactivity, while on the negative side n-3 PUFA may impair fibrinolysis (4). Other potential effects of n-3 PUFA with respect to preventing atherosclerosis and thrombosis include a reduction in leukocyte reactivity, an improvement of vessel wall function, and positive effects on blood rheology (3,4,57).

Most likely a concerted action of several mechanisms accounts for the possible beneficial effect of n-3 PUFA in the prevention and treatment of CAD.

VIII. CONCLUSIONS

Data from epidemiological studies, animal experiments, and clinical trials in humans indicate a beneficial role of n-3 PUFA on CAD. An effect of n-3 PUFA may be mediated through several effects and mechanisms. Among these are (1) a reduction in leukocyte and platelet reactivity, (2) an improvement of the lipid profile, (3) an improvement of vessel wall characteristics, (4) a modest decrease in blood pressure, (5) an improvement of blood rheology, and (6) an antiarrhythmic effect. Further clinical studies in patients with acute myocardial ischemia, post-MI patients, patients undergoing coronary bypass surgery, and patients with arrhythmias should be undertaken, because only results from controlled clinical trials can establish whether supplements with n-3 PUFA should be used to reduce the risk of CAD. In the meantime, it is sound sense to advocate incorporation of fatty and lean fish in the diet.

REFERENCES

1. Fuster V, Badimon L, Badimon JJ, Chesebro JH. The pathogenesis of coronary artery disease and the acute coronary syndromes. N Engl J Med 1992; 326:242–250, 310–318.
2. Davies MJ. Stability and instability: Two faces of coronary atherosclerosis. Circulation 1996; 94:2013–2020.
3. Schmidt EB, Dyerberg J. Omega-3 fatty acids: Current status in cardiovascular medicine. Drugs 1994; 47:405–424.
4. Schmidt EB. n-3 fatty acids and the risk of coronary heart disease. Dan Med Bull 1997; 44:1–22.
5. Hepburn FN, Exler J, Weihrauch JL. Provisional tables on the content of omega-3 fatty acids and other fat components of selected foods. J Am Diet Assoc 1986; 86:788–793.
6. Bjerregaard P, Dyerberg J. Mortality from ischaemic heart disease and cerebrovascular disease in Greenland. Int J Epidemiol 1988; 17:514–519.
7. Mulvad G, Pedersen HS, Jul E, et al. Atherosclerosis in Greenland natives. An autopsy study. Poster at IX International Congress on Circumpolar Health. Reykjavik, Iceland, June 20–25, 1993.
8. Newman III WP, Propst MT, Middaugh JP. Atherosclerosis in Alaska natives and non-natives. Lancet 1993; 341:1056–1057.

9. Hamazaki T, Urakaze M, Sawazaki S, Yamazaki K, Taki H, Yano S. Comparison of pulse wave velocity of the aorta between inhabitants of fishing and farming villages in Japan. Atherosclerosis 1988; 73:157–160.
10. Kromhout D, Feskens EJM, Bowles CH. The protective effect of a small amount of fish on coronary heart disease mortality in an elderly population. Int J Epidemiol 1995; 24:340–345.
11. Rodriguez BL, Sharp DS, Abbott RD, et al. Fish intake may limit the increase in risk of coronary heart disease morbidity and mortality among heavy smokers. Circulation 1996; 94:952–956.
12. Daviglus ML, Stamler J, Orencia AJ, et al. Fish consumption and the 30-year risk of fatal myocardial infarction. N Engl J Med 1997; 336:1046–1053.
13. Rapp JH, Connor WE, Lin DS, Porter JM. Dietary eicosapentaenoic acid and docosahexaenoic acid from fish oil. Their incorporation into advanced human atherosclerotic plaques. Arterioscler Thromb 1991; 11:903–911.
14. Seidelin KN, Myrup B, Fischer-Hansen B. n-3 Fatty acids in adipose tissue and coronary artery disease are inversely related. Am J Clin Nutr 1992; 55:1117–1119.
15. Soei LK, Lamers JMJ, Sassen LMA, et al. Fish oil: A modulator of experimental atherosclerosis in animals. In: Kristensen SD, Schmidt EB, De Caterina R, Endres S, eds. n-3 Fatty Acids: Prevention and Treatment of Vascular Disease. New York: Springer-Verlag, 1995:55–75.
16. Hornstra G. The significance of fish and and fish-oil enriched food for prevention and therapy of cardiovascular disease. In: Vergroesen A, Crawford M, eds. The Role of Fats in Human Nutrition. New York: Academic Press, 1989:152–235.
17. Lam JYT, Badimon JJ, Ellefson RD, Fuster V, Chesebro JH. Cod liver oil alters platelet-arterial wall response to injury in pigs. Circ Res 1992; 71:769–775.
18. Harker LA, Kelly AB, Hanson SR, et al. Interruption of vascular thrombus formation and vascular lesion formation by dietary n-3 fatty acids in fish oil in nonhuman primates. Circulation 1993; 87:1017–1029.
19. Kim D, Schmee J, Baker JE, et al. Dietary fish oil reduces microthrombi over atherosclerotic lesions in hyperlipidemic swine even in the absence of plasma cholesterol reduction. Exp Mol Pathol 1993; 59:122–135.
20. Lee TH, Hoover RL, Williams JD, et al. Effects of dietary enrichment with eicosapentaenoic acid and docosahexaenoic acids on in vitro neutrophil and monocyte leukotriene generation and neutrophil function. N Engl J Med 1985; 312:1217–1224.
21. Schmidt EB, Pedersen JO, Varming K, et al. n-3 Fatty acids and leukocyte chemotaxis: Effects in hyperlipidemia and dose-response studies in healthy men. Arterioscler Thromb 1991; 11:429–435.
22. Lehr H-A, Nolte D, Hübner C, Messmer K. n-3 Fatty acids and leucocyte adhesion. In: Caterina RD, Endres S, Kristensen SD, Schmidt EB, eds. n-3 Fatty Acids and Vascular Disease. New York: Springer-Verlag, 1993:39–47.
23. Entman ML, Ballantyne CM. Inflammation in acute coronary syndromes. Circulation 1993; 88:800–803.
24. Nakamura N, Hamazaki T, Yamazaki K, et al. Intravenous infusion of tridocosahexaenoyl-glycerol emulsion into rabbits. J Clin Invest 1993; 92:1253–1261.
25. Ernst E. Effects of n-3 fatty acids on blood rheology. J Intern Med 1989; 225(suppl 1):129–132.

26. Vanhoutte PM, Shimokawa H, Boulanger C. Fish oil and the platelet-blood vessel wall interaction. World Rev Nutr Diet 1991; 66:233–244.
27. Charnock JS, McLennan PL, Abeywardena MY. Dietary modulation of lipid metabolism and mechanical performance of the heart. Mol Cell Biochem 1992; 116:19–25.
28. McLennan PL. Relative effects of dietary saturated, monounsaturated, and polyunsaturated fatty acids on cardiac arrhythmias in rats. Am J Clin Nutr 1993; 57:207–212.
29. Hallaq H, Smith TW, Leaf A. Modulation of dihydropyridine-sensitive calcium channels in heart cells by fish oil fatty acids. Proc Natl Acad Sci USA 1992; 89: 1760–1764.
30. Kang JX, Leaf A. Antiarrhythmic effects of polyunsaturated fatty acids. Recent studies. Circulation 1996; 94:1774–1780.
31. Saynor R, Verel D, Gillott T. The long term effect of dietary supplementation with fish lipid concentrate on serum lipids, bleeding time, platelets and angina. Atherosclerosis 1984; 50:3–10.
32. Kristensen SD, Schmidt EB, Andersen HR, Dyerberg J. Fish oil in angina pectoris. Atherosclerosis 1987; 64:13–19.
33. Burr ML, Fehily AM, Gilbert JF, et al. Effects of changes in fat, fish, and fibre intakes on death and myocardial reinfarction: diet and reinfarction trial (DART). Lancet 1989; ii:757–761.
34. Hardarson T, Kristinsson A, Skuladottir G, Asvalddottir H, Snorrason SP. Cod liver oil does not reduce ventricular extrasystoles after myocardial infarction. J Intern Med 1989; 226:33–37.
35. Christensen JH, Gustenhoff P, Ejlersen E, et al. n-3 Fatty acids and ventricular extrasystoles in patients with ventricular tachyarrhythmias. Nutr Res 1995; 15:1–8.
36. Sellmayer A, Witzgall H, Lorenz RL, Weber PC. Effects of dietary fish oil on ventricular premature complexes. Am J Cardiol 1995; 76:974–977.
37. Gapinski JP, VanRuiswyk JV, Heudebert GR, Schectman GS. Preventing restenosis with fish oils following coronary angioplasty. A meta-analysis. Arch Intern Med 1993; 153:1595–1601.
38. Leaf A, Jorgensen MB, Jacobs AK, et al. Do fish oils prevent restenosis after coronary angioplasty? Circulation 1994; 90:2248–2257.
39. Cairns JA, Gill J, Morton B, et al. Fish oils and low-molecular-weight heparin for the reduction of restenosis after percutaneous transluminal coronary angioplasty. Circulation 1994; 94:1553–1560.
40. Roy L, Meyer F, Gingras L, Auger L. A double-blind randomized controlled study comparing the efficacy of fish oil and low dose ASA to prevent coronary saphenous vein graft obstruction after CABG. Circulation 1991; 84(suppl II):II-285.
41. Eritsland J, Arnesen H, Grønseth K, Fjeld NB, Abdelnoor M. Effect of dietary supplementation with n-3 fatty acids on coronary artery bypass graft patency. Am J Cardiol 1996; 77:31–36.
42. Fleischhauer FJ, Yan W-D, Fischell TA. Fish oil improves endothelium-dependent coronary vasodilation in heart transplant recipients. J Am Coll Cardiol 1993; 21: 982–989.

43. Barbir M, Hunt B, Kushwaha S, et al. Maxepa versus bezafibrate in hyperlipidemic cardiac transplant recipients. Am J Cardiol 1992; 70:1596–1601.
44. Ventura HO, Milani RV, Lavie CJ, et al. Cyclosporine-induced hypertension. Efficacy of w-3 fatty acids in patients after cardiac transplantation. Circulation 1993; 88:281–285.
45. Andreassen AK, Hartmann A, Offstad J, Geiran O, Kvernebo K, Simonsen S. Hypertension prophylaxis with omega-3 fatty acids in heart transplant recipients. J Am Coll Cardiol 1997; 29:1324–1331.
46. Luostarinen R, Boberg M, Saldeen T. Fatty acid composition in total phospholipids of human coronary arteries in sudden cardiac death. Atherosclerosis 1993; 99:187–193.
47. Siscovick DS, Raghunathan TE, King I, et al. Dietary intake and cell membrane levels of long-chain n-3 polyunsaturated fatty acids and the risk of primary cardiac arrest. JAMA 1995; 274:1363–1367.
48. Albert CM, Hennekens CH, O'Donnell CJ, et al. Fish consumption and risk of sudden cardiac death. JAMA 1998; 279:23–28.
49. Stein PK, Bosner MS, Kleiger RE, Conger BM. Heart rate variability: a measure of cardiac autonomic tone. Am Heart J 1994; 127:1376–1381.
50. Christensen JH, Gustenhoff P, Korup E, et al. Effect of fish oil on heart rate variability in survivors of myocardial infarction: a double blind randomised controlled trial. Br Med J 1996; 312:677–678.
51. Christensen JH, Korup E, Aarøe J. Fish consumption, n-3 fatty acids in cell membranes, and heart rate variability in survivors of myocardial infarction with left ventricular dysfunction. Am J Cardiol 1997; 79:1670–1673.
52. Christensen JH, Aarøe J, Knudsen N, et al. Heart rate variability and n-3 fatty acids in patients with chronic renal failure—a pilot study. Clin Nephrol 1998; 49:102–106.
53. Schmidt EB, Kristensen SD, De Caterina R, Illingworth DR. The effects of n-3 fatty acids on plasma lipids and lipoproteins and other cardiovascular risk factors in patients with hyperlipidemia. Atherosclerosis 1993; 103:107–121.
54. Harris WS. n-3 fatty acids and lipoproteins: Comparison of results from human and animal studies. Lipids 1996; 31:243–252.
55. Morris MC, Sacks F, Rosner B. Does fish oil lower blood pressure? Circulation 1993; 88:523–533.
56. Hamsten A. The hemostatic system and coronary heart diasese. Thromb Res 1993; 70:1–38.
57. Endres S, De Caterina R, Schmidt EB, Kristensen SD. n-3 Polyunsaturated fatty acids update 1995. Eur J Clin Invest 1995; 25:629–638.

8
Lipoic Acid: A Multifunctional Nutraceutical

Aalt Bast and Guido R. M. M. Haenen
Universiteit Maastricht, Maastricht, The Netherlands

I. INTRODUCTION

Lipoic acid is a naturally occurring compound present in most kinds of pro- and eukaryotic cells. In our food, lipoic acid is present in several products, such as meat, liver, and heart. Lipoic acid gained attention in the late 1940s as a growth factor and was shown to be a requirement for pyruvate oxidation in certain microorganisms. In 1951, 30 mg of lipoic acid was purified from 100 kg of liver residue by Reed et al. (1). In the following years the molecular structure was elucidated (3,4) and the compound was identified as 1,2-dithiolane-3-pentanoic acid. It has a chiral center at the C3 carbon atom, which is in the R configuration (Fig. 1). In humans, lipoic acid is part of several 2-oxo acid dehydrogenases, which are involved in energy formation. Linked to lysine residues of the 2-oxo acid dehydrogenase multienzyme complexes, lipoic acid acts as a cofactor (5,6). It binds acyl groups and transfers them from one part of the enzyme complex to another. During this process, lipoic acid is reduced to dihydrolipoic acid, which is subsequently reoxidized by lipoamide dehydrogenase under the formation of NADH. Lipoic acid and dihydrolipoic acid can thus act as a redox couple, carrying electrons from the substrate of the dehydrogenase to NAD^+.

In 1966, German physicians started to administer racemic lipoic acid to patients with liver cirrhosis, mushroom poisoning, heavy metal intoxication, and diabetic neuropathy. Originally, the rationale for this treatment was the observation that patients with liver cirrhosis, diabetes mellitus, and polyneuropathy had lower levels of lipoic acid (7). It was assumed that supplementation with lipoic acid would help to overcome the shortage, thereby restoring the 2-oxo acid oxida-

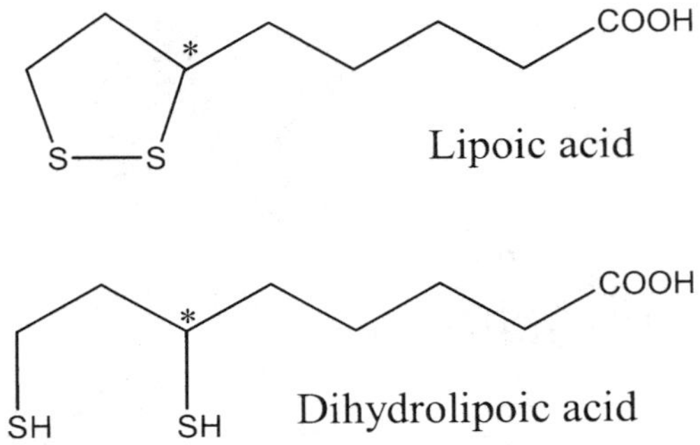

Figure 1 The chemical structures of lipoic acid (1,2-dithiolane-3-pentanoic acid) and dihydrolipoic acid. The chiral centers at the C3 carbon atoms are indicated with asterisks.

tion. Indeed, destruction of the cofactor function of lipoic acid may be involved in pathological processes. In arsenite intoxication, As^{3+} can form a complex with lipoic acid in the 2-oxoacid dehydrogenases, rendering it inactive. In certain types of liver disease, autoantibodies, which recognize lipoylated subunits in the multienzymes, have been demonstrated in patients' sera. Oxidative stress near the dehydrogenase complex can also lead to oxidative destruction, thereby adversely affecting the functioning of lipoic acid as a cofactor (7).

In recent years emphasis has been placed on the antioxidant action of lipoic acid (for review, see Ref. 8) to explain its activity.

II. ANTIOXIDANT ACTION

In contrast to many antioxidants, both the reduced (dihydrolipoic acid) and the oxidized forms of lipoic acid (Fig. 1) can act as antioxidants. Direct scavenging of various reactive oxygen species may occur (8) (Table 1).

Dihydrolipoic acid is a powerful reducer. In 1988 it was found that oxidized glutathione (GSSG) was reduced to its reduced form, GSH, by dihydrolipoic acid (9). In this way an indirect antioxidant activity of dihydrolipoic acid can be observed. This is illustrated using rat liver microsomes. In this system GSH transiently protects against lipid peroxidation (10). This inhibition depends on the presence of vitamin E and has been attributed to an enzymatic regeneration of vitamin E from its free radical form by GSH. This enzymatic factor has been called a vitamin E free radical reductase, although other phenols can take over the role of vitamin E (11). The denomination free radical reductase (Fig. 2) is therefore probably more appropriate. The oxidized form, GSSG, is not active as an inhibitor of lipid peroxidation. However, when GSSG and dihydrolipoic acid

Table 1 Scavenging of Reactive Oxygen Species by Either Lipoic Acid or Dihydrolipoic Acid[a]

	Lipoic acid	Dihydrolipoic acid
$O_2^{\cdot -}$	−	+
H_2O_2	−	−
$^{\cdot}OH$	+	+
HOCl	+	+
$ONOO^-$	+	+
$^1\Delta gO_2$	+	−

[a] The + and −, respectively, indicates that scavenging does or does not occur.
Source: Ref. 6.

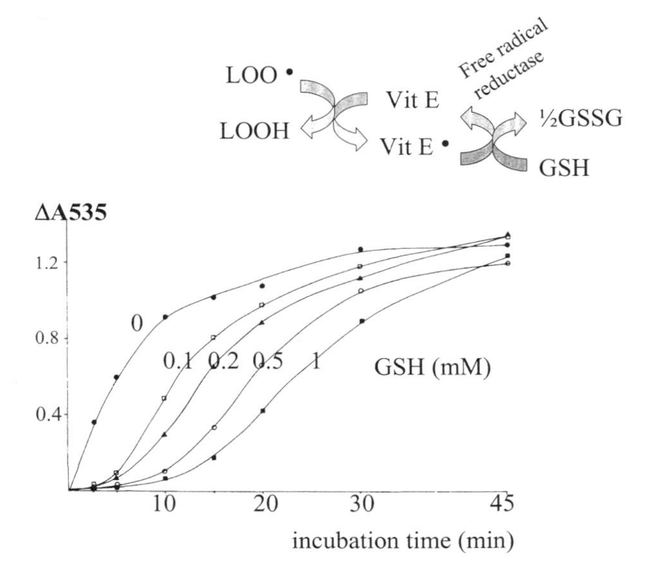

Figure 2 Inhibition of GSH on Fe/vitamin C–induced lipid peroxidation in rat liver microsomes through regeneration of vitamin E.

are combined, lipid peroxidation is inhibited. This indicates that GSSG is reduced to GSH by dihydrolipoic acid (Fig. 3).

Under certain conditions dihydrolipoic acid alone might act as a pro-oxidant, probably via reduction of Fe ions (9).

Not only GSH, but also vitamin C takes part in the water-soluble antioxidant network (6). Vitamin C can also regenerate vitamin E from the vitamin E free radical. Dihydrolipoic acid can reduce dehydroascorbate, giving vitamin C (Fig. 4). Dihydrolipoic acid has a greater reactivity toward dehydroascorbate than GSH, indicating that at certain concentrations dihydrolipoic acid is preferentially used for vitamin C regeneration than GSH. The rate constants k for this reaction are 32 M^{-1} min^{-1} for GSH and 875 M^{-1} min^{-1} for dihydrolipoic acid (6).

The oxidation product of lipoic acid, β-lipoic acid, is also reduced by dihydrolipoic acid (Fig. 5).

There is evidence that regeneration of antioxidants also occurs in vivo. This has been obtained by the measurement of antioxidant levels and by the determination of synergistic protection.

Healthy newborn rats are unable to synthesize vitamin C and are used as a model for oxidative stress (12). In this model, the regeneration of vitamin C

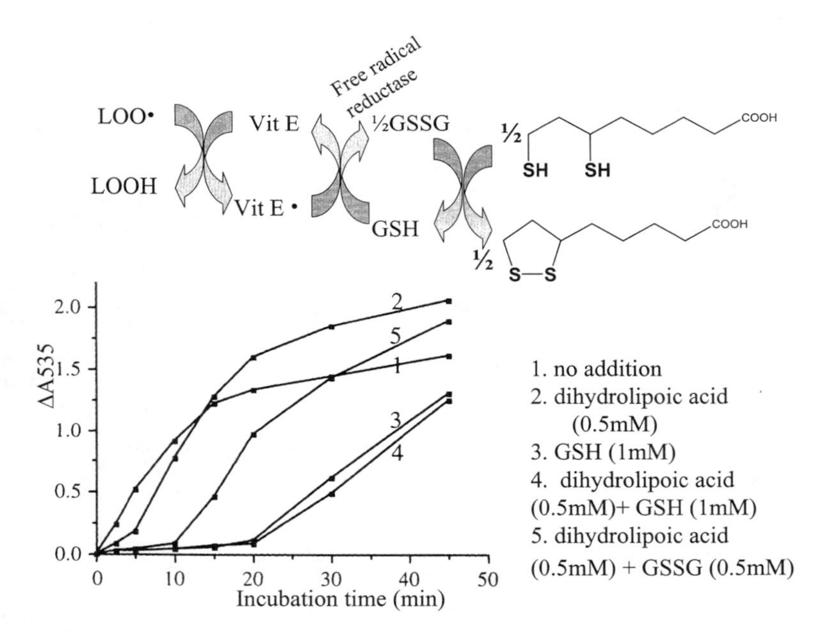

Figure 3 Inhibition of GSSH in combination with dihydrolipoic acid on Fe/vitamin C–induced lipid peroxidation in rat liver microsomes through regeneration of vitamin E.

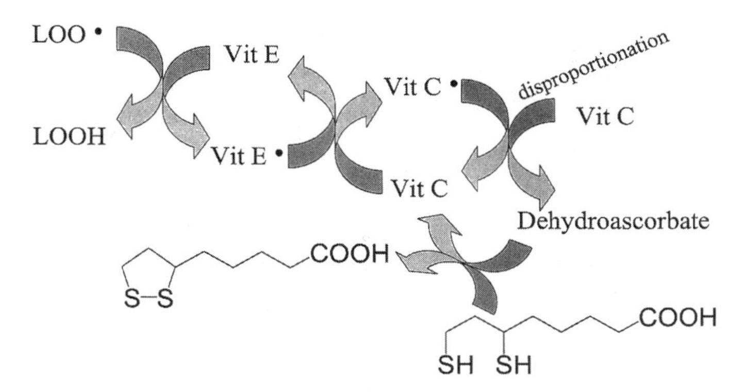

Figure 4 Interaction of dihydrolipoic acid, vitamin C, and vitamin E in the scavenging of lipid hydroperoxide free radicals (LOO•). Dihydrolipoic acid reduces dehydroascorbate to vitamin C.

was studied after treatment of rats with the GSH synthesis inhibitor 1-buthionine-(S,R)-sulfoximine (BSO). Lipoic acid prevented a decrease in vitamin C in the eye lenses. Clearly, lipoic acid can influence vitamin C levels. However, it is not known whether vitamin C regeneration occurs or whether lipoic acid acts as a scavenger, thus sparing vitamin C. BSO treatment of newborn rats resulted in a decreased vitamin E level, which is also prevented by lipoic acid (12).

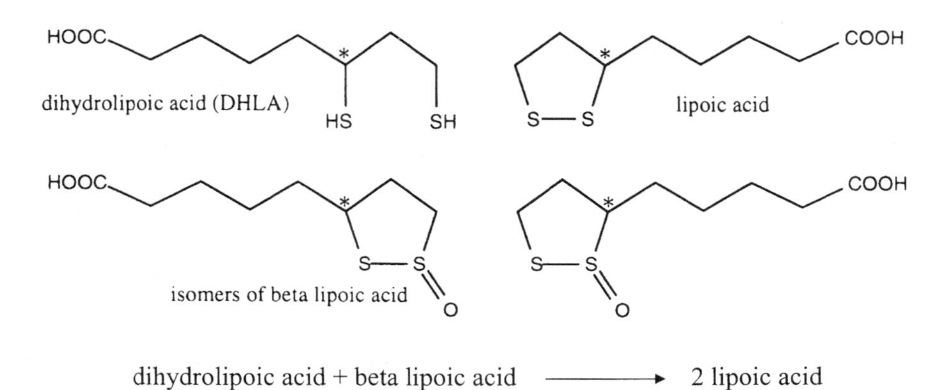

Figure 5 Molecular structures of dihydrolipoic acid, lipoic acid, and the isomers of beta-lipoic acid. The R-configuration is naturally occurring. The reaction between beta-lipoic acid and dihydrolipoic acid is also indicated.

Different reports demonstrated the regeneration of GSH. In mice, total GSH levels were increased in liver, kidney, and lung tissue cells after administration of lipoic acid (13). In contrast, lipoic acid did not influence the GSH or GSSG levels in the sciatic nerve of healthy rats (14). In animals subjected to oxidative stress, lipoic acid prevented depletion of GSH in all reported experiments (see, e.g., Ref. 15).

Another approach to establish in vivo antioxidant regeneration is to study the occurrence of a synergistic effect. In guinea pigs deficient in vitamin C, suboptimal amounts of vitamin C in combination with lipoic acid prevented scurvy symptoms better than either compound alone. For vitamin E–deficient animals a similar synergistic protection was found. The combination of lipoic acid plus vitamin E was more effective than either compound alone against the symptoms of vitamin E deficiency (16). In particular, the latter experiments, which date from 1959, suggest that lipoic acid regenerates vitamin C and vitamin E in vivo.

III. THE ROLE OF LIPOIC ACID IN REPAIR OF OXIDATIVE DAMAGE

Oxidants can damage lipids, DNA, or proteins. Subsequent degradation of these oxidatively damaged molecules may lead to renewal and might thus be envisioned as an important physiological process. Mild oxidative modification of proteins, for example, results in selective recognition and degradation by proteasomes (17). Repair of oxidatively damaged proteins, instead of degradation and renewal, might be of particular importance for proteins with a low turnover rate. Dihydrolipoic acid can play a role in such a protein repair process. This is illustrated by the repair of α_1-antiprotease.

The inactivation of protease inhibitors like α_1-antiprotease alters the protease-antiprotease balance in favor of the protein-degrading enzyme. This is of functional importance for neutrophils and macrophages. These cells secrete oxidants during inflammation. For this reason, methionine residues in proteins can oxidize to methionine sulfoxide. Methionine oxidation in α_1-antiprotease inhibits its action (18). Subsequent increased protease activation facilitates the phagocytosis. This should, however, be restricted to exogenous material. Inactivation of α_1-antiprotease by oxidation leads to increased elastase activity, which may lead to the deterioration of elastin and subsequent lung emphysema (Fig. 6).

The enzyme peptide methionine sulfoxide reductase has been reported to reduce oxidized methionine in a protein structure. The thioredoxin system supplies the enzyme with reducing equivalents (19). Dihydrolipoamide, an analog of dihydrolipoic acid, can reduce thioredoxin (20,21). We reported that dihydrolipoic acid (formed out of lipoic acid via NADH-dependent lipoamide dehydroge-

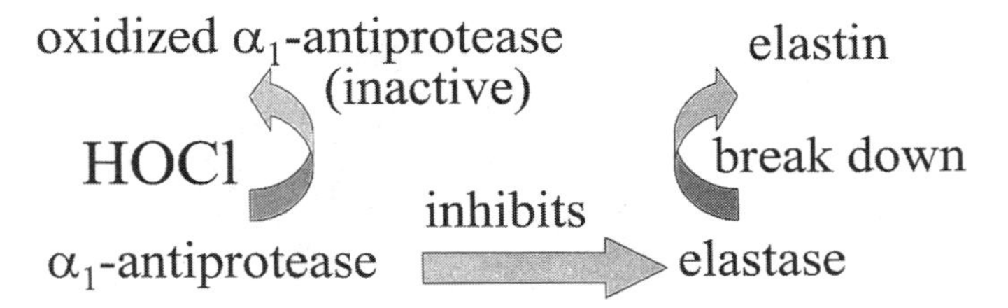

Figure 6 α_1-Antiprotease and elastase balance. Oxidation of α_1-antiprotease by, for example, the oxidant hypochlorous acid (HOCl) leads to inactivation. Consequently, the inhibition of elastase is reduced and elastin will be destroyed. This forms the pathological basis for lung emphysema.

nase activity) can shuttle the reducing equivalents, through thioredoxin, to the enzyme peptide methionine sulfoxide reductase, thereby reducing and activating the oxidized α_1-antiprotease (22) (Fig. 7).

In bacteria, the role of peptide methionine sulfoxide reductase gene in protecting against oxidative damage has been established (23). The promising possibilities of oxidized protein repair in humans and the actual contribution of lipoic acid in this respect for emphysema have to be further explored.

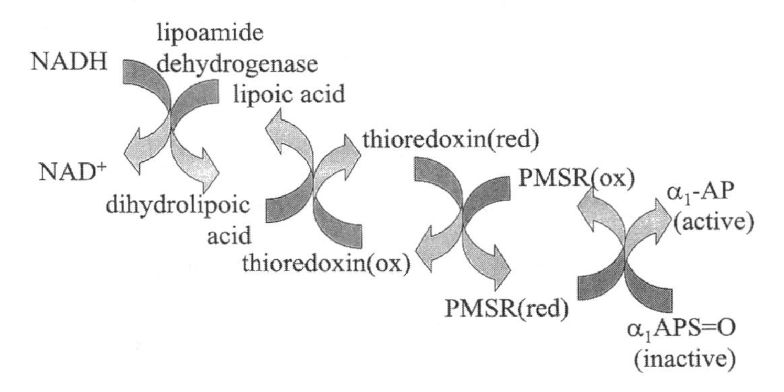

Figure 7 Repair of oxidatively damaged α_1-antiprotease. Lipoic acid is reduced to dihydrolipoic acid via the NADH-dependent lipoamide dehydrogenase. The reducing equivalents are further shuttled from dihydrolipoic acid through thioredoxin, to the enzyme peptide methionine sulfoxide reductase, thereby reducing and activating the oxidized α_1-antiprotease.

IV. OXIDATIVE STRESS IN DIABETES

Ongoing diabetes results in vascular and ocular damage and degeneration of nerves. These complications present a serious problem. It is becoming increasingly clear that oxidative stress is associated with diabetes-induced tissue damage (24). Several sources for increased formation of reactive oxygen species or a decreased antioxidant protection in diabetes can be recognized.

A. The Polyol Pathway

Under normal conditions glucose is phosphorylated to glucose-6-phosphate by a hexokinase. Phosphorylated glucose enters the hexose monophosphate shunt and leads to the formation of NADPH. When high glucose concentrations saturate the hexokinase, glucose is reduced by NADPH to sorbitol. This route is called the polyol pathway. This first reaction is catalyzed by aldose reductase. The second reaction consists of the oxidation of sorbitol to fructose, generating NADH. In the overall reaction, NADPH is exchanged by NADH.

Under hyperglycemic conditions, the polyol pathway activity may account for more than 30% of the glucose utilized. Consequently, the rate of NADPH utilization increases dramatically. The cell cannot compensate for such a loss of NADPH, and a sharp fall in steady-state concentrations of NADPH will take place. Glutathione reductase, the enzyme that reduces oxidized glutathione (GSSG), depends on NADPH for reducing equivalents. Reduction of GSSG to GSH is important for the overall cellular antioxidant activity (25).

B. The Formation of Glycation End Products

The formation of advanced glycation end products (AGE) starts with coupling of glucose to protein amines (8). As a nucleophile the amine attacks the carbonyl function of the sugar, and after enolization Amadori products are formed. Subsequent Amadori rearrangements occur, leading to the uncoupling of deoxyglucosomes. These deoxyglucosomes are very reactive toward proteins, resulting in protein cross-linking, browning, and fluorescence products.

The binding of AGE proteins to endothelial cells results in intracellular oxidative stress. This can promote the expression of genes. This is the result of activation of transcription factors such as NF-κB. The activation of this transcription factor is controlled by oxidants, and antioxidants can inhibit the activation of this transcription factor.

C. Metal-Catalyzed Oxidative Stress

Glucose induced damage can also be initiated by metal catalyzed oxidative reactions (8). In these reactions, reactive oxygen species and reactive aldehydes are generated. Glucose, but also Amadori products may undergo metal catalyzed oxidation. Antioxidants may prevent the damage that results.

V. THE MULTIFUNCTIONAL ROLE OF LIPOIC ACID IN DIABETES

The metabolic functions of lipoic acid are manifold. This is best demonstrated by explaining its protective effect in diabetes (8).

Several studies have shown an increased glucose uptake in skeletal muscle by lipoic acid (e.g., Refs. 26, 27). In streptozotocin-induced diabetic rats, lipoic acid reduces the blood glucose concentration by enhancing the muscle glucose transporter protein GLUT4 (27). This leads to an increase in insulin-stimulated glucose uptake. In another study, the direct stimulating effect of skeletal muscle glucose transport was shown to be largely insulin independent (26).

It has been found that lipoic acid reduces acetyl CoA and HSCoA levels (28). This will impair the influx of acetyl CoA in the citric acid cycle and the subsequent formation of citric acid. Because citric acid is an inhibitor of phosphofructokinase, which is involved in glycolysis, the impaired influx of acetyl CoA eventually stimulates the glycolysis. In addition, under conditions of a low acetyl CoA concentration, gluconeogenesis is impaired because the inhibition of pyruvate carboxylase (which occurs by acetyl CoA) is prevented (8,29).

The polyol pathway shifts the reducing equivalents from NADPH to NADH. This leads to a decreased antioxidant capacity and the successive loss of GSH, because the enzyme GSSG reductase receives its reducing equivalents from NADPH. The shift from NADPH to NADH may favor the reduction of lipoic acid to dihydrolipoic acid by the enzyme lipoamide dehydrogenase, which derives its reducing equivalents from NADH. Dihydrolipoic acid in turn reduces GSSG and can thus replenish the antioxidant GSH (Fig. 8).

Lipoic acid may prevent the AGE formation and their effects in several ways. Lipoic acid can react with reactive aldehydes, thus preventing the formation of AGE. Incubation of cultured bovine aortic endothelial cells with AGE albumin reduced intracellular GSH and vitamin C levels. The resulting oxidative stress gave activation of NF-κB. Cellular supplementation with lipoic acid prevented the AGE albumin–dependent depletion of reduced glutathione and vitamin C (30). It was further demonstrated that lipoic acid acted by inhibiting the translocation of NF-κB from the cytoplasm into the nucleus. As a result lipoic

$$NADPH + H^+ + glucose \xrightarrow{\text{aldose reductase}} sorbitol + NADP^+$$

$$NAD^+ + sorbitol \xrightarrow{\text{sorbitol dehydrogenase}} fructose + NADH + H^+$$

$$NADH + H^+ + \text{lipoic acid} \xrightarrow{\text{lipoamide dehydrogenase}} \text{dihydrolipoic acid} + NAD$$

$$\text{dihydrolipoic acid} + GSSG \longrightarrow \text{lipoic acid} + 2\ GSH$$

Figure 8 The aldose reductase pathway results in a shift of reducing equivalents from NADPH to NADH. This will lead to a decreased activity of the NADPH-dependent enzyme GSSG reductase and successive loss of GSH. At the same time the NADH-dependent enzyme lipoamide dehydrogenase activity will increase and the reduction of lipoic acid to dihydrolipoic acid will be enhanced. Dihydrolipoic acid can regenerate GSH from GSSG. In other words, although NADPH loss occurs, the GSSG can still be reduced to GSH, albeit indirectly, via dihydrolipoic acid.

acid reduced AGE albumin–induced NF-κB mediated expression of endothelial genes as for endothelin-1 (30). Inhibition of NF-κB by lipoic acid has been found in various studies (e.g., Ref. 31).

Glucose is known to initiate metal-catalyzed oxidative stress. Lipoic acid prevents damage by complexing the transition metals or directly by scavenging the reactive oxygen species (Table 1).

VI. RACEMATE, R-ENANTIOMER OR METABOLITE?

Until now most studies on lipoic acid have been performed with the racemic mixture of the compound. In recent years several studies showed some advantage in action of the naturally occurring R-enantiomer over the S-enantiomer.

Streeper et al. (32) corroborated earlier findings that lipoic acid enhances insulin-stimulated glucose transport and glucose metabolism in insulin-resistant rat skeletal muscle. Moreover, they found that the R-enantiomer was more effective than the S-enantiomer (32). Also, the pharmacokinetics was slightly different for both enantiomers (33). R-lipoic acid showed a somewhat higher oral bioavailability compared to the S-enantiomer (33).

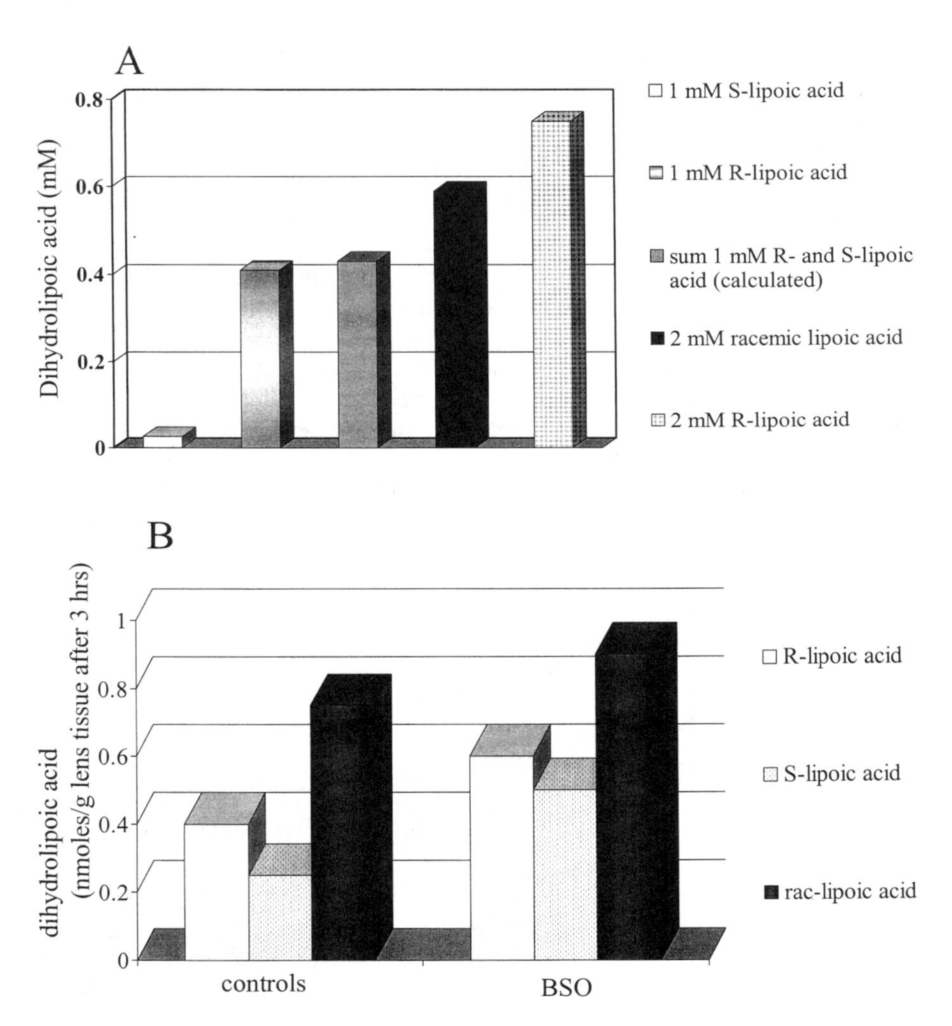

Figure 9 (A) The amount of dihydrolipoic acid formed after 15-minute incubation of both enantiomers and racemic mixture of lipoic acid in the presence of NADH and lipoamide dehydrogenase. (B) Dihydrolipoic acid levels in the lens tissue 3 hours after treatment with either R-, S-, or racemic lipoic acid in control or buthionine sulfoximine treated newborn rats. (Adapted from Ref. 36.)

Although both the reduced and the oxidized forms show biological activity (see, e.g., Table 1), the dihydrolipoic acid is regarded as the biologically most active form. Interestingly two enzymes involved in the reduction of lipoic acid show opposite stereospecificity (34). The NADPH-dependent GSSG reductase reduces S-lipoic acid two times faster than R-lipoic acid. In contrast, the NADH-dependent lipoamide dehydrogenase reduces the R form 28 times faster than the S form (34).

We have found that actually a synergistic antioxidant effect on the simultaneous administration of both enantiomers might occur (35). This is explained as follows. R-dihydrolipoic acid, formed by the preferential reduction of the R-lipoic acid by lipoamide dehydrogenase, can nonenzymatically reduce S-lipoic acid into S-dihydrolipoic acid. In other words, indirectly, through R-dihydrolipoic acid, the S-form is also reduced by lipoamide dehydrogenase (Fig. 9A). This synergistic action, due to a catalyst function of R-lipoic acid in the reduction of S-lipoic acid, may in fact also be suggested from in vivo experiments (36). Maitra et al. (36) studied the stereospecific effects of lipoic acid on cataract formation in newborn rats that were treated with the glutathione synthesis inhibitor BSO. It appeared that 3 hours after treatment with equimolar dosages of either R-,

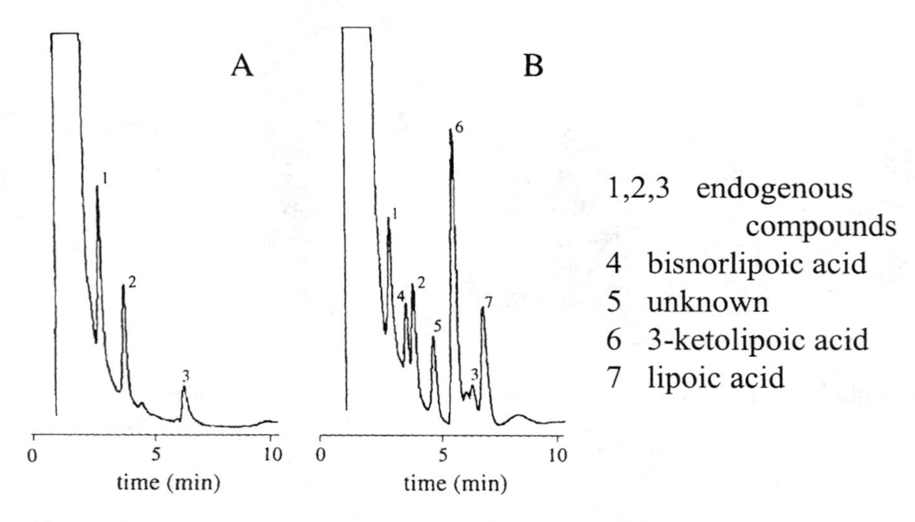

Figure 10 HPLC chromatogram of a plasma sample before oral administration of lipoic acid (A) and the HPLC chromatogram of a plasma sample 119 minutes after oral administration of 1 g of R-lipoic acid to a healthy male volunteer (B). Peaks 1, 2, and 3 were from endogenous compounds in the plasma. Peak 4 was identified as bisnorlipoic acid; 5 is an unidentified metabolite of lipoic acid; 6 was identified by GC/MS as 3-ketolipoic acid; 7 is lipoic acid.

S-, or racemic lipoic acid, the dihydrolipoic acid level in the lens tissue was the highest after administration of the racemic mixture of lipoic acid (Fig. 9B).

Further studies on the need to develop the R-enantiomer of lipoic acid for human use are clearly needed. The possible stereoselective activity of a recently cloned Na^+-dependent mammalian vitamin transporter should also be taken into account here (37).

After oral administration of 1 g of R-lipoic acid to a male volunteer, 3-ketolipoic acid was found as a major metabolite (38) (Fig. 10). It appeared in relatively high concentrations in the plasma and has the structural characteristics of an antioxidant. This metabolite might largely contribute to the therapeutic activity of lipoic acid. It is probably formed during beta-oxidation and needs further research.

VII. CONCLUSION

A remarkably diverse range of actions can be ascribed to lipoic acid (Fig 11). Lipoic acid prevents oxidative damage. Interestingly, both the reduced as well as the oxidized form of the molecule can react with oxidants (39). This is nicely illustrated by the reaction of both compounds with hypochlorous acid (18).

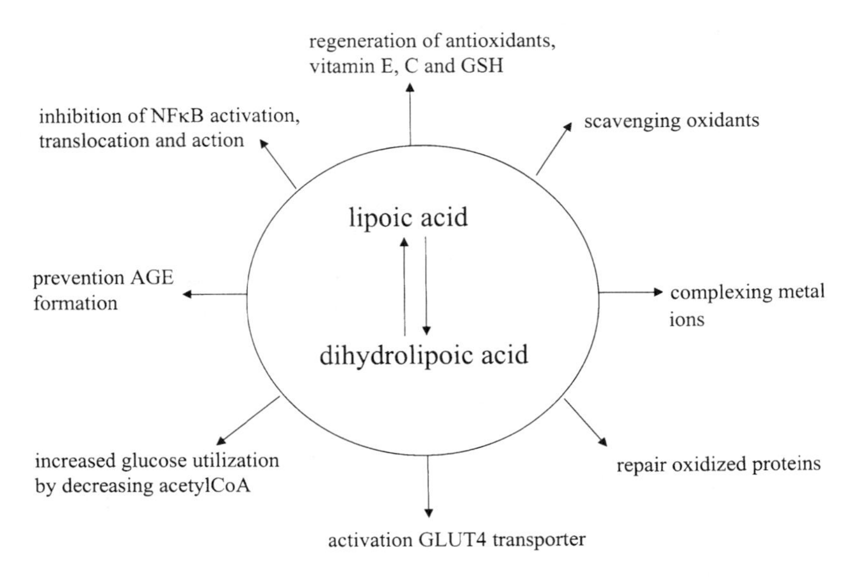

Figure 11 Many modes of action have been established for the redox couple dihydrolipoic acid–lipoic acid.

Dihydrolipoic acid regenerates the antioxidants vitamin C and E and GSH from their oxidized forms. Dihydrolipoic acid can shuttle reducing equivalents via thioredoxin to peptide methionine sulfoxide reductase and is thus involved in the repair of oxidized proteins.

Lipoic acid is used in the treatment of type II diabetes and has been shown to increase the glucose uptake and utilization. Because oxidative stress plays a role in the development of long-term diabetic late complications, the antioxidant action of lipoic acid is of benefit here. Lipoic acid prevents the potential harmful effects of a shift of NADPH into NADH, because it may make possible the use of NADH for the reduction of GSSG to GSH, which at a relative NADPH lack would otherwise not occur. Lipoic acid may prevent toxic AGE formation, and it inhibits NF-κB activation, translocation, and action.

R-lipoic acid is the naturally occurring form of lipoic acid. Further studies on the putative therapeutic advantage of this enantiomer are needed, as is further research on the possible role of lipoic acid metabolites in the therapeutic actions of lipoic acid.

REFERENCES

1. Reed LJ, de Busk BG, Gunsalus IC, Schnakenberg GHF. Crystalline a-lipoic acid: a catalytic agent associated with pyruvate dehydrogenase. Science 1951; 114:93.
2. Bullock MW, Brockamann JA, Patterson EL, Pierce JV, von Saltza MH, Sanders F, Stokstad ELR. Synthesis in the thioctic acid series. J Am Chem Soc 1954; 76: 1828–1832.
3. Bullock MW, Brockmann JA, Patterson EL, Pierce JV, Macchi ME. Proposed structures for protogen-A and protogen-B. J Am Chem Soc 1954; 76:1827–1828.
4. Morris TW, Reed KE, Cronan JE. Lipoic acid metabolism in *Escherichia coli*: the lplA and lipB genes define redundant pathways for ligation of lipoyl groups to apoprotein. J Bacteriol 1995; 177:1–10.
5. Fujiwara K, Okamura-Ikeda K, Motokawa Y. In: Packer L, ed. Assay for Protein Lipoylation Reaction. Methods in Enzymology, Vol. 251. London: Academic Press 1995:333–350.
6. Biewenga GPh, Haenen GRMM, Bast A. The pharmacology of the antioxidant lipoic acid. Gen Pharmacol 1997; 29:315–331.
7. Gutierrez Correa JG, Stoppani AOM. Catecholamines enhance dihydrolipoamide dehydrogenase inactivation by the copper Fenton system. Enzyme protection by copper chelators. Free Rad Res 1996; 24:311–322.
8. Biewenga GPh, Haenen GRMM, Bast A. The role of lipoic acid in the treatment of diabetic polyneuropathy. Drug Metab Rev 1998; 29:1025–1054.
9. Bast A, Haenen GRMM. Interplay between glutathione and lipoic acid in the protection against microsomal lipid peroxidation. Biochim Biophys Acta 1988; 963:558–561.

10. Haenen GRMM, Bast A. Protection against lipid peroxidation by a microsomal glutathione-dependent labile factor. FEBS Lett 1983; 159:24–28.
11. Aarts L, van der Hee R, Dekker I, de Jong J, Langemeijer H, Bast A. The widely used anesthetic agent propofol can replace α-tocopherol as an antioxidant. FEBS Lett 1995; 357:83–85.
12. Maitra I, Serbinova E, Tritschler H, Packer L. Alpha-lipoic acid prevents buthionine sulfoximine-induced cataract formation in newborn rats. Free Rad Biol Med 1995; 18:823–829.
13. Busse E, Zimmer G. Schopohl B, Kornhuber B. Influence of α-lipoic acid on intracellular glutathione in vitro and in vivo. Arzneim-Forsch Drug Res 1992; 42:829–831.
14. Nagamatsu M, Nickander KK, Schmelzer JD, Raya A, Rohwer DA, Tritschler H, Low PA. Lipoic acid prevents endoneurial ischemia and improves experimental diabetic neuropathy. Pharm Res 1995; 31S:163.
15. Sumathi R, Jayanthi S, Varalakshmi P. DL α-lipoic acid as a free radical scavenger in glyoxylate-induced lipid peroxidation. Med Sci 1993; 21:135–137.
16. Rosenberg HR, Culik R. Effect of α-lipoic acid on vitamin C and vitamin E deficiencies. Arch Biochem Biophys 1959; 80:86–93.
17. Grune T, Blasig IE, Sitte N, Roloff B, Haseloff R, Davies KJ. Peroxynitrite increases the degradation of aconitase and other cellular proteins by proteasome. J Biol Chem 1998; 273:10857–10862.
18. Haenen GRMM, Bast A. Scavenging of hypochlorous acid by lipoic acid. Biochem Pharmacol 1991; 42:2244–2246.
19. Brot N, Fliss H, Coleman T, Weissbach H. Enzymatic reduction of methionine sulfoxide residues in proteins and peptides. Proc Natl Acad Sci 1981; 78:2155–2158.
20. Holmgren A. Thioredoxin catalyses the reduction of insulin disulfides by thiothreitol and dihydrolipoamide. J Biol Chem 1979; 254:9627–9632.
21. Spector A, Huang R-RC, Yan G-Z, Wang R-R. Thioredoxin fragment 31–36 is reduced by dihydrolipoamide and reduces oxidized protein. Biochem Biophys Res Commun 1988; 150:156–162.
22. Biewenga GPh, Veening-Griffioen DH, Nicastia AJ, Haenen GRMM, Bast A. A new antioxidant property of dihydrolipoic acid: Repair of oxidatively damaged alpha-1 antiprotease. Drug Res 1998; 48:144–148.
23. Moskovitz J, Rahman MA, Strassman J, Yancey SO, Kushner SR, Brot N, Weisbach H. *Escherichia coli* peptide methionine sulfoxide reductase gene: regulation of expression and role in protecting against oxidative damage. J Bacteriol 1995; 177: 502–507.
24. Wolff SP, Jiang ZY, Hunt JV. Protein glycation and oxidative stress in diabetes mellitus and ageing. Free Rad Biol Med 1991; 10:339–352.
25. Gonzalez AM, Sochor M, Hothersall JS, McLean P. Effect of aldose reductase inhibitor (sorbinil) on integration of polyol pathway and glycolytic route in diabetic lens. Diabetes 1986; 35:1200–1205.
26. Henriksen EJ, Jacob S, Streeper RS, Fogt DL, Hokama JY, Tritschler HJ. Stimulation by α-lipoic acid of glucose transport activity in skeletal muscle of lean and obese zucker rats. Life Sci 1997; 61:805–812.

27. Khamaisi M, Potashnik R, Tirosh A, Demshchak E, Rudich A, Tritschler H, Wessel K, Bashan N. Lipoic acid reduces glycemia and increases muscle GLUT4 content in streptozotozin-diabetic rats. Metabolism 1997; 46:763–768.
28. Blumenthal SA. Inhibition of gluconeogenesis in rat liver by lipoic acid. Evidence for more than one site of action. Biochem J 1984; 219:773–780.
29. Wagh SS Natraj CV, Menon KKG. Mode of action of lipoic acid in diabetes. J Biosci 1987; 11:59–74.
30. Bierhaus A, Chevion S, Chevion M, Hofmann M, Quehenberger P, Illmer T, Luther T, Berentshtein E, Tritschler H, Müller M, Wahl P, Ziegler R, Nawroth PP. Advanced glycation end product-induced activation of NF-κB is suppresses by α-lipoic acid in cultured endothelial cells. Diabetes 1997; 46:1481–1490.
31. Packer L, Suzuki YJ, Vitamin E and alpha-lipoate: the role in antioxidant recycling and activation of NF-kappa B transcription factor. Mol Aspects Med 1993; 14:229–239.
32. Streeper RS, Henriksen EJ, Jacob S, Hokama JY, Donovan LF, Tritschler HJ. Differential effects of lipoic acid stereoisomers on glucose metabolism in insulin-resistant skeletal muscle. Am J Physiol 1997; 273:E185–E191.
33. Hermann R, Niebch G, Borbe HO, Fieger-Büschges H, Ruus P, Nowak H, Riethmüller-Winzen, Peukert M, Blume H. Enantioselective pharmacokinetics and bioavailability of different racemic α-lipoic acid formulations in healthy volunteers. Eur J Pharm Sci 1996; 4:167–174.
34. Biewenga GPh, Dorstijn MA, Verhagen JV, Haenen GRMM, Bast A. The reduction of lipoic acid by lipoamide dehydrogenase. Biochem Pharmacol 1996; 51:233–238.
35. Biewenga GPh, Haenen GRMM, Groen BH, Biewenga JE, van Grondelle R, Bast A. Combined non-enzymatic and enzymatic reduction favours bioactivation of racemic lipoic acid. An advantage of a racemic drug? Chirality 1997; 9:362–366.
36. Maitra I, Serbinova E, Tritschler HJ, Packer L. Stereospecific effects of R-lipoic acid on buthionine sulfoximine-induced cataract formation in newborn rats. Biochem Biophys Res Commun 1996; 221:422–429.
37. Prasad PD, Wang H, Kekuda R, Fujita T, Fei Y-J, Devoe LD, Leibach FH, Ganapathy V. Cloning and functional expression of a cDNA encoding a mammalian sodium-dependent vitamin transporter mediating the uptake of pantothenate, biotin, and lipoate. J Biol Chem 1998; 273:7501–7506.
38. Biewenga G, Haenen GRMM, Bast A (inventors). Thioctic acid metabolites and methods of use thereof. U.S. Patent 5,925,668 (Assignee, ASTA Medica AG, Dresden). Date of patent, July 20, 1999.
39. Biewenga GPh, de Jong J, Bast A. Lipoic acid favors thiolsulfinate formation after hypochlorous acid scavenging: a study with lipoic acid derivatives. Arch Biochem Biophys 1994; 312:114–120.

9
R-α-Lipoic Acid

Klaus Krämer
BASF Aktiengesellschaft, Ludwigshafen, Germany

Lester Packer
University of Southern California School of Pharmacy, Los Angeles, California

I. INTRODUCTION

R-α-Lipoic acid is a naturally occurring substance that offers health benefits beyond plain nutrition. It plays a pivotal role in cellular metabolism by acting as a coenzyme in energy production and by functioning as an ideal antioxidant. R-α-lipoic acid also offers protection against the sequelae of diabetes, such as neuropathy, cataract, and cardiovascular disease. R-α-lipoic acid ameliorates insulin sensitivity in type 2 diabetes. In addition, there is evidence that R-α-lipoic acid delays the aging process, improves brain function and memory, stimulates immune function, and supports liver health.

This information has been compiled to provide a comprehensive review about this unique biological compound. If not otherwise specified in the text, the term lipoic acid refers to the racemic mixture of R- and S-α-lipoic acid or either of both enantiomers.

II. DESCRIPTION

R-Lipoic acid (CAS-No. 1200-22-2, thioctic acid, 1,2-dithiolane-3-pentanoic acid) has a chiral center at C6 carbon atom (Fig. 1). Lipoic acid produced by BASF has an R-configuration and is identical to the form found in nature. Characteristic for the molecule is the 1,2-dithiolane-ring system containing a disulfide.

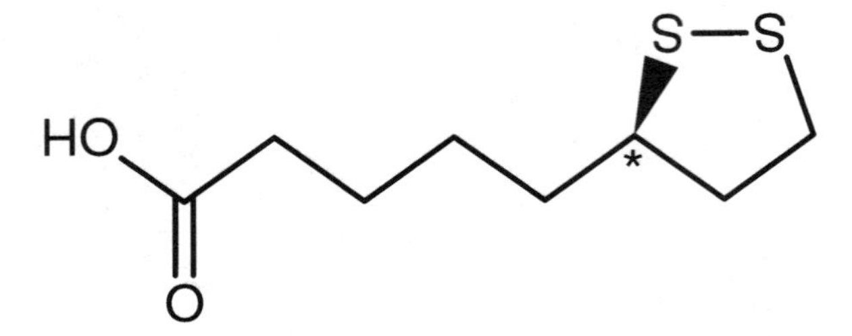

Figure 1 Structure of R-lipoic acid.

R-lipoic acid is a crystalline, yellowish powder. Its purity is guaranteed to be higher than 99%. Enantiomeric purity of the R-configuration is higher than 99%.

R-lipoic acid as a bulk material is stable at room temperature for 24 months if sealed in a container. It should not be exposed to sunlight. Its melting point is 46–48°C.

III. PRODUCTION PROCESS

Conventional chemical synthesis of lipoic acid yields a racemic mixture of R- and S-enantiomers. Lipoic acid from BASF is manufactured by a proprietary process applying an enantioselective synthesis that gives rise to the active R-isomer only (11). In contrast to racemate separation, this ensures an economic advantage and a high enantiomeric purity.

IV. DISCOVERY AND BRIEF HISTORY

R-Lipoic acid was first discovered in 1937 by Snell and coworkers (100), who found that certain bacteria needed a compound from potato extract for growth. However, it was not before 1951 that the so-called ''potato growth factor'' was isolated and characterized (Fig. 1) by Lester Reed (79,81). Reed and his group used 10 tons of beef liver residue for the purification of only 30 mg of crystalline R-lipoic acid. Initially, R-lipoic acid was tentatively regarded a vitamin, but later it turned out that R-lipoic acid is synthesized both by plants and animals (79,85). Although the biosynthetic pathway of R-lipoic acid is not well understood, it seems that R-lipoic acid is synthesized in mitochondria from octanoic acid and a sulfur source (46,112).

An antioxidant action of lipoic acid was proposed for the first time by

Rosenberg and Culik in 1959 (85). The authors observed that lipoic acid reduced scurvy in vitamin C–depleted guinea pigs and prevented vitamin E deficiency in rats. More recently, in the work of Bast and Packer, the antioxidant function of lipoic acid was fully recognized (for reviews, see Refs. 6, 72). In 1991, Packer and his group showed that vitamin E, vitamin C, lipoic acid, and glutathione act synergistically in the so-called ''antioxidant network.'' In the following years many contributions demonstrated the synergistic action of lipoic acid with other antioxidants.

R,S-lipoic acid has been used for the treatment of diabetic neuropathy in Germany for almost 4 decades. Recently, enhancement of glucose disposal by lipoic acid in type II diabetic patients was discovered (40). Since this pioneering work, the insulin-sensitizing activity of lipoic acid has been confirmed in several animal and human trials.

V. PHYSIOLOGICAL FUNCTION OF R-LIPOIC ACID

R-lipoic acid naturally occurs in plant and animal tissues, where it is covalently bound to the ε-amino group of lysine residues. As lipoamide, lipoic acid functions as a cofactor of mitochondrial enzymes, catalyzing oxidative decarboxylation of

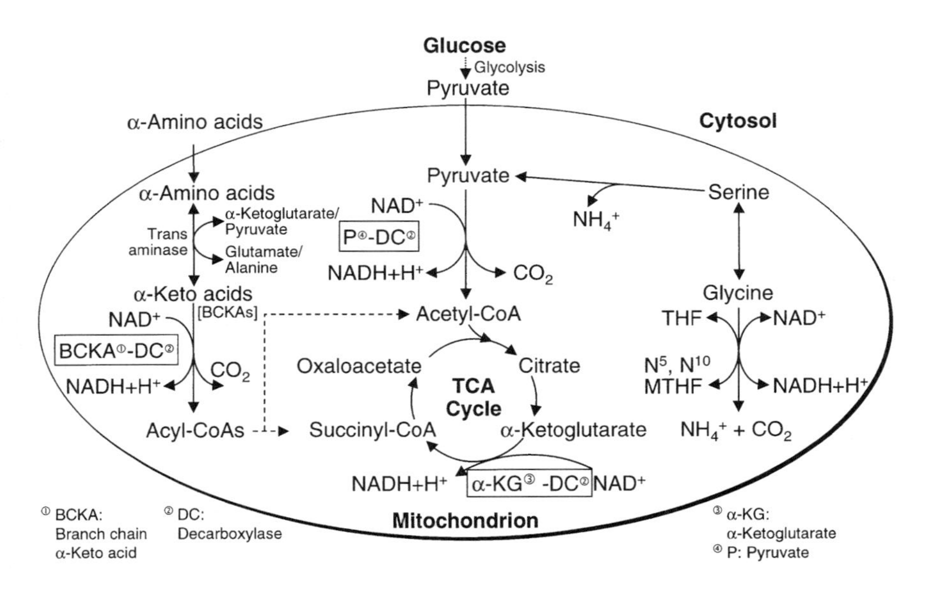

Figure 2 R-lipoic acid is a cofactor in major metabolic pathways.

pyruvate, α-ketoglutarate, and branched chain α-keto acids (80). The pyruvate dehydrogenase is a multienzyme complex composed of four subunits. Subunit E2 contains two-lipoyl and subunit X one-lipoyl residues. Lipoic acid is of vital importance for energy production (ATP) and branched-chain amino acid degradation (Fig. 2). Interestingly, in the glycine cleavage system lipoic acid is interlinked with folate metabolism (73). This lipoamide-dependent enzyme oxidizes glycine to CO_2 and ammonia, forming NADH and 5,10-methylenetetrahydrofolate.

VI. ANALYSIS OF LIPOIC ACID AND OCCURRENCE

Gas chromatography (GC), gas chromatography mass spectroscopy (GC-MS), and HPLC have been widely used for the determination of lipoic acid in biologi-

Table 1 Lipoyllysine Content of Various Sources

Source	μg/g dry weight[a]
Garden pea	0.39 ± 0.07
Brussel sprouts	0.39 ± 0.21
Rice bran	0.16 ± 0.02
Banana	nd
Orange peel	nd
Soybean	nd
Horseradish	nd
Egg yolk	0.05 ± 0.07
Yeast	0.27 ± 0.05
E. coli	8.07
Kidney	2.64 ± 1.23
Heart	1.51 ± 0.75
Liver	0.86 ± 0.33
Spleen	0.36 ± 0.08
Brain	0.27 ± 0.08
Pancreas	0.12 ± 0.05
Lung	0.12 ± 0.08
Spinach	3.15 ± 1.11
Broccoli	0.94 ± 0.25
Tomato	0.56 ± 0.23

[a] Lipoyllysine × 0.62 = lipoic acid. Values represent mean ± SD.

Source: Ref. 58.

cal and food samples (for review, see Ref. 48). Among these, GC and GC-MS methods are highly specific but require derivatization and acidic or alkaline hydrolysis with the risk of low recovery. Moreover, GC-MS requires expensive equipment. HPLC methods are more practical for routine analyses. With a new HPLC method specific for lypoyllysine, it is possible to determine lipoic acid in tissues and food samples (58). This method involves protease digestion for sample preparation.

HPLC with electrochemical or fluorescence detection has also been used for the determination of lipoic acid in human plasma (34,65,96,108,109,114). In addition to the separate analysis of the R- and S-enantiomers (34,65), oxidized and reduced lipoic acid have been determined (96,114).

In plants lipoyllysine content is highest in spinach (3.15 μg/g dry weight). In animal tissues lipoyllysine is most abundant in kidney, followed by heart (Table 1).

VII. BIOAVAILABILITY

Bioavailability of racemic lipoic acid has extensively been studied in humans using single dose administration (10,22,33,34,108). Lipoic acid is absorbed with a T_{max} of 0.5–1 hour and exhibits dose-proportionality between 50 and 600 mg (10). There was no difference between R- and S-lipoic acid concentrations in plasma after intravenous administration. However, after oral intake of the racemic mixture, a higher response was found for R-lipoic acid than for the S-form (33). Means for AUC and C_{max} were at least 60% higher for the R-form, and this difference was highly significant (Fig. 3). Lipoic acid was better absorbed from an aqueous solution than from galenical preparations. Food intake resulted in reduced bioavailability of lipoic acid (22). Therefore, it has been recommended to take up the compound after fasting and 30 minutes before a meal. In diabetic patients gastric emptying is usually delayed. In insulin-dependent diabetics, delayed gastric emptying had no substantial influence on lipoic acid bioavailability (35).

The absolute bioavailability (oral vs. intravenous) of 200 mg lipoic acid in aqueous solution has been estimated to be 38% for the R- and 28% for the S-form (34). Galenical forms had lower absolute bioavailabilities—25% for R- and 20% for S-lipoic acid. In a later study not distinguishing between the enantiomers, a similar absolute bioavailability of 29% was found after ingestion of 200 mg tablets (108).

The relative low bioavailability of lipoic acid may be due to a high first-pass effect. In preclinical work on the pharmacokinetics of lipoic acid in rats applying [7,8-^{14}C]rac-α-lipoic acid, the AUC of radioactivity in plasma averaged 66% after oral administration as compared to the intravenous route (74). How-

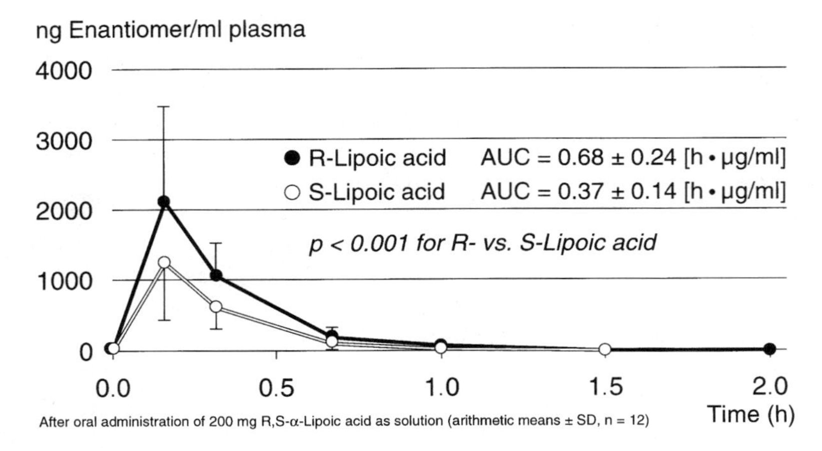

Figure 3 Plasma concentration time curves (Ref. 33).

ever, radioactivity recovered over 168 hours in the urine amounted to 93% of the administered dose. In dogs, urinary radioactivity amounted to 93% of the applied dosage (75). These data indicate that lipoic acid is extensively metabolized in the liver. Indeed, in a study with radiolabeled lipoic acid in rats analyzing the composition or urinary radioactivity, it was found that much of the radioactivity came from shorter-chain homologs, including bisnorlipoic acid, tetranorlipoic acid, and β-hydroxybisnorlipoic acid, formed through β-oxidation of lipoic acid (101). β-Oxidation of lipoic acid also occurs in humans. After supplying a single dose of 1 g R-lipoic acid to a male volunteer, 3-ketolipoic acid and bisnorlipoic acid were detected in plasma (6).

VIII. ANTIOXIDANT PROPERTIES OF LIPOIC ACID

In order to be considered a powerful antioxidant, a compound must meet several criteria. In addition to displaying antioxidant features such as radical quenching, metal chelation, interaction with other antioxidants, amphiphilic character, metabolic regeneration, and gene regulation, the substance needs to be bioavailable and safe. The latter criteria are indispensable for being classified as a nutraceutical. It is noteworthy to mention that lipoic acid and its reduced form, dihydrolipoic acid (DHLA), meet all the above criteria. This renders lipoic acid an ideal antioxidant. For comparison, vitamin E, which is regarded as one of the most important biological antioxidants, scavenges only peroxyl radicals in membranes.

The predominant form that interacts with reactive oxygen species is DHLA, but the oxidized form of lipoic acid can also inactivate free radicals. Table 2 gives an overview on the broad array of reactive oxygen species scavenged by lipoic acid and DHLA. Transition metals such as iron, copper, mercury, or cadmium can induce free radical damage in biological systems by catalyzing decomposition of hydroperoxides and, thus, generating highly toxic hydroxyl radicals. Lipoic acid and DHLA may exhibit antioxidant activity by metal chelating (72), which also explains the usefulness of lipoic acid for the detoxification in heavy metal poisoning (1,24,69).

An interaction of lipoic acid with other antioxidants in vivo was indicated by the initial observation by Rosenberg and Culik (85) that lipoic acid prevented symptoms of vitamin C and vitamin E deficiency. This was confirmed in 1994 by the Packer lab in vitamin E–deficient hairless mice (77). Lipoic acid and its reduced form, DHLA, appeared in tissues in free form, demonstrating that lipoic acid is activated metabolically to DHLA in vivo. DHLA is a strong reductant and thus can regenerate oxidized antioxidants. When antioxidants scavenge radicals, they become radicals themselves. DHLA can directly and indirectly recycle ascorbate, glutathione, coenzyme Q_{10}, and vitamin E (18,55,72). These observations have coined the idea of an antioxidant network (Fig. 4). When vitamin E scavenges a peroxyl radical, a vitamin E radical is formed. The vitamin E radical may be reduced at the lipid/water interface by several antioxidants, such as ascorbate, ubiquinol, and reduced glutathione (GSH). DHLA is able to reduce all these antioxidants and can be regenerated by several enzymes, including lipoamide reductase, glutathione reductase, and thioredoxin reductase (Fig. 5). Therefore,

Table 2 R-Lipoic Acid/Dihydrolipoic Acid—The Most Versatile Antioxidant Pair

	Scavenged by	
Oxidant	Lipoic acid	Dihydrolipoic acid
Hydrogen peroxide	Yes	Yes
Singlet oxygen	Yes	No
Hydroxyl radical	Yes	Yes
Nitric oxide radical	Yes	Yes
Superoxide radical	No	Yes
Hypochlorous acid	Yes	Yes
Peroxynitrite	Yes	Yes
Peroxyl radical	No	Yes

Source: Ref. 57.

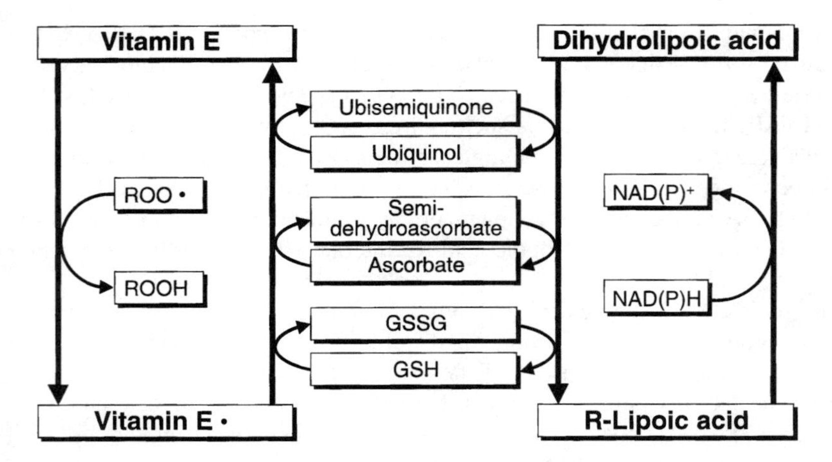

Figure 4 R-lipoic acid/dihydrolipoic acid antioxidant network.

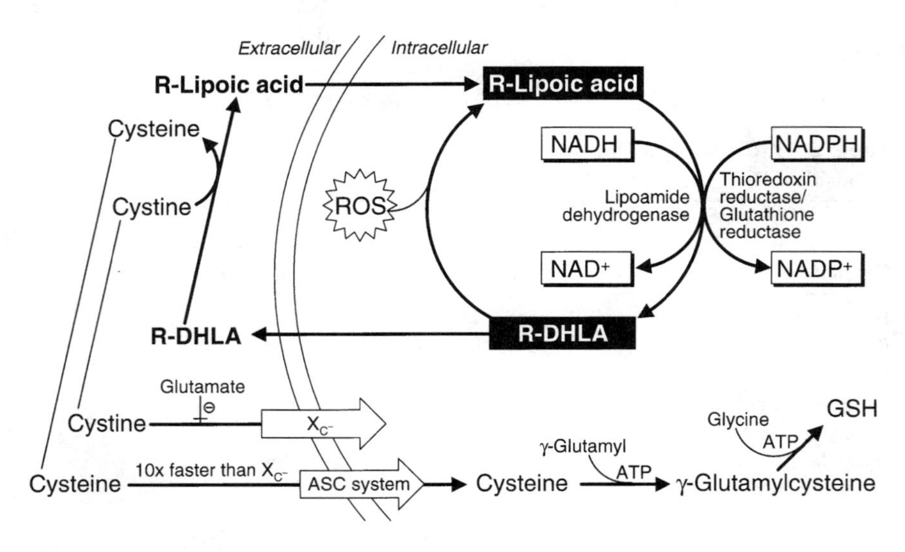

Figure 5 Lipoic acid increases cellular glutathione (GSH) levels (97).

lipoic acid and DHLA take a central position in the antioxidant network. In addition, lipoic acid has both water-soluble and membrane-soluble characteristics, enabling it to reduce oxidized antioxidants at the lipid/water interphase.

Furthermore, treatment with lipoic acid increases glutathione (GSH) levels in vivo and in vitro (13,29,77,95). Glutathione is the most important water-soluble endogenous antioxidant. It occurs in reduced thiol (GSH) and oxidized disulfide (GSSG) form. Glutathione is linked to many physiological processes, including detoxification of xenobiotics, modulation of signal transduction, prostaglandin metabolism, regulation of immune response, control of enzyme activity and peptide hormones, etc. Studies with human cells have provided insights into the mechanism how lipoic acid increases GSH levels (Fig. 5). Cysteine availability is known as the rate-limiting factor in glutathione synthesis. Lipoic acid is taken up rapidly by the cell and reduced to DHLA, which is released into the medium. Subsequently DHLA reduces cystine to cysteine. The cell takes up cysteine about 10 times faster than cystine, leading to an accelerated biosynthesis of GSH (97).

The standard redox potential of the R-lipoic acid/DHLA pair is −320 mV. Hence, DHLA is able to reduce oxidized glutathione (GSSG) chemically (redox potential GSSG/GSH pair is 250/mV) (45).

Redox regulation of signal transduction and gene expression is emerging as a novel fundamental mechanism in biology. Recent research has pinpointed the effects of antioxidants beyond mere protection from oxidative damage. Oxidants and antioxidants are involved in the regulation of key mechanisms related to metabolism, immune and arterial function, cell proliferation, aging, and cell death. Oxidation and reduction (redox) emerges as the principle underlying mechanism. Thiol antioxidants such as glutathione and lipoic acid appear to play a predominant role in the redox-dependent regulation of numerous cellular targets (for a review, see Ref. 94).

Redox-sensitive transcription factors of the nuclear factor kappa B (NF-kappa B) family play an important role in the regulation of genes related to several pathologies. These include atherosclerosis, arthritis, cancer, ischemia-reperfusion injury, apoptosis, and HIV infection, all involving inflammation (2,70,93, 105,106). In several cell lines, lipoic acid and DHLA showed a strong inhibitory effect on phorbol ester (PMA)–tumor necrosis factor-α (TNF-α)–and hydrogen peroxide–induced NF-kappa B activation (70,94). This effect seems to be mediated by a calcium-responsive element of lipoic acid. Recently, it has been shown that lipoic acid at clinically relevant dosages downregulated the expression of the cell adhesion molecules ICAM-1 and VCAM-1 in a dose-dependent way (50–250 μM) (86). The expression of ICAM-1 and VCAM-1 is NF-kappa B–dependent. These observations may be of preventive and/or therapeutic benefit in arteriosclerosis and other inflammatory disorders.

IX. DIABETES MELLITUS

A. Characteristics of Disease

Diabetes mellitus is a very common disease. Recent estimates indicate that around 135 million people are affected by the disease worldwide (113). This figure is expected to increase to almost 300 million by the year 2025. In the United States a total of 15.7 million people (5.9% of the population) have diabetes (16). Among them are 5.4 million with yet undiagnosed diabetes.

There are two forms of diabetes: in type I insulin-dependent diabetes mellitus (IDDM), the pancreas fails to produce insulin. This form, known as juvenile diabetes, usually develops during childhood and adolescence. More than 90% of all cases are type II or non–insulin-dependent diabetes mellitus (NIDDM). NIDDM emerges in middle and late life and is characterized by an increase in blood sugar, even though at first the pancreas produces sufficient insulin. In some cases the β cells of the pancreas become exhausted and insulin-replacement therapy becomes indispensable.

An unhealthy lifestyle, usually characterized by inappropriate diet and lack of exercise leading to obesity, is highly correlated with NIDDM, which is thought to be a most important contribution to accelerated aging. However, genetic factors such as a family history of diabetes, previous gestational diabetes, and advanced age also increase the risk for the disease. Although the causal factors for NIDDM are not yet fully understood, insulin resistance plays an important role in the development of the disease (17,78,98). Several molecular defects have been associated with insulin resistance. These include reduced expression of insulin receptors, altered signal transduction, and disturbances of insulin-responsive metabolic pathways, such as glucose uptake and glycogen synthesis.

Not all people with insulin resistance develop diabetes. An increase in abdominal and visceral fat (obesity) is an important risk factor for the development of NIDDM. This type of adipose tissue is less responsive to insulin but more highly sensitive to lipolytic hormones, with a concomitant increase in free fatty acids. In the muscle, this leads to elevated β-oxidation of fatty acids, followed by inhibition of glycolysis and glycogen synthesis resulting in impaired glucose uptake. In the liver, free fatty acids provoke β-oxidation and gluconeogenesis. Both stimulation of hepatic glucose production and impaired muscular glucose utilization are responsible for hyperglycemia in NIDDM. Moreover, by an increase in free fatty acids, VLDL synthesis in the liver is stimulated (hypertriglyceridemia), hepatic insulin clearance is slowed down, and pancreatic insulin secretion is enhanced (hyperinsulinemia). Insulin secretion is three-to-four times higher in obese people compared to normal-weight controls (78). Taken together, obesity accounts for almost all major metabolic alterations of the metabolic syndrome (Fig. 6).

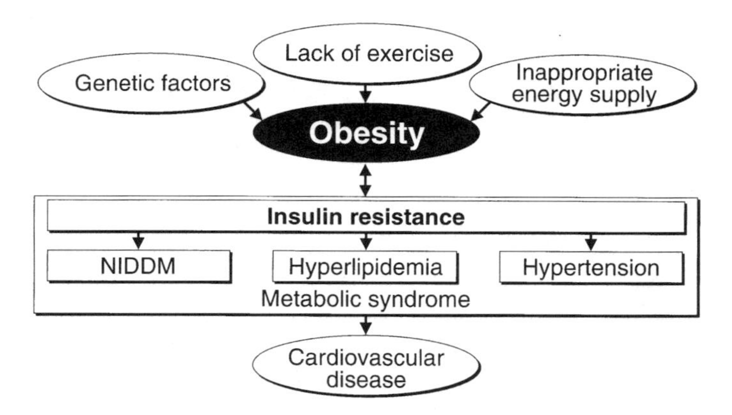

Figure 6 Causes and consequences of obesity.

Because diabetes is a (micro- and macrovascular) chronic disease causing severe late complications including heart disease, stroke, kidney failure, blindness, and amputations, prevention and control of the disease is a top priority (16,113). Cardiovascular disease (CVD) is the leading cause of death among western communities. In adults, diabetes increases the risk of CVD two- to fourfold. Polyneuropathy, a damage of sensory nerves, is the most common complication in diabetes. Peripheral vascular disease and neuropathy give rise to ulcer and necrosis of the limbs (''diabetic foot''), a frequent cause of amputations. In addition, neuropathy is a common reason for male impotence. Kidney failure causes disability due to dialysis therapy and transplantation. After 15 years of diabetes, about 2% of diabetics become blind and approximately 10% severely visually handicapped due to retinopathy and cataract.

B. Treatment of Diabetes

1. Hyperglycemia and Oxidative Stress

Several lines of evidence underscore the benefits of lipoic acid in diabetes prevention and treatment. Oxidative stress is widely observed in diabetes (3,9,21,66,67,82,111,115). Diabetic patients have increased levels of lipid peroxidation products, measured as TBARS (thiobarbituric acid reactive substances), lipid peroxides, F_2-isoprostanes, and oxidatively damaged DNA bases and decreased levels of protecting antioxidants, including α-tocopherol, ascorbic acid, and reduced glutathione (GSH). It has been suggested that oxidative stress deter-

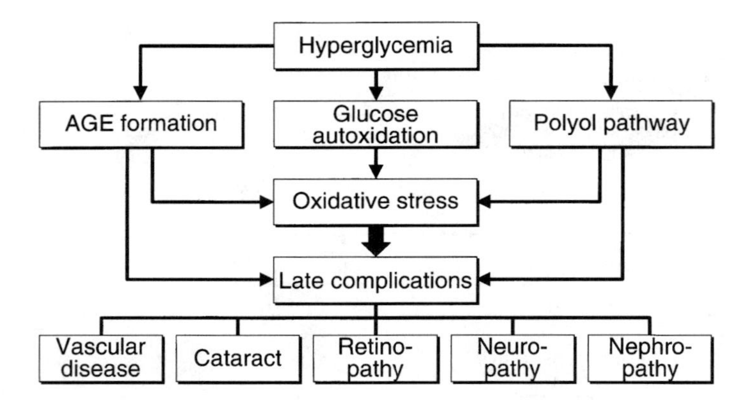

Figure 7 Proposed mechanism for the development of diabetic late complications.

mines onset and progression of late diabetes complications (Fig. 7) (66). The main reason for increased oxidative stress in diabetes appears to be hyperglycemia, resulting in the stimulation of the polyol pathway and the formation of advanced glycation end products (AGEs), with a resultant formation of reactive oxygen species and free radicals.

Lipoic acid reduces oxidative stress in healthy adults and diabetic patients (9,44) (Table 3). A daily supplement of 600 mg lipoic acid for 3 months significantly reduced lipid hydroperoxide formation (9). In a recent study with 31

Table 3 Lipoic Acid Attenuates Lipid Peroxidation in Diabetic Patients

	Control	Lipoic acid
Number of patients	74	33
Type 1	45	19
Type 2	29	14
HbA_1 (%)	8.1 ± 1.7	8.8 ± 1.8
Urinary albumin concentration (mg/L)	102.2 ± 397.5	277.3 ± 511.4
ROOH (μmol/L)	7.1 ± 3.2	4.7 ± 2.4*
α-Tocopherol (μmol/mL)	17.7 ± 6.2	19.7 ± 5.3
Cholesterol (mmol/L)	5.1 ± 1.0	5.4 ± 1.2
α-Tocopherol/cholesterol	3.5 ± 1.0	3.7 ± 1.2
ROOH/(α-tocopherol/cholesterol)	2.1 ± 1.1	1.3 ± 0.7*

Subject received lipoic acid (600 mg/d) for >3 months.
Data are given as mean ± SD. Significant differences between groups: * <0.0005.
Source: Ref. 9.

healthy adults, supplementation with 600 mg of lipoic acid per day for 2 months significantly enhanced lag time for LDL oxidation and decreased urinary F_2-isoprostane excretion (44). A combination with 400 IU of vitamin E did not improve antioxidant status further.

2. Cataract Formation

Under normal conditions glucose is phosphorylated by the enzyme hexokinase to glucose-6-phosphate. Glucose-6-phosphate is oxidized via glycolysis and via hexosemonophosphate shunt or is used for glycogen synthesis. In hyperglycemia, when glucose-utilizing enzymes become saturated, glucose is irreversibly reduced to sorbitol by aldose reductase at the expense of NADPH. This reaction is called the polyol pathway (Fig. 8). Sorbitol is then oxidized to fructose, using NAD^+ as a receptor for the reduction equivalents. The overall reaction leads to a shortage of intracellular NADPH and a surplus of NADH, i.e., a reductive imbalance. Because glutathione reductase is NADPH-dependent, reduced glutathione becomes depleted, resulting in oxidative stress. In addition, fructose and sorbitol lead to osmotic swelling of the eye lens. Further, glycosylating compounds such as sorbitol-3-phosphate or fructose-3-phosphate are formed (6).

The polyol pathway is known as the primary cause of cataractogenesis in diabetes. Lipoic acid may exert protective effects in different ways. The reduction of R-lipoic acid by lipoamide reductase is NADH dependent. Accordingly, intramitochondrial reduction of R-lipoic acid can alleviate NADH surplus in diabe-

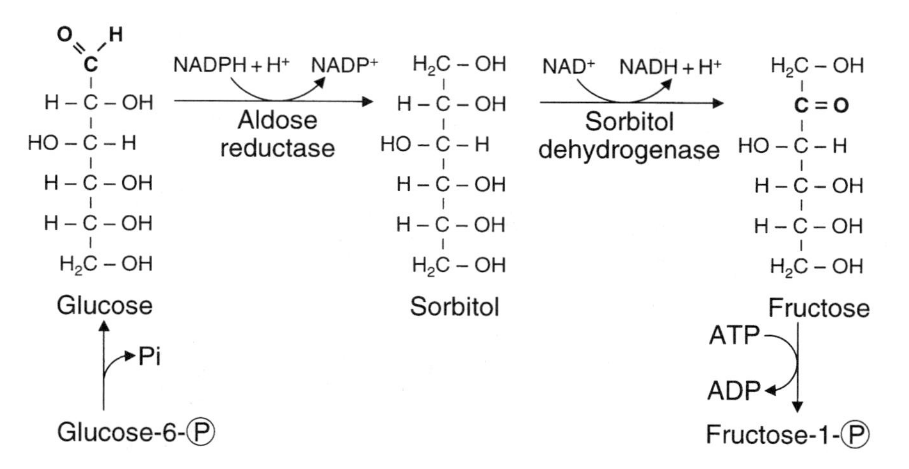

Figure 8 The polyol pathway results in a shift of reducing equivalents from NADPH to NADH and potent glycosylation agents.

tes. In a model of glucose-induced lens opacity in vitro, stereospecific protection by lipoic acid has been observed (52,53). While R-lipoic acid resulted in complete protection of the lens, addition of racemic lipoic acid decreased damage only by about one half, whereas S-lipoic acid potentiated deterioration of the lens. This is consistent with the specific reduction of R-lipoic acid in mitochondria and its effect in enhancing GSH synthesis. In newborn rats treated with buthionine sulfoximine (BSO), a known inhibitor of glutathione synthesis, lipoic acid prevented cataract formation in 60% of animals (62). In streptozotocin-induced diabetes in rats, lipoic acid ameliorated GSH levels, prevented the reduction of the $NAD^+/NADH$ ratio, and improved energy (ATP) status in the lens, while the $NADP^+/NADPH$ ratio remained unaffected (68).

3. Vascular Damage

The formation of AGEs has also been implicated in diabetic pathologies, particularly in vascular complications (12). AGEs are nonenzymatic reaction products of the aldehyde or keto group of sugars with the terminal amino group of proteins. This reaction generates superoxide and hydroxyl radicals by the autooxidation of glucose (39). AGEs exert their damaging effects by binding to specific receptors on the cell surface. One of these receptors (RAGE) occurs on endothelial cells, macrophages, neurons, and smooth muscle cells. Binding of AGE to RAGE causes oxidative stress and, thus, leads to the activation of NF-κB (Fig. 9). NF-κB

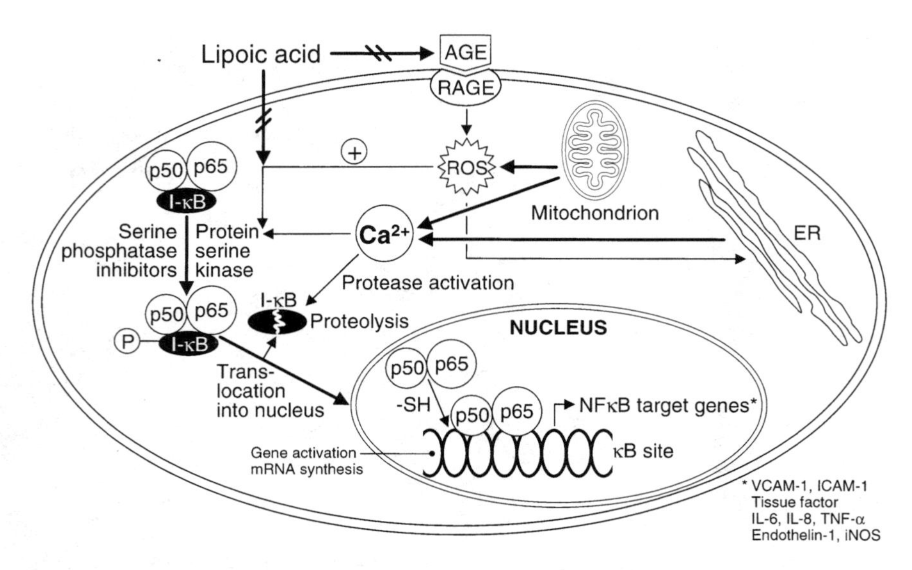

Figure 9 Lipoic acid inhibits NF-κB activation in vascular endothelial cells.

regulates gene expression of adhesion molecules, cytokines, nitric oxide synthase, and inner tissue factors known to be involved in vascular disease. As described above, lipoic acid is a potent inhibitor of NF-κB activation (68,70,94), including AGE-induced NF-κB activation and subsequent expression of adhesion factors (4,56). In addition to the inhibition of NF-κB activation by AGEs, lipoic acid has also been shown to prevent protein glycation in vitro (107). NF-κB–binding activity in mononuclear cells from patients with nephropathy correlated with microalbuminuria and thrombomodulin plasma concentrations. Treatment for 3 days with 600 mg of lipoic acid improved measures of oxidative stress and reduced NF-κB activation (37), indicating that lipoic acid may be useful in the treatment of vascular dysfunction in diabetes.

4. Polyneuropathy

Hyperglycemia and endoneural hypoxia causing oxidative stress have been implicated in the development of diabetic neuropathy. Recently it was shown that hyperglycemia-induced oxidative stress induces programmed cell death of nerves and, thus, may contribute to the pathologies in diabetic neuropathy (23). The role of oxidative stress and antioxidants in nerve damage have been studied extensively in experimental diabetes and diabetes patients (60,111). Motor nerve and sensory nerve conduction velocity (NCV) are the principal endpoints in studying the therapeutic effectiveness of lipoic acid on nerve function. Lipoic acid has been reported to improve motor NCV in experimental diabetic neuropathy in rats (15,64) and has also been shown to protect peripheral nerves from ischemia-reperfusion injury in rats (63). Animal data are supported by cell culture studies in neuroblastoma cells, showing that lipoic acid stimulated sprouting of neurites (20). Diabetic neuropathy is a major cause of male impotence. Interestingly, in a recent study lipoic acid corrected corpus cavernosum function in streptozotocin-induced diabetes in male rats (49).

Treatment of painful neuropathic symptoms and improving quality of life are of outstanding importance in the management of diabetic late complications. Clinical trials have been undertaken to study the efficacy of lipoic acid in the treatment of diabetic polyneuropathy (Table 4) (19,26,47,83,89,92,118–122). For the therapy of this condition, R,S-lipoic acid is approved in Germany.

Patients with diabetic polyneuropathy have an impaired neurovascular reflex. This is detected as a delayed decrease in microcirculation of the ipsilateral hand after a cold stimulus is applied to the contralateral hand. In patients with diabetic polyneuropathy, capillary blood cell flow velocity (CEV) was measured by nailfold capillaroscopy before, during, and after cooling of the contralateral hand (26). Infusion of 600 mg of lipoic acid for 3 weeks resulted in significant improvement of the microcirculatory response to the cold stimulus, and symptoms of neuropathy were significantly improved.

Table 4 Monocenter Human Trials on the Efficacy of R,S-Lipoic Acid in Diabetic Polyneuropathy

Study (Ref.)	Number of patients	Dose	Duration of treatment	Findings
Double-blind studies				
Sachse and Willms, 1980 (89)	10	300 mg p.o.	3 weeks	No effect
Schulz et al., 1986 (92)	31	200 mg i.v.	2 weeks	DML improved
Jörg et al., 1988 (47)	35	600 mg p.o.	12 weeks	Trends for improvement
Single-blind studies				
Delcker et al., 1989 (19)	25	400 mg i.v./p.o.	7 months	No effect
Reschke et al., 1989 (83)	28	400 mg i.v./p.o.	7 months	HRV improved
Ziegler et al., 1993 (122)	23	600 mg i.v./p.o.	15 weeks	PP improved
Haak et al., 1999 (26)	10	600 mg i.v.	3 weeks	Neurovascular reflex arc and NSS improved

DML, distal motor latency; HRV, heart rate variability; PP, pain paresthesia; NSS, neuropathy symptom score.

Results from multicenter clinical trials on diabetic polyneuropathy are summarized in Table 5. In the ALADIN study (Fig. 10), 3-week intravenous lipoic acid administration of 600 and 1200 mg significantly improved clinical symptoms of neuropathy (pain, numbness, paresthesias, burning) (121). In patients with cardiac autonomic neuropathy (DEKAN study), a daily oral dose of 800 mg of lipoic acid for 4 months significantly improved heart rate variability (118). More recently, the ALADIN III study has been completed (120). Injections with 600 mg of lipoic acid for 3 weeks significantly improved the Neuropathy Impairment Score (NIS), and there was a trend for a better NIS after 7 months in response to an oral daily supplement of 1800 mg of lipoic acid. However, there was no effect on neuropathic symptoms. According to the authors, failing effect may be due to intercenter variability in symptom scoring.

5. Glucose Disposal

Insulin resistance is typical for type II diabetes. Therapeutic intervention aimed at enhancing glucose uptake by skeletal muscle is of potential importance for the prevention and treatment of NIDDM. Pharmaceutical companies have recently launched the thiazolinediones, a new class of drugs that enhance glucose disposal. However, one of these compounds, troglitazone, has already been withdrawn in the United Kingdom due to severe side effects. There is good evidence that R-lipoic acid may also increase glucose disposal in the peripheral vasculature without the risk of adverse effects.

There were reports as early as 1970 showing that lipoic acid enhances glucose uptake into rat tissues (31,99). Later, obese Zucker rats, an animal model of insulin resistance, were used to investigate the effects of acute and chronic intravenous treatment with R,S-lipoic acid on glucose transport in isolated skeletal muscle (measured as 2-deoxyglucose uptake) in the absence or presence of insulin (43). Lipoic acid markedly increased net glucose uptake. This was associated with a significant enhancement of glycogen synthesis and a significant reduction in plasma insulin and free fatty acids. There was no effect on the glucose transporter GLUT-4. This observation was supported by a separate experiment in vitro from the same group (33), showing an increased glucose uptake into muscle from either lean (insulin-sensitive) or obese (insulin-resistant) Zucker rats (Fig. 11). The effect of lipoic acid was only partially mediated via the insulin signal transduction pathway. The major effect of lipoic acid on glucose uptake was insulin independent.

In the same model, the contribution of the individual enantiomers of lipoic acid on glucose disposal, hyperinsulinemia, and dyslipidemia was also studied (104). Obese Zucker rats were treated acutely or chronically by intraperitoneal injection with R- or S-lipoic acid. Acute treatment with R-lipoic acid increased insulin-mediated glucose transport by 64%, while the S-form showed no signifi-

Table 5 Multicenter, Double-Blind Placebo-Controlled Human Trials on the Efficacy of R,S-Lipoic Acid in Diabetic Polyneuropathy

Ziegler et al. Study (Ref.)	Number of patients	Design	Dose	Duration of treatment	Findings
1995[a] (121)	328	Parallel group	1200/600/100 mg i.v.	3 weeks	TSS and NDS improved
1997[b] (118)	73	Parallel group	800 mg p.o.	4 months	HRV and QTc improved
1999[c] (120)	509	Parallel group	600 mg i.v. → 1800 mg p.o. 600 mg i.v. → placebo p.o. placebo i.v. → placebo p.o.	3 weeks (i.v.) 6 months (p.o.)	TSS no change, NIS improved after 19 d, trend for improved NIS at end

HRV, heart rate variability; NCV, nerve conduction velocity; NDS, neuropathy disability score; NIS, neuropathy impairment score; QTc, corrected QT interval; TSS, total symptom score (pain, burning, paresthesias, numbness).

[a] ALADIN study—α-lipoic acid diabetic neuropathy study.

[b] DEKAN study—Deutsche Kardinale Autonome Neuropathie Studie.

[c] ALADIN III study—α-lipoic acid diabetic neuropathy study.

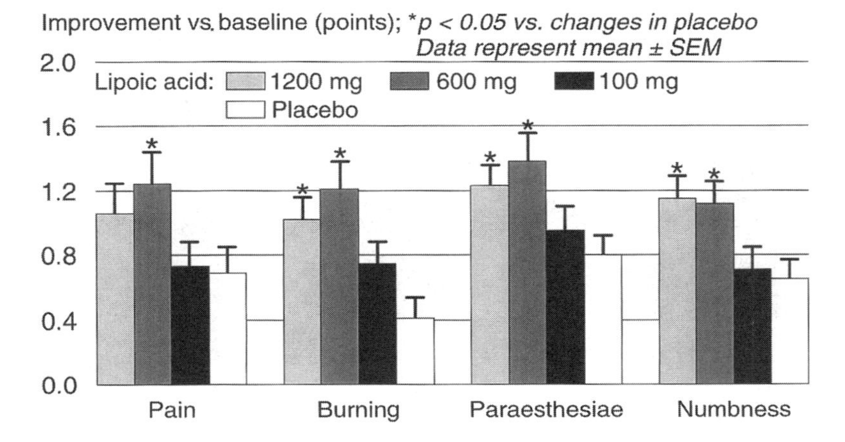

Figure 10 Improvement in the individual scores for diabetic neuropathy (ALADIN study). (Ref. 121.)

cant effect (Fig. 12). Chronic R-lipoic acid administration reduced plasma insulin and free fatty acids, whereas S-lipoic acid increased insulin and had no effect on free fatty acids. Furthermore, R-lipoic acid improved insulin-stimulated glycogen synthesis and glucose oxidation. Glucose transporter (GLUT 4) protein was not altered after chronic R-lipoic acid treatment but was reduced by S-lipoic acid.

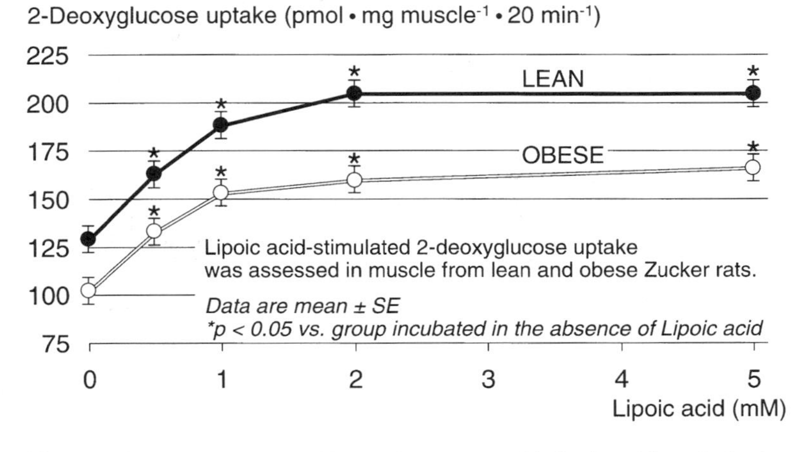

Figure 11 Dose-response effect of incubation with lipoic acid on skeletal muscle glucose transport activity. (Ref. 32.)

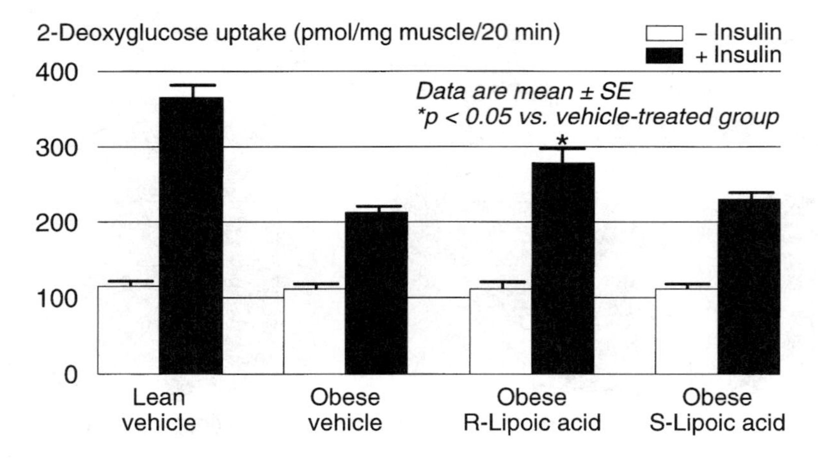

Figure 12 Effect of chronic parenteral treatment with R- or S-lipoic acid on skeletal muscle glucose transport. (Ref. 104.)

More recently, in fasting nondiabetic or streptozotocin-induced diabetic rats, intravenous injection of high doses of R,S-lipoic acid led to a rapid reduction of blood glucose at unaltered insulin levels (50). This was attributed to the inhibition of gluconeogenesis from alanine and pyruvate. The influence of lipoic acid on glucose transport into heart muscle has also been investigated (84). Glucose uptake into Langendorff hearts of insulin-resistant Zucker rats was measured with the [^{14}C] 3-O-methylglucose washout method. Glucose uptake rate increased 1.6-fold with R,S-lipoic acid, 1.8-fold with the R-form, and was negatively influenced by the S-enantiomer (−50%).

There is only one study in which the favorable effects of lipoic acid on glucose disposal were not reproduced (7).

NADH levels are increased in diabetes, which is attributable to a stimulation of the polyol pathway. R-Lipoic acid uses NADH for the reduction to DHLA (87), resulting in increased NAD^+/NADH ratio and, thus, stimulating glycolysis (Fig. 13). Enhanced glucose uptake into tissues may also be attributed to a reduction of acetyl-CoA levels in tissues due to sequestration as lipoyl-CoA, bisnorlipoyl-CoA, or tetranorlipoyl-CoA (8). A reduction in acetyl-CoA leads to decreased citrate levels and, thus, via the activation of phosphofructokinase, to enhanced glycolysis. Moreover, lipoic acid has been shown to inhibit gluconeogenesis in rat liver (8). In addition, gluconeogenesis may be reduced by an inhibitory effect of lipoic acid on biotin-dependent carboxylases (117) because the initial step in gluconeogenesis, the pyruvate carboxylase reaction, is biotin-dependent.

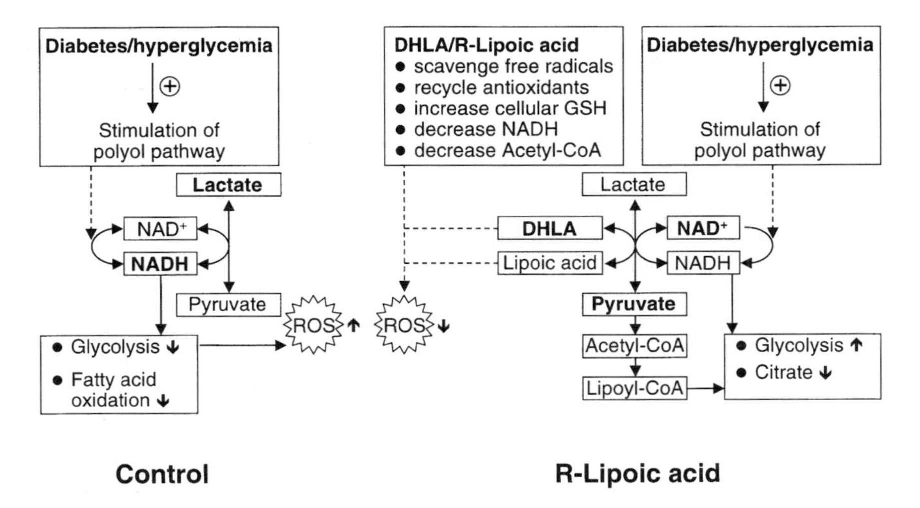

Figure 13 Proposed mechanism for R-lipoic acid-stimulated enhancement in glucose disposal. (Ref. 87.)

Mechanistic studies in cell culture found a superior glucose uptake in response to R-lipoic acid compared to R,S- and S-lipoic acid in L6 myotubes. Similar effects of R-lipoic acid and insulin were demonstrated in 3T3-L1 adipocytes (110). R-Lipoic acid stimulated glucose uptake in L6 myotubes that were made insulin resistant through cytokine treatment and exposure to oxidative stress (51,88). In 3T3-L1 adipocytes, R-lipoic acid caused a translocation of the glucose transporters GLUT 1 and GLUT 4 to the plasma membrane, thereby mediating the R-lipoic acid effect on glucose uptake (116). In this experiment, the stimulation of glucose uptake into cells was blocked by wortmannin, an inhibitor of phosphatidylinositol-3-kinase (PI3-K). PI3-K is also involved in insulin action, which suggests that R-lipoic acid uses parts of the insulin-signaling cascade.

Studies on the use of R,S-lipoic acid in insulin-stimulated glucose disposal have also been carried out in patients with type 2 diabetes (Table 6). Acute intravenous administration of 1000 mg of lipoic acid significantly improved insulin-stimulated glucose disposal assessed by a glucose clamp technique by 50% (40). The amount of glucose required to maintain isoglycemia is an indirect measure of insulin sensitivity. After a bolus injection of insulin, plasma glucose concentration was held constant throughout a glucose infusion. Under steady-state conditions either lipoic acid or saline (placebo) was given as a short infusion. Thereafter, a second steady state was established. The difference between the two steady-state conditions is a measure of the lipoic acid effect. Improved insulin-stimulated glucose uptake of similar magnitude was also found in 20 patients

Table 6 Human Trials on the Efficacy of R,S-Lipoic Acid in Insulin-Stimulated Glucose Disposed in NIDDM

Study (Ref.)	Number of patients	Dose	Duration of treatment	Findings
Jacob et al., 1995 (40)	13	1000 mg i.v.	Single dose	50% increased MCR of glucose
Jacob et al., 1996 (41)	20	500 mg i.v.	10 days	40% increased MCR of glucose
Jacob et al., 1999 (42)	74	600 mg p.o. 1200 mg p.o. 1800 mg p.o.	4 weeks 4 weeks 4 weeks	27% increased MCR of glucose, no dose effect of lipoic acid
Konrad et al., 1999 (54)	20	1200 mg p.o.	4 weeks	Glucose effectiveness after OGTT improved, decrease of serum, lactate, and pyruvate

MCR, metabolic clearance rate; OGTT, oral glucose tolerance test.

with NIDDM after 10 days of 500 mg lipoic acid injections, again applying the hyperinsulinemic, isoglycemic glucose-clamp technique (41). In a recent multicenter trial from the same group, a 4-week oral treatment with lipoic acid increased insulin sensitivity in patients with type II diabetes (42). Furthermore, a daily supplement of 1200 mg of lipoic acid over 4 weeks improved glucose effectiveness after oral glucose tolerance tests in type 2 diabetic patients (54). In addition, lipoic reduced serum levels of pyruvate and lactate.

Lipoic acid seems to be unique among other oral antidiabetes drugs (acarbose, sulfonylureas, metformin, thiazolidinediones) in its ability to stimulate glucose uptake and its simultaneous antioxidant activity.

These data provide a rationale for the use of R-lipoic acid for the prevention and treatment of diabetic late complications and for the use as an insulin sensitizer, which will be studied in clinical trials.

X. AGING

Mitochondrial function declines with age and leads to lowered membrane potential, decreased substrate transport, altered phospholipid composition, decreased oxygen utilization, and increased oxidant production and consequently reduced GSH levels. This enhances DNA damage and increases the variability in size and shape of mitochondria (28). Mitochondrial deterioration is regarded as one of the most important principles underlying aging. Staining of rat liver mitochondria with a fluorescent dye (rhodamine 123) is used for measuring the mitochon-

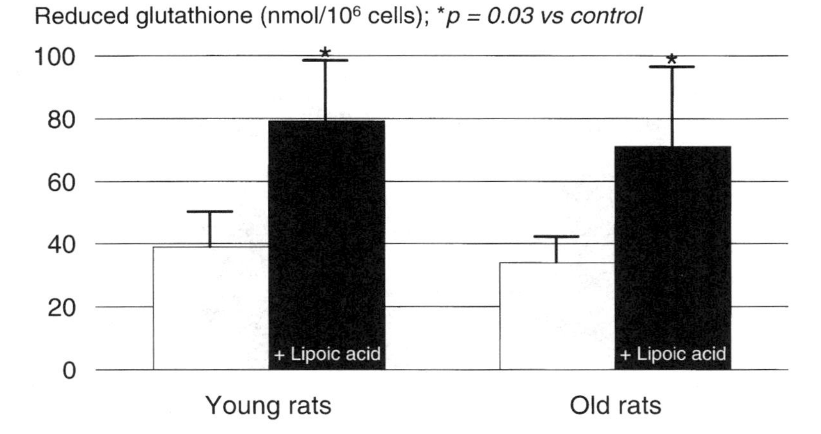

Figure 14 Hepatocellular glutathione (GSH) levels increase after R-lipoic acid supplementation. (Ref. 27.)

drial membrane potential. Mitochondria from young rats show higher fluorescence than mitochondria from older animals, demonstrating that the membrane potential of mitochondria is higher in young animals. The decline in mitochondrial membrane potential during aging is mainly due to a decline in the mitochondrial phospholipid cardiolipin. Cardiolipin functions as translocator of ADP/ATP, is an essential cofactor for several catalytic activities, but is also prone to oxidative damage.

Feeding old rats with a diet containing 0.5% R-lipoic acid (w/w) reversed much of the mitochondrial decay (27,61). Lipoic acid reversed the age-related decline in oxygen consumption, improved mitochondrial membrane potential, attenuated radical formation, and increased ascorbic acid and GSH levels (Fig. 14). Rats also showed more physical activity following R-lipoic acid administration (Fig. 15).

Age-associated decline in memory and cognitive function may also be improved by lipoic acid supplementation (102,103). Old but otherwise healthy mice were given lipoic acid over 15 days before cognitive tests started. Lipoic acid improved longer-term habituation in the open field test, probably by partial compensation for NMDA receptors. A test in the Morris water maze also supported the attenuating effect of lipoic acid on learning and memory. Interestingly, there was no improvement in performance in young mice. These results may also have implications for the use of lipoic acid in Alzheimer's and Parkinson's diseases, as well as ischemia/reperfusion-induced brain damage (for review, see Ref. 71).

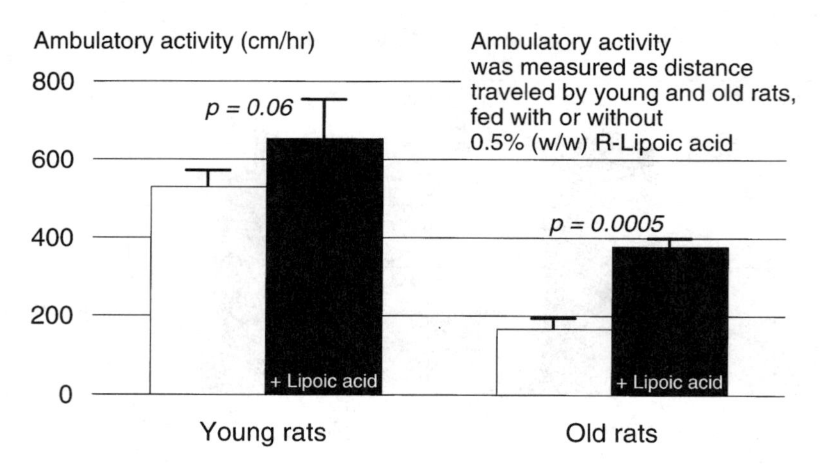

Figure 15 R-lipoic acid increases ambulatory activity in young and old rats. (Ref. 27.)

XI. NATURAL VERSUS R,S- AND S-LIPOIC ACID

Until recently, chemical synthesis of lipoic acid has yielded a racemic mixture of the optically active enantiomers, the R- and S-forms, in a 50:50 ratio. The biopotency of the R- versus S-form has not yet been fully established. In-depth studies that address the exchange rate of R- versus R,S-lipoic acid are underway. However, there is enough evidence supporting superior effects of the R-form.

Only the naturally occurring R-lipoic acid is a cofactor of α-keto acid dehydrogenases. Mammalian α-keto acid dehydrogenases are multienzyme complexes composed of four subunits. Lipoic acid is covalently linked to the E2- and X-subunit in the case of the pyruvate dehydrogenase complex. Mammalian lipoic acid–reducing enzymes exhibit different subcellular distribution. The enzyme glutathione reductase occurs in the cytosol and the lipoamide reductase is localized in the mitochondrion, the major site of free radical generation. Studies in vitro using porcine heart lipoamide reductase indicate a high specificity for the R-form (90). The racemate showed only 40% of the activity compared to the R-form, while the S-form yielded no reduced lipoic acid.

While S-lipoic acid is reduced two times faster than R-lipoic acid by cytosolic glutathione reductase using NADPH, the R-form is preferentially reduced by the intramitochondrial NADH-dependent lipoamide reductase 18-fold faster than S-lipoic acid (76). This was confirmed in other studies, where a 24- or 28-fold faster reduction with lipoamide reductase of R-lipoic acid as compared to the S-form was shown (5,59). The Michaelis constants of both enantiomers for the mammalian lipoamide reductase are comparable (K_m = 3.7 and 5.5 mM for

R- and S-lipoic acid, respectively). This indicates that the S-form inhibits the R-lipoic acid regeneration, and thus, S-lipoic acid may act as an antimetabolite (59). This may reduce the body's antioxidant capacity under oxidative stress conditions.

Figure 16 shows the NADH- or NADPH-dependent reduction of lipoic acid enantiomers by rat liver cytosol (a) and mitochondrial matrix (b) (30). Oxidized

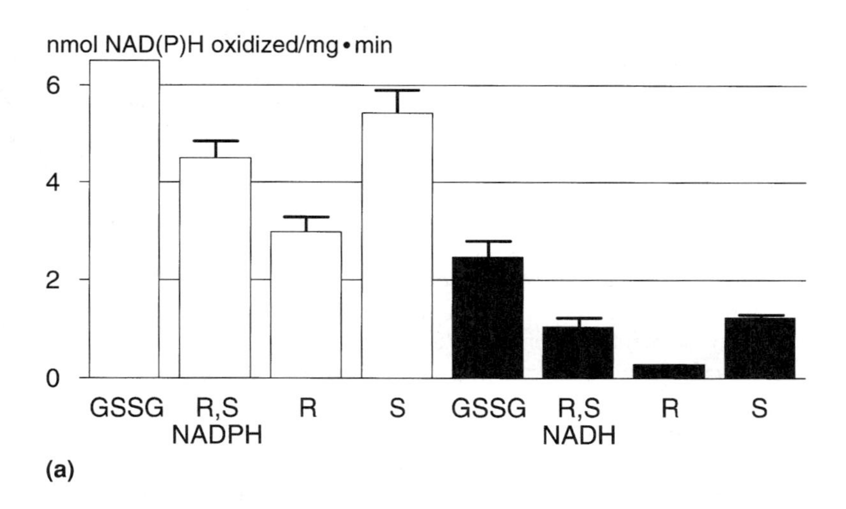

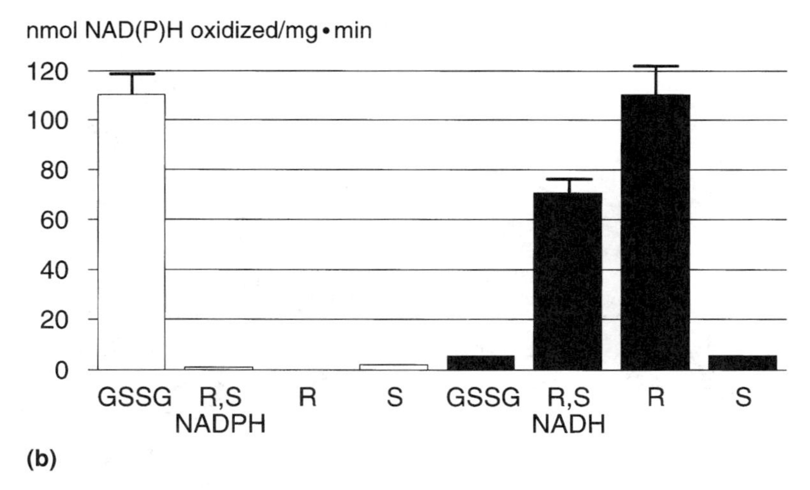

Figure 16 (a) Reduction of lipoic acid by rat liver cytosolic fraction. (b) Reduction of lipoic acid by mitochondrial matrix fraction. (Ref. 30.)

glutathione (GSSG) was used as a reference substance. In cytosol GSSG was rapidly reduced by NADPH, demonstrating a high activity of glutathione reductase. The NADPH-dependent reduction in the cytosol showed preferential reduction of S-lipoic acid. In the mitochondrial matrix, the major site of free radical generation, the reduction of lipoic acid by NADH is by far more active and specific for R-lipoic as compared to the S-form.

Both enantiomers of lipoic acid inhibited purified mammalian pyruvate dehydrogenase activity; in particular the acyltransferase moiety of the enzyme complex was affected (38). However, R-lipoic acid, in contrast to S-lipoic acid, did not inhibit pyruvate decarboxylation in HepG2 cells.

There is also evidence for superiority of R-lipoic acid from studies with perfused hearts. In the working rat heart during reoxygenation, R-lipoic acid improved aortic flow, reaching 70% of normoxic conditions at nM concentrations, whereas 1 μM of the S-form was needed to achieve only 60% (123). In the same study, R-lipoic acid added to perfusion medium increased mitochondrial ATP synthesis of the working rat heart, while ATP synthesis remained unaltered in response to S-lipoic acid. Furthermore, much higher concentrations of R-DHLA compared to S-DHLA were detected in the effluent buffer of isolated perfused rat heart using the Langendorff technique (30) (Fig. 17). This indicates the high concentration of mitochondria in rat heart responsible for R-lipoic acid reduction.

Membrane fluidity of red blood cells is reduced under hyperglycemic conditions. Lipoic acid counteracted the glucose-induced decrease in fluidity of red blood cells in vitro (36). S-Lipoic acid increased fluidity at low concentrations.

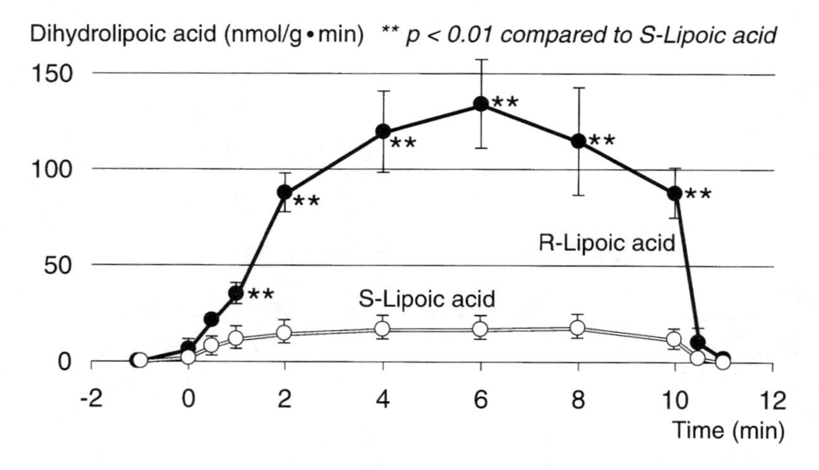

Figure 17 Lipoic acid reduction by isolated perfused rat heart. (Ref. 30.)

However, R-lipoic acid was more effective over a wider range of concentrations. This is also commensurate with the distinctive effects of the lipoic acid forms in cataractogenesis, discussed above (52,53).

The favorable effects of R-lipoic acid compared to the S-form in relation to glucose utilization are discussed in Sec. IX.B.5. Acute treatment of obese Zucker rats with R-lipoic acid increased insulin-mediated glucose transport, while the S-form showed no significant effect. In addition, chronic R-lipoic acid treatment reduced plasma insulin and free fatty acids, whereas S-lipoic acid increased insulin and had no effect on free fatty acids. These effects were also supported by mechanistic studies in L6 myotubes.

REFERENCES

1. Anuradha B, Varalakshmi P. Protective role of DL-α-lipoic acid against mercury-induced neural lipid peroxidation. Pharmacol Res 1999; 39:67–80.
2. Barnes PJ, Karin M. Nuclear factor-κB—a pivotal transcription factor in chronic inflammatory diseases. N Engl J Med 1997; 336:1066–1071.
3. Baynes JW. Role of oxidative stress in development of complications in diabetes. Diabetes 1991; 40:405–412.
4. Bierhaus A, Chevion S, Chevion M, Hofmann M, Quehenberger P, Illmer T, Luther T, Berentshtein E, Tritschler H, Müller M, Wahl P, Ziegler R, Nawroth PP. Advanced glycation end product-induced activation of NF-κB is suppressed by α-lipoic acid in cultured endothelial cells. Diabetes 1997; 46:1481–1490.
5. Biewenga GPH, Dorstijn MA, Verhagen JV, Haenen GRMM, Bast A. The reduction of lipoic acid by lipoamide reductase. Biochem Pharmacol 1996; 51:233–238.
6. Biewenga GPH, Haenen GRMM, Bast A. The role of lipoic acid in the treatment of diabetic polyneuropathy. Drug Metabol Rev 1997; 29:1025–1054.
7. Black K, Qu XQ, Seale JP, Donnelly R. Metabolic effects of thioctic acid in rodent models of insulin resistance and diabetes. Clin Exp Pharmacol Physiol 1998; 25: 712–714.
8. Blumenthal SA. Inhibition of gluconeogenesis in rat liver by lipoic acid. Biochem J 1984; 219:773–780.
9. Borcea V, Nourooz-Zadeh J, Wolff SP, Klevesath M, Hofmann M, Ulrich H, Wahl P, Ziegler R, Tritschler H, Halliwell B, Nawroth PP. α-Lipoic acid decreases oxidative stress even in diabetic patients with poor glycemic control and albuminuria. Free Rad Biol Med 1999; 22:1495–1500.
10. Breithaupt-Grögler K, Niebch G, Schneider E, Erb K, Hermann R, Blume HH, Schug BS, Belz GG. Dose-proportionality of oral thioctic acid—coincidence of assessments via pooled plasma and individual data. Eur J Pharmaceut Sci 1999; 8: 57–65.
11. Bringmann G, Herzberg D, Adam G, Balkenhohl F, Paust J. A short and productive synthesis of (R)-α-lipoic acid. Z Naturforsch 1999; 54b:655–661.

12. Brownlee M, Cerami A, Vlassara H. Advanced glycation end products in tissue and the diabetic basis of diabetic complications. N Engl J Med 1988; 318:1315–1321.
13. Busse E, Zimmer G, Schopohl B, Kornhuber B. Influence of α-lipoic acid on intracellular glutathione in vitro and in vivo. Arzneim-Forsch/Drug Res 1992; 42:829–832.
14. Bustamente J, Lodge J, Marcocci L, Tritschler HJ, Packer L, Rihn BT. α-Lipoic acid in liver metabolism and disease. Free Rad Biol Med 1998; 24:1023–1039.
15. Cameron NE, Cotter MA, Horrobin DH, Tritschler HJ. Effects of α-lipoic acid on neurovascular function in diabetic rats: interaction with essential fatty acids. Diabetologia 1998; 41:390–399.
16. CDC. National Diabetes Fact Sheet. Centers for Disease Control and Prevention, 1998. http://www.cdc.gov/nccdphp/ddt/pubs/facts98.htm
17. Cline GW, Petersen KF, Krssak M, Shen J, Hundal RS, Trajanoski Z, Inzucchi S, Dresner A, Rothman DL, Shulman GI. Impaired glucose metabolism as a cause of decreased insulin-stimulated muscle glycogen synthesis in type 2 diabetes. N Engl J Med 1999; 341:240–246.
18. Constantinescu A, Han D, Packer L. Vitamin E recycling in human erythrocyte membranes. J Biol Chem 1993; 268:10906–10913.
19. Delcker A, Fischer P-A, Ulrich H. Randomisierte Studie Thioctsäure gegenüber Vitamin-B-Kombinationspräparat bei Patienten mit diabetischer Polyneuropathie unter besonderer Berücksichtigung des peripheren Nervensystems. In: Borbe HO, Ulrich H, eds. Neue biochemische, pharmazeutische und klinische Erkenntnisse zur Thioctsäure. Frankfurt: Verlag, 1989:335–344.
20. Dimpfel W, Spüler M, Pierau F-K, Ulrich H. Thioctic acid induces dose-dependent sprouting of neurites in cultured rat neuroblastoma cells. Dev Pharmacol Ther 1990; 14:193–199.
21. Giugliano D, Ceriello A, Paolisso G. Oxidative stress and diabetic vascular complications. Diabetes Care 1996; 19:257–267.
22. Gleiter CH, Schug BS, Hermann R, Elze M, Blume HH, Gundert-Remy U. Influence of food intake on the bioavailability of thioctic acid enantiomers [letter]. Eur J Clin Pharmacol 1996; 50:513–514.
23. Greene DA, Stevens MJ, Obrosova I, Feldman EL. Glucose-induced oxidative stress and programmed cell death in diabetic neuropathy. Eur J Pharmacol 1999; 375:217–223.
24. Gregus Z, Stein AF, Varga F, Klaassen CD. Effect of lipoic acid on biliary excretion of glutathione and metals. Toxicol Appl Pharmacol 1992; 114:88–96.
25. Gries FA. Alternative therapeutic principles in the prevention of microvascular and neuropathic complications. Diabet Res Clin Pract 1995; 28 (suppl):S201–S207.
26. Haak ES, Usadel KH, Kohleisen M, Yilmaz A, Kusterer K, Haak T. The effect of alpha-lipoic acid on the neurovascular reflex arc in patients with diabetic neuropathy assessed by capillary microscopy. Microvasc Res 1999; 58:28–34.
27. Hagen TM, Ingersoll RT, Lykkesfeldt J, Liu J, Wehr CM, Vinarsky V, Bartholomew JC, Ames BN. (R)- α-Lipoic acid-supplemented old rats have improved mitochondrial function, decreased oxidative damage, and increased metabolic rate. FASEB J 1999; 13:411–418.

28. Hagen TM, Yowe DL, Bartholomew JC, Wehr CM, Do KL, Park J-Y, Ames BN. Mitochondrial decay in hepatocytes from old rats: membrane potential declines, heterogeneity and oxidants increase. PNAS 1997; 94:3064–3069.
29. Han D, Handelman G, Marcocci L, Sen CK, Roy S, Kobuchi H, Flohé L, Packer L. Lipoic acid increases de novo synthesis of cellular glutathione by improving cysteine utilization. Biofactors 1997; 6:321–338.
30. Haramaki N, Handelman GJ. Tissue-specific pathways of α-lipoate reduction in mammalian systems. In: Packer L, Cadenas E, eds. Biothiols in Health and Disease. New York: Marcel Dekker, 1997:145–162.
31. Haugaard N, Haugaard ES. Stimulation of glucose utilization by thioctic acid in rat diaphragm incubated in vitro. Biochim Biophys Acta 1970; 222:583–586.
32. Henriksen EJ, Jacob S, Streeper RS, Fogt DL, Hokama JY, Tritschler HJ. Stimulation by alpha-lipoic acid of glucose transport activity in skeletal muscle of lean and obese Zucker rats. Life Sci 1997; 61:805–812.
33. Hermann R, Niebch G. Human pharmacokinetics of α-lipoic acid. In: Packer L, Cadenas E, eds. Biothiols in Health and Disease. New York: Marcel Dekker, 1997; 337–360.
34. Hermann R, Niebch G, Borbe HO, Fieger-Büschges, Ruus P, Nowak H, Riethmüller-Winzen H, Peukert M, Blume H. Enantioselective pharmacokinetics and bioavailability of different racemic α-lipoic acid formulations in healthy volunteers. Eur J Pharmaceut Sci 1996; 4:167–174.
35. Hermann R, Wildgrube HJ, Ruus P, Niebch G, Nowak H, Gleiter CH. Gastric emptying in patients with insulin dependend diabetes mellitus and bioavailability of thioctic acid-enantiomers. Eur J Pharmaceut Sci 1998; 6:27–37.
36. Hofmann M, Mainka P, Tritschler H, Fuchs J, Zimmer G. Decrease in red blood cell membrane fluidity and- SH groups due to hyperglycemic conditions is counteracted by α-lipoic acid. Arch Biochem Biophys 1995; 324:85–92.
37. Hofmann MA, Schiekofer S, Isermann B, Kanitz M, Henkels M, Joswig M, Treusch A, Morcos M, Weiss T, Borcea V, Abdel Khalek AKM, Amiral J, Tritschler H, Ritz E, Wahl P, Ziegler R, Bierhaus A, Nawroth PP. Peripheral blood mononuclear cells isolated from patients with diabetic nephropathy show increased activation of the oxidative-stress sensitive transcription factor NF-κB. Diabetologia 1999; 42: 222–232.
38. Hong YS, Jacobia SJ, Packer L, Patel MS. The inhibitory effects of lipoic compounds on mammalian pyruvate dehydrogenase complex and its catalytic components. Free Rad Biol Med 1999; 26:685–694.
39. Hunt JV, Dean RT, Wolff SP. Hydroxyl radical production and autooxidative glycosylation. Biochem J 1988; 256:205–212.
40. Jacob S, Henriksen EJ, Schiemann AL, Simon I, Clancy DE, Tritschler HJ, Jung WI, Augustin HJ, Dietze GJ. Enhancement of glucose disposal in patients with type 2 diabtes by alpha-lipoic acid. Arzneim-Forsch/Drug Res 1995; 8:872–874.
41. Jacob S, Henriksen EJ, Tritschler HJ, Augustin HJ, Dietze GJ. Improvement of insulin-stimulated glucose disposal in type 2 diabetes after repeated parenteral administration of thioctic acid. Exp Clin Endocrinol Diabetes 1996; 104:284–288.

42. Jacob S, Ruus P, Hermann R, Tritschler HJ, Maerker E, Renn W, Augustin HJ, Dietze GJ, Rett K. Oral administration of rac-α-lipoic acid modulates insulin sensitivity in patients with type-2 diabetes mellitus: a placebo-controlled pilot trial. Free Rad Biol Med 1999; 27:309–314.
43. Jacob S, Streeper RS, Fogt DL, Hokama JY, Tritschler HJ, Dietze GJ, Henriksen EJ. The antioxidant alpha-lipoic acid enhances insulin-stimulated glucose metabolism in insulin resistant rat skeletal muscle. Diabetes 1996; 45:1024–1029.
44. Jialal I, Marangon K, Devaraj S. A comparison of the effect of α-lipoic acid and α-tocopherol supplementation on plasma, LDL and whole body oxidation. Oxygen Club of California 1999 World Congress, March 3–6, 1999, Santa Barbara.
45. Jocelyn PC. The standard redox potential of cysteine-cystine from the thiol-disulfide exchange reaction with glutathione and lipoic acid. Eur J Biochem 1967; 2: 327–331.
46. Jordan SW, Cronan JE. Biosynthesis of lipoic acid and posttranslational modification with lipoic acid in *Escherichia coli*. Meth Enzymol 1997; 279:176–183.
47. Jörg J, Metz F, Scharafinski H. Zur medikamentösen Behandlung der diabetischen Polyneuropathie mit der alpha-Liponsäure oder Vitamin-B-Präparaten. Nervenarzt 1988; 59:36–44.
48. Kataoka H. Chromatographic analysis of lipoic acid and related compounds. J Chromatogr 1998; B717:247–262.
49. Keegan A, Cotter MA, Cameron NE. Effects of diabetes and treatment with the antioxidant α-lipoic acid on endothelial and neurogenic responses of corpus cavernosum in rats. Diabetologia 1999; 42:343–350.
50. Khamaisi M, Rudich A, Potashnik R, Tritschler HJ, Gutman A, Bashan N. Lipoic acid acutely induces hypoglycemia in fasting nondiabetic and diabetic rats. Metabol Clin Exp 1999; 48:504–510.
51. Khanna S, Roy S, Packer L, Sen CK. Cytokine-induced glucose uptake in skeletal muscle: redox regulation and the role of α-lipoic acid. Am J Physiol 1999; 276: R1327–R1333.
52. Kilic F, Handelman GJ, Serbinova E, Packer L, Trevithick JR. Modelling cortical cataractogenesis 17: in vitro effect of α-lipoic acid on glucose-induced lens membrane damage, a model of diabetic cataractogenesis. Biochem Mol Biol Int 1995; 37:361–370.
53. Kilic F, Handelman GJ, Traber K, Tsang K, Packer L, Trevithick JR. Modelling cortical cataractogenesis XX: in vitro effect of alpha-lipoic acid on glutathione concentration in lens in model diabetic cataractogenesis. Biochem Mol Biol Int 1998; 46:585–595.
54. Konrad T, Vicini P, Kusterer K, Hoflich A, Assadkhani A, Bohles HJ, Sewell A, Tritschler HJ, Cobelli C, Usadel KH. Alpha-lipoic acid treatment decreases serum lactate and pyruvate concentrations and improves glucose effectiveness in lean and obese patients with type 2 diabetes. Diabetes Care 1999; 22:280–287.
55. Kozlov AV, Gille L, Staniek K, Nohl H. Dihydrolipoic acid maintains ubiquinone in the antioxidant active form by two-electron reduction of ubiquinone and one-electron reduction of ubisemiquinone. Arch Biochem Biophys 1999; 363:148–154.
56. Kunt T, Forst T, Wilhelm A, Tritschler H, Pfuetzner A, Harzer O, Engelbach M,

Zschaebitz A, Stofft E, Beyer J. α-Lipoic acid reduces expression of vascular cell adhesion molecule-1 and endothelial adhesion of human monocytes after stimulation with advanced glycation end products. Clin Sci 1999; 96:75–82.
57. Landvik SV, Packer L. Alpha-lipoic acid in health and disease. In: Papas AM, ed. Antioxidant status, diet, nutrition, and health. Boca Raton, FL: CRC Press, 1999: 591–598.
58. Lodge JK, Youn H-D, Handelman GJ, Konishi T, Matsugo S, Mathur VV, Packer L. Natural sources of lipoic acid: determination of lipoyllysine released from protease-digested tissues by high performance liquid chromatography incorporating electrochemical detection. J Appl Nutr 1997; 49:3–11.
59. Löffelhardt S, Bonaventura C, Locher M, Borbe HO, Bisswanger H. Interaction of α-lipoic acid enantiomers and homologues with the enzyme components of the mammalian pyruvate dehydrogenase complex. Biochem Pharmacol 1995; 50:637–646.
60. Low PA, Nickander KK, Tritschler HJ. The roles of oxidative stress and antioxidant treatment in experimental diabetic neuropathy. Diabetes 1997; 46 (suppl 2):S38–S42.
61. Lykkesfeldt J, Hagen TM, Vinarsky V, Ames BN. Age-associated decline in ascorbic acid concentration, recyling, and biosynthesis in rat hepatocytes—reversal with (R)- α-lipoic acid supplementation. FASEB J 1998; 12:1183–1189.
62. Maitra I, Serbinova E, Tritschler H, Packer L. α-Lipoic acid prevents buthionine sulfoximine-induced cataract formation in newborn rats. Free Rad Biol Med 1995; 18:823–829.
63. Mitsui Y, Schmelzer J, Zollman PJ, Mitsui M, Tritschler HJ, Low PA. Alpha-lipoic acid improves neuroprotection from ischemia-reperfusion injury of peripheral nerve. J Neurol Sci 1999; 163:11–16.
64. Nagamatsu M, Nicklander KK, Schmelzer JB, Raya A, Wittrock DA, Tritschler H, Low PA. Lipoic acid improves nerve blood flow, reduces oxidative stress and improves distal nerve conduction in experimental diabetic neuropathy. Diabetes Care 1995; 18:1160–1167.
65. Niebch G, Buchele B, Blome J, Grieb S, Brandt G, Kampa P, Raffel HH, Locher M, Borbe HO, Nubert I, Fleischhauer I. Enantioselective high-performance liquid chromatography assay of (+)R- and (−)S-alpha-lipoic acid in human plasma. Chirality 1997; 9:32–36.
66. Nourooz-Zadeh J, Rahimi A, Tajaddini-Sarmadi J, Tritschler H, Rosen P, Halliwell B, Betteridge DJ. Relationship between plasma measures of oxidative stress and metabolic control in NIDDM. Diabetologia 1997; 40:647–653.
67. Oberley LW. Free radicals and diabetes. Free Rad Biol Med 1988; 5:113–124.
68. Obrosova I, Cao X, Greene DA, Stevens MJ. Diabetes-induced changes in lens antioxidant status, glucose utilization and energy metabolism: effect of DL-α-lipoic acid. Diabetologia 1998; 41:1442–1450.
69. Ou P, Tritschler HJ, Wolff SP. Thioctic (lipoic) acid: a therapeutic metal-chelating antioxidant? Biochem Pharmacol 1995; 50:123–126.
70. Packer L, alpha-Lipoic acid: a metabolic antioxidant which regulates NF-kappa B signal transduction and protects against oxidative injury. Drug Metabol Rev 1998; 30:245–275.

71. Packer L, Tritschler HJ, Wessel K. Neuroprotection by the metabolic antioxidant α-lipoic acid. Free Rad Biol Med 1997; 22:359–378.
72. Packer L, Witt EH, Tritschler HJ, Wessel K, Ulrich H. Antioxidant properties and clinical implications of α-lipoic acid. In: Packer L, Cadenas E, eds. Biothiols in Health and Disease. New York: Marcel Dekker, 1995:479–516.
73. Patel MS, Roche TE. Molecular biology and biochemistry of pyruvate dehydrogenase. FASEB J 1990; 4:3224–3233.
74. Peter G, Borbe HO. Absorption of [7,8-^{14}C]rac-α-lipoic acid from in situ ligated segments of the gastrointestinal tract of the rat. Arzneim-Forsch/Drug Res 1995; 45:293–299.
75. Peter G, Borbe HO. Untersuchungen zur Absorption und Verteilung der Thioctsäure als Grundlage der klinischen Wirksamkeit bei der Behandlung der diabetischen Polyneuropathie. Diabetes Stoffwechsel 1996; 5(suppl 3):12–16.
76. Pick U, Haramaki N, Constantinescu A, Handelman GJ, Tritschler HJ, Packer L. Glutathione reductase and lipoamide dehydrogenase have opposite stereospecificities for α-lipoic acid enantiomers. Biochem Biophys Res Commun 1995; 206:724–730.
77. Podda M, Tritschler HJ, Ulrich H, Packer L. α-Lipoic acid supplementation prevents symptoms of vitamin E deficiency. Biochem Biophys Res Commun 1994; 204:98–104.
78. Polonsky KS, Sturis J, Bell GI. Non-insulin-dependend diabetes mellitus—a genetically programmed failure of the beta cell to compensate for insulin resistance. N Engl J Med 1996; 334:777–783.
79. Reed LJ. The chemistry and function of lipoic acid. Adv Enzymol 1957; 18:319–347.
80. Reed LJ. Multienzyme complexes. Acc Chem Res 1974; 7:40–46.
81. Reed LJ, DeBusk BG, Gunsalus IC, Hornberger CS. Crystalline α-lipoic acid: a catalytic agent associated with pyruvate dehydrogenase. Science 1951; 114:93–94.
82. Rehman A, Nourooz-Zadeh J, Moller W, Tritschler H, Pereira P, Halliwell B. Increased oxidative damage to all DNA bases in patients with type II diabetes. FEBS Lett 1999; 448:120–122.
83. Reschke B, Zeuzem S, Rosak C, Petzoldt R, Althoff P-H, Ulrich H, Schöffling K. Hochdosierte Langzeitbehandlung mit Thioctsäure bei der diabetischen Polyneuropathie: Ergebnisse einer kontrollierten, randomisierten Studie unter besonderer Berücksichtigung der autonomen Neuropathie. In: Borbe HO, Ulrich H, eds. Neue biochemische, pharmazeutische und klinische Erkenntnisse zur Thioctsäure. Frankfurt: Verlag, 1989:318–334.
84. Rett K, Maerker E, Tritschler HJ, Wessel K, Wicklmayr, Standl E. Einfluss von alpha-Liponsäure (Thioctsäure) auf den Glucosetransport in Langendorff-Herzen insulinresistenter Zucker-Ratten. Diabetes Stoffwechsel 1996; 5(suppl 3):55–58.
85. Rosenberg HR, Culik R. Effect of α-lipoic acid on vitamin C and vitamin E deficiencies. Arch Biochem Biophys 1959; 80:86–93.
86. Roy S, Sen CK, Kobuchi H, Packer L. Antioxidant regulation of phorbol ester-induced adhesion of human Jurkat T-cells to endothelial cells. Free Rad Biol Med 1998; 25:229–241.

87. Roy S, Sen CK, Tritschler H, Packer L. Modulation of cellular reducing equivalent homeostasis by alpha-lipoic acid: mechanisms and implications for diabetes and ischemic injury. Biochem Pharmacol 1997; 53:393–399.
88. Rudich A, Tirosh A, Potashnik R, Khamaisi M, Bashan N. Lipoic acid protects against oxidative stress induced impairment in insulin stimulation of protein kinase B and glucose transport in 3T3-L1 adipocytes. Diabetologia 1999; 42:949–957.
89. Sachse G, Willms B. Efficacy of thioctic acid in the therapy of peripheral diabetic neuropathy. In: Gries FA, Freund HJ, Rabe F, Berger H, eds. Aspects of Autonomic Neuropathy in Diabetes. New York: Thieme, 1980:105–108.
90. Schempp H, Ulrich H, Elstner EF. Stereospecific reduction of R (+)-thioctic acid by porcine heart lipoamide dehydrogenase/diaphorase. Z Naturforsch 1994; 49c: 691–692.
91. Schneider A, Martin-Villalba A, Weih F, Vogel J, Wirth T, Schwaninger M. NF-κB is activated and promotes cell death in focal cerebral ischemia. Nature Med 1999; 5:554–559.
92. Schulz B, Reichel G, Hüttl I, Zander E, Runge U. Zur Wirksamkeit der Thioctsäuretherapie bei Typ-I-Diabetikern. Wiss Z Ernst-Moritz-Arndt-Universität Greifswald, Med Reihe 1986; 35:48–50.
93. Schulze-Osthoff K, Los M, Baeuerle PA. Redox signalling by transcription factors NF-κB and AP-1 in lymphocytes. Biochem Pharmacol 1995; 50:735–741.
94. Sen CK. Redox signaling and the emerging therapeutic potential of thiol antioxidants. Biochem Pharmacol 1998; 55:1747–1758.
95. Sen CK, Roy S, Han D, Packer L. Regulation of cellular thiols on human lymphocytes by alpha-lipoic acid: a flow cytometric analysis. Free Rad Biol Med 1997; 22:1241–1257.
96. Sen CK, Roy S, Khanna S, Packer L. Determination of oxidized and reduced lipoic acid using high-performance liquid chromatography and coulometric detection. Meth Enzymol 1999; 299:239–246.
97. Sen CK, Roy S, Packer L. α-Lipoic acid: cell regulatory function and potential therapeutic implications. In: Packer L, Hiramatsu M, Yoshikawa T, eds. Antioxidant Food Supplements in Human Health. San Diego: Academic Press, 1999:111–119.
98. Shepherd PR, Kahn BB. Glucose transporters and insulin action. Implications for insulin resistance and diabetes mellitus. N Engl J Med 1999; 341:248–257.
99. Singh HPP, Bowman R. Effect of DL-alpha lipoic acid on the citrate concentration and phosphofructokinase activity of perfused hearts from normal and diabetic rats. Biochem Biophys Res Commun 1970; 41:551–561.
100. Snell EE, Strong FM, Peterson WH. Growth factors for bacteria. VI: Fractionation and properties of an accessory factor for lactic acid bacteria. Biochem J 1937; 31: 1789–1799.
101. Spence JT, McCormick DB. Lipoic acid metabolism in the rat. Arch Biochem Biophys 1976; 174:13–19.
102. Stoll S, Hartmann H, Cohen SA, Müller WE. The potent free radical scavenger α-lipoic acid improves memory in aged mice: putative relationship to NMDA receptor deficits. Pharmacol Biochem Behav 1993; 46:799–805.
103. Stoll S, Rostock A, Bartsch R, Korn E, Meichelböck A, Müller WE. The potent

free radical scavenger α-lipoic acid improves cognition in rodents. Ann NY Acad Sci 1994; 717:122–128.
104. Streeper RS, Henriksen EJ, Jacob S, Hokama JY, Fogt DL, Tritschler HJ. Differential effects of lipoic acid stereoisomers on glucose metabolism in insulin-resistant skeletal muscle. Am J Physiol 1997; 273:E185–E191.
105. Suzuki YJ, Aggarwal BB, Packer L. α-Lipoic acid is a potent inhibitor of NF-κB activation in human T cells. Biochem Biophys Res Commun 1994; 189:1709–1715.
106. Suzuki YJ, Packer L, Mizuno M, Ulrich H. Regulation of gene expression by lipoic acid. In: Packer L, Cadenas E, eds. Biothiols in Health and Disease. New York: Marcel Dekker, 1995:455–466.
107. Suzuki YJ, Tsuchiya M, Packer L. Lipoate prevents glucose-induced protein modifications. Free Rad Res Commun 1992; 17:211–217.
108. Teichert J, Kern J, Tritschler HJ, Ulrich H, Preiss R. Investigations on the pharmacokinetics of alpha-lipoic acid in healthy volunteers. Int J Clin Pharmacol Therapeut 1998; 36:625–628.
109. Teichert J, Preiss R. Determination of lipoic acid in human plasma by high-performance liquid chromatography with electrochemical detection. J Chromatogr 1995; B672:277–281.
110. Tsakiridis T, Ewart HS, Ramlal T, Volchuk A, Kilp A, Estrada ED, Tritschler HJ. Alpha-lipoic acid stimulates glucose transport into muscle cells in culture: comparison with the actions of insulin and dinitrophenol. In: Packer L, Cadenas E, eds. Biothiols in Health and Disease. New York: Marcel Dekker, 1997:87–98.
111. Van Dam PS, van Asbeck BS, Erkelens DW, Marx JJM, Gispen W-H, Bravenboer B. The role of oxidative stress in neuropathy and other diabetic complications. Diabetes/Metabol Rev 1995; 11:181–192.
112. Wada H, Shintani D, Ohlrogge J. Why do mitochondria synthesize fatty acids? Evidence for involvement in lipoic acid production. Proc Natl Acad Sci 1997; 94: 1591–1596.
113. WHO. The World Health Report 1997. Geneva: World Health Organization.
114. Witt W, Rustow B. Determination of lipoic acid by precolumn derivatization with monobromobimane and reversed-phase high-performance liquid chromatography. J Chromatogr 1998; B705:127–131.
115. Wolff SP. Diabetes mellitus and free radicals. Br Med Bull 1993; 49:642–652.
116. Yaworsky K, Somwar R, Ramal T, Sweeney G, Bilan P, Tritschler H, Klip A. In vivo activation of insulin signalling pathways by R (+) α-lipoic acid leads to translocation of glucose transporter to the plasma membrane of 3T3-L1 adipocytes. Oxygen Club of California 1999 World Congress, March 3–6, 1999, Santa Barbara.
117. Zempleni J, Trusty TA, Mock DM. Lipoic acid reduces the activities of biotin-dependent carboxylases in rat liver. J Nutr 1997; 127:1776–1781.
118. Ziegler D, Conrad F, Ulrich H, Reichel G, Schatz H, Gries FA. Effects of treatment with the antioxidant α-lipoic acid on cardiac autonomic neuropathy in NIDDM patients: a 4-months randomized controlled multicenter trial (Dekan study). Diabetes Care 1997; 20:369–373.
119. Ziegler D, Gries FA. α-Lipoic acid acid in the treatment of diabetic peripheral and cardiac autonomic neuropathy. Diabetes 1997; 46(suppl 2):S62–S66.
120. Ziegler D, Hanefeld M, Rahnau KJ, Hasche H, Lobisch M, Schutte K, Kerum G,

Malessa R. Treatment of symptomatic diabetic polyneuropathy with the antioxidant alpha-lipoic acid—a 7-month multicenter randomized controlled trial (ALADIN III study). Diabetes Care 1999; 22:1296–1301.

121. Ziegler D, Hanefeld M, Ruhnau KJ, Meissner HP, Lobisch M, Schütte K, Gries FA. Treatment of symptomatic peripheral neuropathy with the anti-oxidant α-lipoic acid. Diabetologia 1995; 38:1425–1433.
122. Ziegler D, Mayer P, Mühlen H, Gries FA. Effekte einer Therapie mit α-Liponsäure gegenüber Vitamin B_1 bei der diabetischen Neuropathie. Diab Stoffw 1993; 2:443–448.
123. Zimmer G, Beikler T-K, Schneider M, Ibel J, Tritschler H, Ulrich H. Dose/response curves of lipoic acid R- and S-forms in the working rat heart during reoxygenation: superiority of the R-enantiomer in the enhancement of aortic flow. J Mol Cell Cardiol 1995; 27:1895–1903.

10
Creatine: Physiology and Exercise Performance

Klaus Krämer
BASF Aktiengesellschaft, Ludwigshafen, Germany

Michael Weiss and Heinz Liesen
Institute of Sports Medicine, University of Paderborn, Paderborn, Germany

I. INTRODUCTION

Throughout history sportsmen have employed nutritional supplements as ergogenic aids to give them an edge over their competitors. In ancient times athletes and soldiers preparing for a battle consumed specific animal parts believed to confer the strength and speed of that animal (1). Today we know that flesh, in particular from game animals, is rich in creatine. Creatine is a physiological compound that plays a pivotal role in energy metabolism of skeletal muscle and brain. The first well-known athletes to announce that they were taking creatine to enhance performance were the British sprinter Linford Christie and hurdler Colin Jackson. Thereafter, creatine became the nutritional watchword of the 1996 Summer Olympic Games. Supposedly three out of four medal winners were taking creatine. This may explain why creatine is now the blockbusting nutritional supplement in sports.

The short-term use of creatine as a performance enhancer seems to be based on sound science. However, it is not known if taking large quantities over a longer period may bear risks. The aim of this literature survey, therefore, is to give an overview on creatine metabolism and its use in sports nutrition, to address dosing and safety, and to discuss further indications for the medical use of creatine.

II. BIOCHEMISTRY AND PHYSIOLOGY

Creatine [*N*-(aminoiminomethyl)*N*-methyl glycine] is a natural constituent of a mixed diet and is most abundant in fish and meat (Table 1). Vegetable food is almost devoid of creatine. Some traces are found, for instance, in cranberries. Dietary intake in normal individuals averages 1 g per day (2). Creatine intake in vegetarians is extremely low. Total body creatine content of a 70 kg man is around 120 g, with more than 95% in skeletal muscle (3). Lower concentrations are found in brain, liver, kidney, and testes. Daily turnover is estimated to be approximately 2 g (3). The loss needs to be substituted by endogenous synthesis and/or dietary sources.

De novo biosynthesis of creatine in humans takes place in the pancreas, liver, and kidney (Fig. 1). Three amino acids (glycine, arginine, methionine in the form of S-adenosylmethionine) serve as precursors. Two enzymes, a transaminidase and a transmethylase, are involved in creatine synthesis (3). The rate-limiting step (site of regulation) is the transaminidase reaction. Creatine is recognized as a negative feedback regulator of the transaminidase. There is no enzyme activity for creatine synthesis in muscle. Therefore, muscle creatine must be obtained from blood against a concentration gradient that may reach 200:1 (4).

Reference values for muscle creatine (from *m. quadriceps femoris*) obtained from 81 young male and female untrained subjects are (as mmol/kg dry matter) 124.4 (SD 11.2) for total creatine, 49.0 (SD 7.6) for free creatine, and 75.5 (SD 7.6) for creatine phosphate, respectively (5). Type II fibers (fast-twitch)

Table 1 Creatine Content of Food

Food	Creatine (g/kg)
Fish	
Shrimp	Trace
Cod	3
Herring	6.5–10
Plaice	2
Salmon	4.5
Tuna	4
Meat	
Beef	4.5
Pork	5
Other	
Milk	0.1
Cranberries	0.02

Source: Ref. 5.

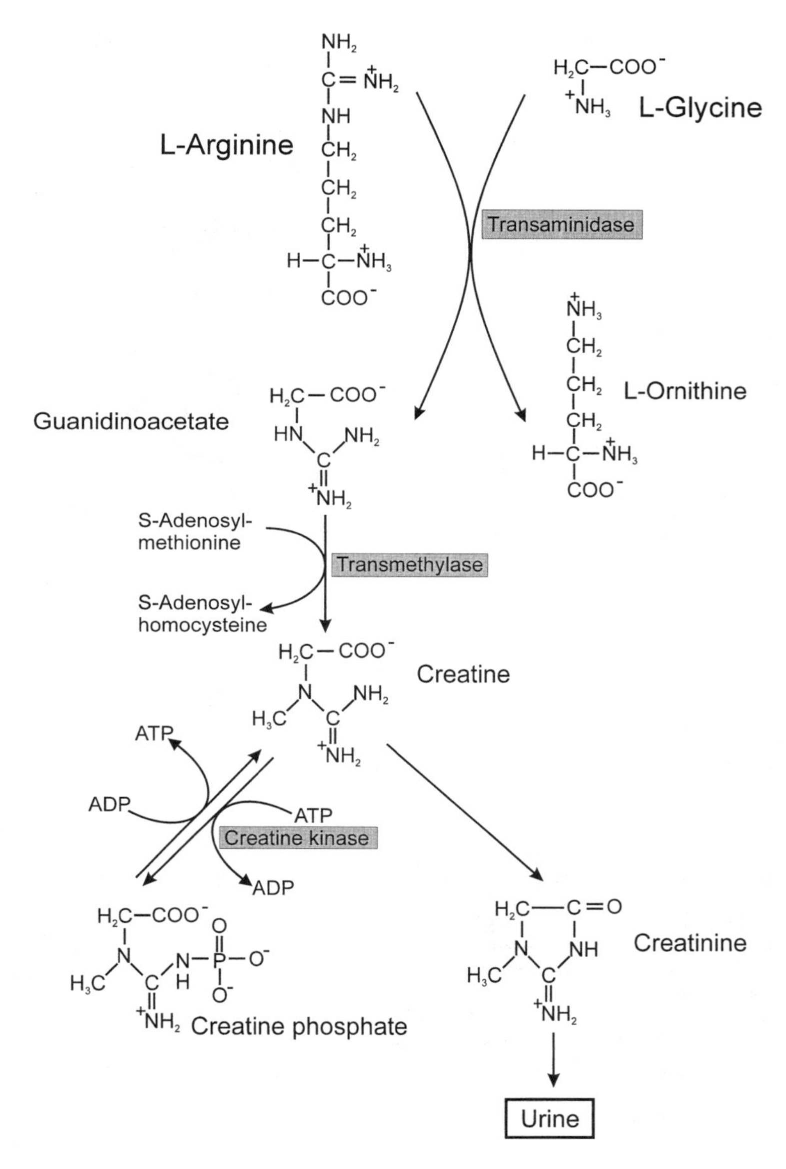

Figure 1 Creatine metabolism.

of human skeletal muscle have been demonstrated to contain more creatine phosphate than type I fibers (slow-twitch) (5). Females have been reported to have higher total creatine in muscle, but the results are inconsistent. Creatine phosphate concentrations in muscle seem to decline during aging (5).

The physiological function of creatine is to maintain muscular ATP levels. ATP is required for muscle contraction and maintenance of ion gradients and syntheses. Creatine is phosphorylated by the action of creatine kinase (Figs. 1

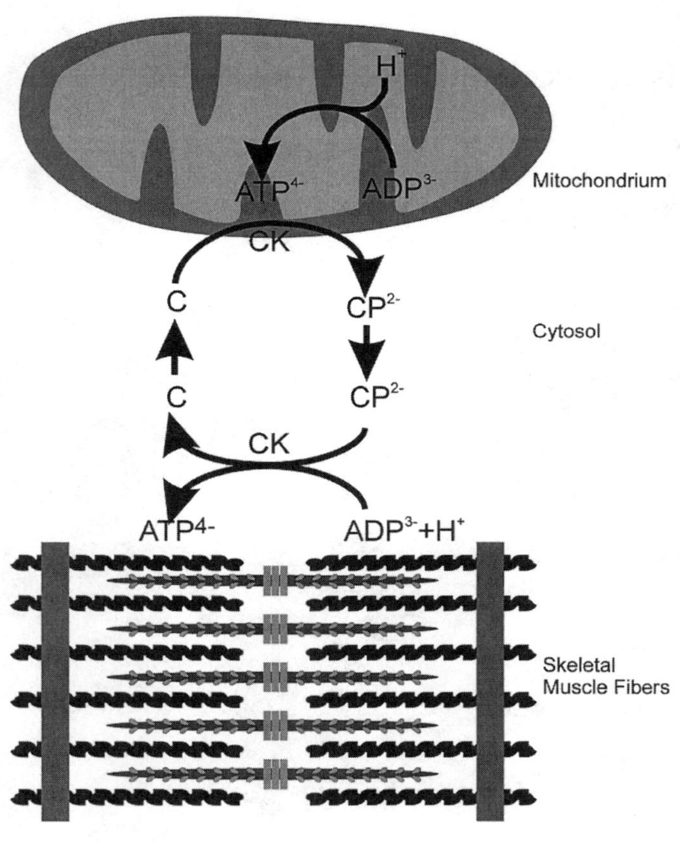

Figure 2 Model of mitochondrial-cytosolic energy shuttle and pH buffer function of the creatine kinase reaction.

Table 2 Reference Values for Creatine and Creatinine in Vegetarians and a Reference Population

	Vegetarians				Reference population			
	Males (n = 55)		Females (n = 44)		Males (n = 25)		Females (n = 35)	
	Mean	SD	Mean	SD	Mean	SD	Mean	SD
Serum								
Creatine, µmol/L	25.1	9.1	32.4	21.4	40.8	19.0	50.2	20.6
Creatine, mg/L	7.7	0.6	7.8	0.8	8.1	1.0	7.6	1.0
Urine								
Creatinine, mg/24 h per 1.73 m^2	1062	263	925	305	1595	269	1231	216
Creatinine clearance, mL/min	96.2	23.5	74.6	18.1	103	17	86	20
Erythrocyte								
Creatine, µmol/L	270	41	281	47	370	72	408	74

Conversion factor: mg/dL × 76.25 = µmol/L.
Source: Ref. 8.

and 2). Isoenzymes of creatine kinase are located in mitochondria (site of energy production in the form of ATP) and cytosol (6). Creatine phosphate functions as an energy shuttle between mitochondria and the cytosolic sites of ATP consumption (3,6) (Fig. 2). During exercise ATP is resynthesized from ADP and creatine phosphate (7):

$$\text{ADP} + \text{creatine phosphate} \rightarrow \text{ATP} + \text{creatine}$$
$$\Delta G^{o'} = -12.6 \text{ kJ/mol}$$

Creatine and creatine phosphate are degraded to creatinine and excreted in the urine (Fig. 1, Table 2) (8). Under physiological conditions creatinine is formed at a constant rate. Hence, plasma creatinine and creatinine clearance are used to measure kidney function.

III. BIOAVAILABILITY

Oral creatine is readily absorbed into the bloodstream and taken up by skeletal muscle. In the first study systematically investigating creatine bioavailability in humans, the intake of 1 g resulted in an increase of plasma concentration from 30 to 100 μmol/L (4). Following 5 g creatine as a single dose, peak plasma levels of 690–1000 μmol/L were achieved within 1 hour of administration. Thereafter, plasma concentration normalized within 7 hours.

Reference values for creatine and creatinine concentrations are given in Table 2. Vegetarians have lower serum concentrations than nonvegetarians (reference population).

Ingestion of 20–30 g creatine per day elevated skeletal muscle total creatine by up to 30%, 20% of which was present as creatine phosphate (4,9,10). In one of these studies, one hour of intensive exercise per day increased creatine uptake by muscle (4). The increase in skeletal muscle creatine depends on its content prior to supplementation (4,9). Subjects with the lowest initial values showed the largest increase in response to creatine administration. Even after consumption of large doses of creatine, muscle creatine concentration increases only to a certain degree. The upper limit of muscle creatine appears to be about 150–160 mmol/kg dry matter (4,9,10). In recent studies simultaneous creatine and glucose ingestion increased whole body creatine retention (measured by urinary creatine and creatinine excretion) (11,12). The authors' explanation is an augmented insulin level in response to carbohydrate intake because in an earlier study (13) insulin increased creatine transport into rat skeletal muscle. However, the stimulatory effect of exercise on creatine retention observed earlier (4) is not seen in combination with carbohydrates.

IV. EXERCISE PERFORMANCE

Several reports have shown that supplementation with creatine improves muscular strength. In a double-blind study, 9 male and 3 female volunteers performed 5 maximal exercise bouts before and after 5 days of supplementation (4 times 5 g creatine monohydrate plus 1 g glucose per day, $n = 6$) and placebo (4 times 6 g glucose per day, $n = 6$) (14). In the creatine group isokinetic torque production determined on a Cybex II dynamometer was increased by 5–7%. No difference in performance was observed in the placebo group. However, randomization of the participants was inadequate, because only men were allocated to the creatine group, and therefore mean initial peak torque production was higher in the creatine group.

In another double-blind placebo-controlled study using 16 participants (15) the exercise protocol comprised 10 consecutive 6-second bouts of high-intensity exercise on a Wingate cycle ergometer. Subjects taking 20 g/day of creatine monohydrate for 6 days were better able to maintain the target pedaling frequency of 140 rev/min than the placebo group (20 g glucose for 6 days) (Fig. 3). Simi-

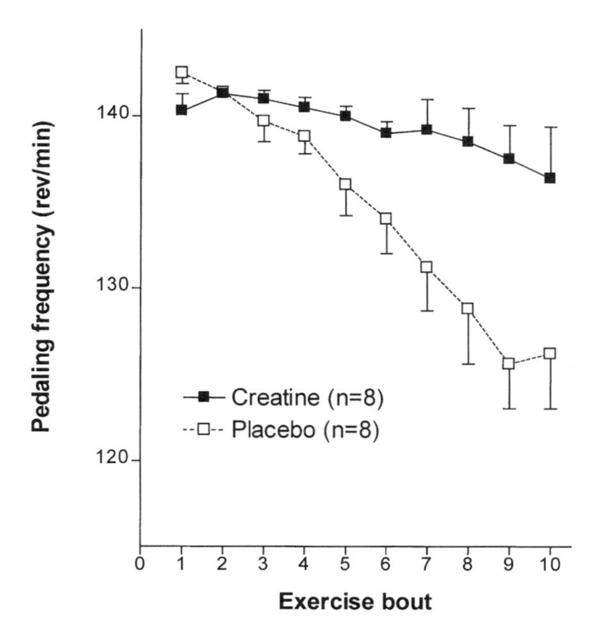

Figure 3 Pedaling frequency (mean and SEM) during 10 bouts of 6-second duration interspersed by 30-second recovery periods. (Ref. 15.)

larly, increases of peak power output, mean power output, and total work output after creatine supplementation for 5 days (20 g per day) during repeated bouts of maximal cycling were observed by Birch et al. (16).

In a study by Earnest et al. (17) trained athletes received either glucose (placebo) or creatine for 28 days in a double-blind manner. Unfortunately, the dosing regime was not reported and only four subjects per treatment completed the experimental protocol. Total anaerobic work performed in a 30-second period (3 Wingate tests) was significantly increased in subjects consuming creatine for 2 weeks by 13, 18, and 18%, respectively. After 4 weeks there was a 6% increase in their one repetition maximum free weight bench press. However, after correction for body weight this effect dissipated because body weight in the creatine group increased during the course of supplementation. In other studies combinations of creatine (20 g/day) with carbohydrates, protein, RNA, and taurine resulted in similar improvements of peak bench press power after 7 days (18) but not after 28 days (19).

In an open study, 7 physically active males performed repeated bouts of high-intensity exercise on a cycle ergometer and squat jumps before and after 6 days of creatine supplementation (20 g/day) (10). While the participants were able to maintain power output longer, there was no effect of creatine intake on jump performance. However, in a double-blind study with 14 well-trained athletes, creatine supplementation (20 g/day for 5 days) improved jumping performance and extended time to exhaustion in a treadmill run (20).

In an unpublished experiment (H. Liesen, K. Hemschemeier, D. Mechau, K. Klöpping-Menke, M. Weiss, 1998), performance and clinical lab parameters were studied in a maximal cycle ergometer interval test. Eleven physically active but not specially trained students of physical education (26 ± 2 years, 178 ± 7 cm height) were evaluated for their maximal power output in a vita max test with increasing workload of 50 W every 30 seconds until exhaustion (step test). The interval test was done after 7 days on their normal diet plus 4 times 10 g maltodextrin per day and reduced physical activity (week 1). It consisted of 10 minutes warming up at 50 W, 5 bouts of 30 seconds at maximal power output and 2 minutes rest (50 W) within the intervals, and one further bout until exhaustion. Thereafter, the subjects were supplemented four times daily with 5 g maltodextrin plus 5 g creatine for 7 days, and then the test was repeated (week 2). At that time plasma creatine had increased 10-fold. Venous blood was taken before the step test one hour before as well as 35 minutes and 24 hours after the interval tests in the first and second week. Capillary blood samples from the hyperemic ear lobe were taken immediately before and after warming up, each interval bout, and up to 30 minutes into recovery.

There was no influence of creatine supplementation on body weight. The performance time in the last interval was not significantly increased after creatine supplementation (1.05 ± 0.5 vs. 1.14 ± 0.5 min). Heart frequencies were somewhat lower after the fifth compared to the first bout (not significantly), but there was no difference between the sixth and first exercise bout. Results of metabolic substrates are shown in Table 3 and Figures 4 and 5.

Briefly, higher blood lactate levels were observed during the recovery period, and lower blood ammonia levels immediately and 3 minutes after the sixth bout in week 2, i.e., the differences between postexercise and resting values were higher in lactate and smaller in ammonia with a decreased ammonia/lactate ratio

Table 3 Blood Parameters Before, During, and After Bicycle Exercise[a] Without[b] and With Preceding Creatine Supplementation

Parameter	Time	Week 1—Maltodextrin (Mean ± SD)	Week 2—Maltodextrin + Creatine (Mean ± SD)	Significance
Creatine	1 h before	22 ± 9	237 ± 147	***
(μmol/L)	35 min after	24 ± 11	215 ± 102	***
	24 h after	40 ± 26	66 ± 49	—
Creatinine	1 h before	81 ± 11	92 ± 10	*
(μmol/L)	35 min after	86 ± 13	97 ± 12	***
	24 h after	80 ± 9	92 ± 10	**
Urea	1 h before	5 ± 1	5 ± 1	—
(mmol/L)	35 min after	6 ± 1.4	5.7 ± 1	—
	24 h after	5.3 ± 1	5.5 ± 1	—
Ammonia	before	31 ± 7	32 ± 11	—
(μmol/L)	after first interval	35 ± 12	32 ± 8	—
	after 5th interval	115 ± 67	84 ± 35	—
	after 6th interval	181 ± 47	137 ± 25	**
	3 min after	215 ± 46	166 ± 67	*
Uric acid	1 h before	327 ± 88	266 ± 40	*
(μmol/L)	before warm-up	342 ± 84	270 ± 47	*
	after 5th interval	333 ± 77	269 ± 40	*
	after 6th interval	337 ± 77	274 ± 39	*
	15 min after	371 ± 81	303 ± 41	*
	30 min after	428 ± 80	382 ± 63	—
	35 min after	411 ± 115	388 ± 66	—
	24 h after	292 ± 131	327 ± 54	—
CK	1 h before	87 ± 56	128 ± 90	—
(U/L)	35 min after	120 ± 167	129 ± 88	—
	24 h after	121 ± 99	142 ± 92	—

[a] 5 × 30 sec vita max with 2-min pause time and sixth exercise bout until exhaustion.
[b] 1st week.
* $p \leq 0.05$; ** $p \leq 0.01$; *** $p \leq 0.001$.

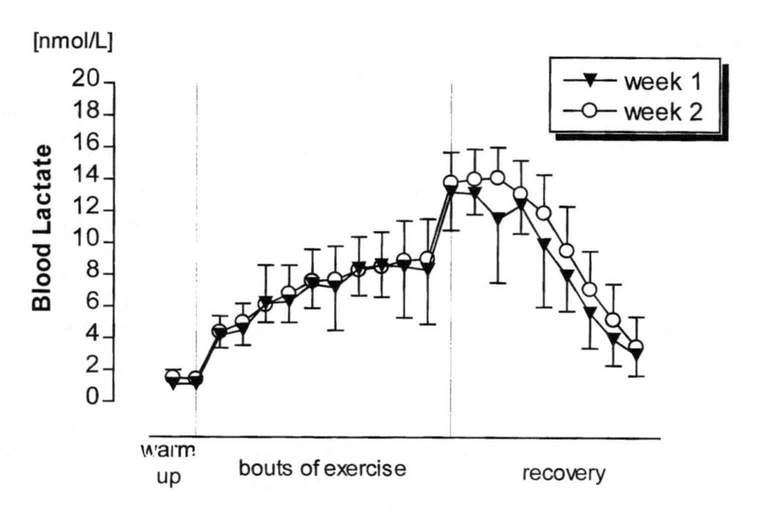

Figure 4 Blood lactate levels during and after bicycle vita max interval exercise without (first week) and with preceding creatine supplementation (second week). Measurements were done immediately before and after each bout of exercise (W vita max from a pretest). The first to fifth bout lasted 30 seconds, pause time was 2 minutes. The sixth bout was performed until exhaustion. Measurements during recovery: 1, 3, 5, 7, 10, 15, 20, 30 minutes.

after the fifth and sixth bouts and 3 minutes of recovery. Uric acid values were lower before, during, and up to 15 minutes after exercise in week 2 in comparison to week 1, but the exercise-induced elevation was the same. Creatinine resting values were slightly increased after creatine supplementation, but the exercise-induced elevation was not different. Uric acid and creatine were correlated with performance in the sixth interval in a different manner before (week 1) and after (week 2) creatine supplementation.

Creatine values after exercise and time to exhaustion were correlated only in week 1 ($r = 0.8685$, $p < 0.001$), whereas the correlation of uric acid and time was only significant in week 2 (Fig. 5). Correlations between parameters of different anaerobic metabolic pathways were only found in the second week after creatine supplementation but not before: ammonia and lactate after the fifth interval ($r = 0.7414$, $p < 0.001$), uric acid and lactate after the sixth interval and at 15 minutes of recovery ($r = 0.7213$, $p < 0.05$ and $r = 0.6154$, $p < 0.05$).

In summary, Liesen et al. found a nonsignificant improvement of high-intensity working capacity after preceding interval exercise by creatine supplementation and a significant shift in the anaerobic energy metabolism with reduced activation of the myoadenylate deaminase reaction. It can be concluded that with-

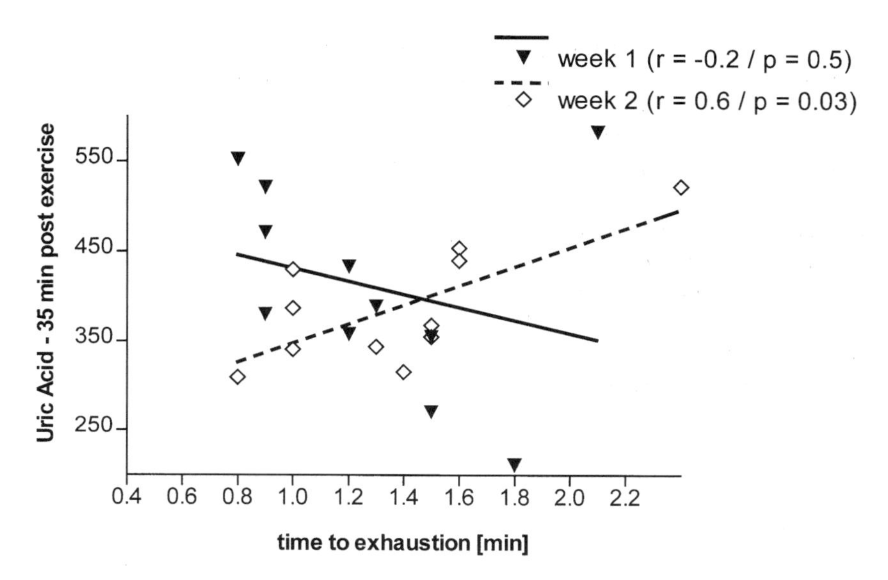

Figure 5 Correlation of plasma uric acid and time to exhaustion in a bicycle interval test of 5 × 30 sec vita max work (pause time 2 min) and a sixth bout of exercise until exhaustion without (first week) and with preceding creatine supplementation (second week).

out creatine supplementation rephosphorylation of creatine phosphate in resting intervals is limiting for further high-intensity exercise, while during creatine supplementation other factors are limiting, despite reduced ammonia production and higher blood lactate accumulation. Those other unknown factors may be responsible for the missing further (significant) improvement of performance time in the last interval of the test after creatine supplementation.

In contrast to studies employing high-intensity, short-term exercise, the effect of oral creatine is not well documented for studies applying endurance exercise protocols. Balsom et al. (21) examined the effect of creatine (four times 5 g creatine monohydrate plus 1 g glucose per day, $n = 9$) versus placebo (four times 6 g glucose per day, $n = 9$) over 6 days on performance during a supramaximal treadmill run and a 6 km cross-country run. A double-blind design was used. For the treadmill run there was no change in performance in either group, comparing the values before and after administration. For the cross-country run the creatine group showed a significant increase in running time, while performance of the placebo group did not change. The authors argue that the increase in body weight in the creatine group may have had a negative impact on performance in this type of exercise. Also, in other trials employing either a continuous incremental test running at 50–90% of maximal oxygen uptake or an exercise protocol with a workload above VO_{2max}, creatine supplementation had no effect on performance (22,23). In well-trained runners performance of two 700 m maximal running bouts lasting 90–120 seconds was not improved after creatine supplementation (24). However, in oarsmen on a 1000 m simulated rowing competition, creatine significantly reduced rowing time from 211 to 208.7 seconds (25). Further evidence that creatine supplementation may increase performance above VO_{2max} originates from a recent study in which anaerobic capacity was measured by determining maximum accumulated oxygen deficit (MAOD) (26). In 26 subjects assigned to placebo and four daily 5 g doses of creatine for 5 days, creatine treatment increased MAOD significantly by approximately 10%. In addition, time to exhaustion on a cycle ergometer was increased.

V. MODE OF ACTION

The improvement of performance in high-intensity exercise by creatine has been explained by an enhanced resynthesis of creatine phosphate during recovery (9,10). In addition, Greenhaff et al. (27) suggested that the level of improvement depends on the muscle creatine concentration prior to supplementation. In a previous study, this group found that only subjects with muscle creatine concentration below 120 mmol/kg of dry muscle weight responded with a marked increase of muscle creatine and that only such volunteers had an improved creatine phosphate resynthesis after a short bout of high-intensity exercise (9). In a subsequent study these results were confirmed by a positive correlation between increases in peak and total work production with the elevation in muscle total creatine of subjects performing two bouts of 30-second maximal, isokinetic cycling, before and after creatine ingestion (28). This may explain why some athletes experience no improvement in performance after creatine ingestion. The improved performance was mediated by an increase of creatine phosphate concentration in type II fibers.

Furthermore, the creatine kinase reaction may increase intramuscular buffering capacity, which is likely due to proton consumption for ATP synthesis, so that the drop of muscular pH is delayed, which has been shown to be the major cause of muscle fatigue (29) (Fig. 2). During short-term, high-intensity exercise (anaerobic conditions), one third of ATP is resynthesized from creatine phosphate and two thirds are produced by glycolysis (30). Glycolysis leads to the formation of lactate and a concomitant drop in muscle pH. After creatine supplementation and intense exercise, plasma lactate was either decreased (15), unaltered (14,10,17), or increased (9). However, studies determining creatine and lactate in muscle established a significant reduction of lactate by 70 and 35%, respectively (10,15). These experiments demonstrate that fatigue is delayed after short-term, high-intensity exercise by increased resynthesis of ATP through creatine phosphate and that under these conditions plasma lactate does not reflect glucose flux through glycolysis in the muscle. This may also explain the varying effects of creatine in short-term and prolonged exercise because during the latter energy is mainly generated by aerobic mechanisms (15), while some anaerobic energy is also supplied, particularly during onset of exercise, at a workload above VO_{2max} and in sports with varying intensity, e.g., ball games.

In a study by Liesen et al. (unpublished) with maximal short-term interval exercise, a shift in anaerobic energy metabolism after creatine supplementation was verified, which may be explained by the scheme of metabolic pathways in Figure 6. By supplementation of 4 × 5 g creatine per day for one week, serum creatine increased approximately 10-fold. There was a slight but significant increase of plasma creatinine, indicating creatine catabolism. At the same time, resting levels of uric acid decreased. In comparison to presupplementation during the same exercise bouts from first to fifth interval at the first bout lactate turnover seemed to be accelerated, thereafter unchanged. At the same time ammonia turn-

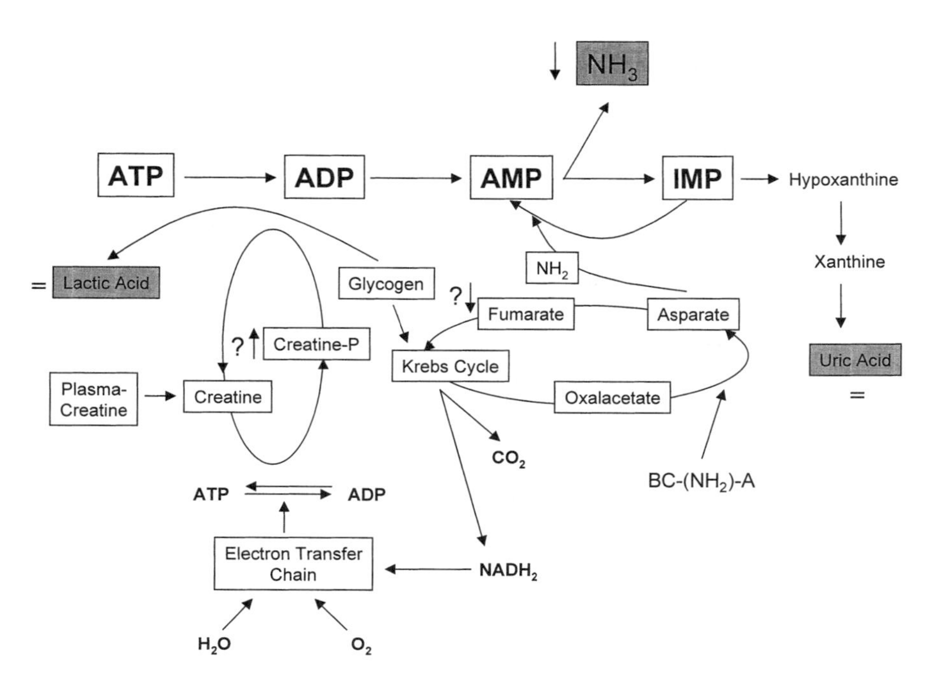

Figure 6 Possible metabolic effects of creatine supplementation. Shadowed metabolic substrates were measured. Increased plasma creatine resulted in decreased blood ammonia levels after exercise. Blood lactic acid was higher at the first bout of exercise; thereafter it remained unchanged. The last exercise bout was maintained for a somewhat longer time, and lactate levels thereafter were significant.

over was reduced. This can only be explained by enhanced ATP rephosphorylation by creatine phosphate. The question arises if a yet unexplored creatine phosphate shuttle is involved in the P transfer from 1,3-bis-phosphoglycerate and/or phosphoenolpyruvate to ATP and in the rephosphorylation from AMP to ADP. Creatine supplementation enhanced the restoration of creatine phosphate in the interval pause, resulting in a sparing effect on ammonia turnover (reduced adenylate deaminase reaction) in the sixth interval with slightly longer performance time until exhaustion. Together with the reduced resting plasma uric acid levels (differences between postexercise and resting values were the same under supplementation and before supplementation), it can be assumed that the total adenosine pool is stabilized. Provided that the above proposed creatine phosphate shuttle in glycolysis exists and thereby the dephosphorylation of 1,3-bis-phosphoglycerate and phosphoenolpryuvate is enhanced, lactate turnover may be enhanced too (higher blood lactate levels after the first interval and in the recovery phase). Whether this benefits aerobic metabolism needs to be clarified in further experiments.

Finally an anabolic effect of creatine has been suggested. In a long-lasting study using creatine as a treatment for gyrate atrophy of the choroid and retina, an increased diameter of type II muscle fibers was shown (31).

VI. DOSING

Nutritionists from the British Olympic Committee (32) recommend 20 g of creatine for 5 consecutive days. This is in agreement with Greenhaff et al. (27,33), who recommend a loading dose of 20 g of creatine for 5–6 days followed by a maintenance dose of 2 g per day. Creatine is usually dissolved in cold or hot drinks (tea, water, milk) prior to consumption. Similar but more gradual muscle creatine loading is achieved by 3 g per day over a period of 28 days (34). Creatine should not be taken together with caffeine because the ergogenic effect of muscle creatine loading may be counteracted (35).

More popular recommendations for body builders take body weight and workout level into account (36). Recommendations range from 12 to 20 g per day and from 4 to 12 g per day for the loading and the maintenance phase, respectively.

VII. SAFETY

To date, no negative side effects of creatine supplementation have been reported. However, all studies with relevant dosages were of short duration, with a maximum of 56 days. There is only one long-term study, with 1.5 g of creatine per day for over 1 year, an amount equivalent to that found in the regular diet (31).

No adverse effects were reported in this trial. Likewise, in another experiment with a dosing regime of 20 g of creatine for 5 days followed by 10 g daily over 51 days, no harmful effects were observed (37).

A possible side effect observed several times was an increase in body weight of 1–2 kg after creatine intake (9–11,15,17,21,22). This may be due to an increase in fat-free mass (17) or an increase in diameter of muscle type II fibers (38). After short-term creatine feeding, at least part of the weight gain accrues from water retention as urine production appears to decrease during a period of creatine supplementation (P. Balsom, personal communication).

Creatine feeding reduces creatine biosynthesis. There are only data from animal experiments that activity of transamidinase (rate-limiting enzyme of creatine synthesis) normalizes after creatine is taken out of the diet (3).

Anabolic effects from creatine supplementation must be questioned since growth inhibition by guanidino compounds and creatine was observed in some cell lines (39) and in hen egg development (40). Although surviving chickens showed no disorders, creatine should not be used during pregnancy for reasons of caution.

High doses of creatine may tense up skeletal muscles. It has been speculated that creatine binds magnesium, resulting in muscle cramps (41). The author recommends taking magnesium along with creatine.

Although no direct toxicity of creatine can be assumed, there is some evidence for problematic metabolic products of creatine, in particular related to renal dysfunction. Athletes, especially body builders, take large quantities of protein in addition to their regular meals. Excess protein is seen as a risk factor for renal dysfunction so that surplus creatine may be retained in the body. The fate of such creatine is unknown. Creatine is converted spontaneously to creatinine (7), and high creatine ingestion increases creatinine levels (Table 2) (8) even at a normal renal function. Toxic methyl guanidine and other guanidino compounds can be derived from creatinine and urea (42) and methyl guanidine from creatinine either by nonenzymatic conversion from creatinine (43) or from creatol—an intermediate occurring in renal failure (44). In a rat model of chronic renal failure, methyl guanidine caused a dose-dependent decrease in survival rate (45). Guanidino compounds and creatine were shown to be uremic toxins (39), contributing to the neurological complications in uremia (46), and they may cause dose-dependent generalized convulsions (guanidino succinate $>$ methyl guanidine $>$ guanidine $\gg$ creatine), possibly due to GABA antagonism (46). In addition, renal failure may be caused by epileptic seizures (47,48), either due to hyperuricemia (49,48) or by rhabdomyolysis leading to renal insufficiency and marked liver dysfunction (47). Furthermore, acute renal failure may occur after heavy exercise (50,51), in particular, in connection with myoglobinuria and rhabdomyolysis (36,52,53) or in connection with drugs like anabolic hormones (53) and nonsteroidal anti-inflammatory drugs and diuretics (36). During heavy exercise renal function may be impaired by reductions in renal blood flow (about 80%), glomerular perfusion (about 75%), and glomerular filtration (about 50%) (36). If this is combined with other factors that impair the renal hemodynamics and/or the tubular functions [drugs (36), exsiccosis, subclinical nephrosclerosis plus drugs (36), hypopotassemia (52), urate nephropathy (48,49), and myoglobin uria/rhabdomyolysis], excretion of creatine/creatinine may be delayed and synthesis of toxic metabolites may take place. Gonella et al. (43) observed increased urinary excretion of methylguanidine after creatine ingestion in normal subjects and in uremic patients.

Myoglobinuria is not rare among athletes, and single cases of rhabdomyolysis after heavy exercise in athletes were described several times in the literature (54). Myoglobinuria and rhabdomyolysis after exercise appear predominantly in patients with metabolic disorders, i.e., metabolic myopathias like McArdle's disease, or after ingestion of drugs or during electrolyte disturbances (55). Other reasons may be enzyme deficiencies in energy metabolism (56) and thyroid myopathia (57).

In conclusion, creatine supplementation at even low doses is contraindicated as follows:

In renal insufficiency or in disorders that are able to impair renal functions.

In combination with anti-inflammatory or antihypertensive drugs, diuretics and/or anabolic steroids, with drugs affecting renal function or potentially enhancing muscle injury (36,50,53,55). In most cases of acute renal failure after a marathon run, anti-inflammatory drugs were taken (51).

After previous episodes of myoglobinuria/rhabdomyolysis.

In cases of metabolic myopathia/enzyme deficiency in glycolysis/β-oxidation, further studies are indicated to elucidate if creatine supplementation is of risk or of benefit in preventing rhabdomyolysis. The same is true for uric acid disorders/urate nephropathy, since we observed decreased resting uric acid levels after creatine supplementation but the same exercise-induced increase.

As large quantities of creatine are taken over a prolonged period, product impurities should be of concern (58). In an earlier study employing practical grade creatine, an impurity [1,1-dimethylbiguanidide] reportedly modified carbohydrate metabolism (depletion of liver glycogen stores) of rats (59).

Finally, product stability is indispensable. There is evidence that creatine may be dehydrated to creatinine in the upper gastrointestinal tract, yielding methyl urea (60). The probability of intragastric production of cancerogenic form(s) of nitrosourea has to be addressed in further studies.

VIII. DOPING

Ergogenic aids may bear health hazards, are recognized as an unfair advantage, and need to be readily analyzed. The reason why they are banned by the governing bodies of sports are the potential harmful effects.

To date, creatine meets all criteria with the exception of the first and is therefore not on the list of banned compounds. However, within the governing bodies of sports reigns controversy as to whether creatine should be recognized as an illegal ergogenic aid or not.

IX. FURTHER APPLICATIONS

Gyrate atrophy of the choroid retina is a progressive disease related to a defect in creatine synthesis. Due to an effect of an ornithine-catabolizing enzyme, the ornithine level is increased, which in turn inhibits the rate-limiting enzyme of creatine synthesis. Patients suffering from gyrate atrophy treated for over one year with 1.5 g of creatine per day showed a significant increase in the mean diameter of muscle type II fibers of *m. vastus lateralis*, comparing the values before and after administration (31).

In several test models creatine proved to be effective as an anti-inflammatory and an analgesic agent (61). Creatine did not induce gastrointestinal irritation, which is common with the use of nonsteroidal antiphlogistic agents.

An inborn error of creatine synthesis affecting the transmethylation reaction (guanidinoacetate methyltransferase) induces creatine deficiency in the brain that causes extrapyramidal movement disorders (38). In the case of a 22-month-old boy administration of creatine monohydrate (4–8 g/day) for 25 months improved muscle tone and lessened extrapyramidal symptoms (38,62). Both muscular and brain creatine levels became normal.

Creatine phosphate (63) and creatine (64) have been used in the treatment of chronic heart failure. In a study by Ferraro et al. (63), five patients with chronic heart failure received 6 g of creatine phosphate for 5 days intravenously. All patients showed an improvement in clinical symptoms. Gordon et al. (64) did not observe an increase of cardiac output after creatine supplementation (20 g daily for 20 days), but the patients showed an increase in muscle creatine and improved muscle strength and endurance. This study had a double-blind, placebo-controlled design with 17 patients.

Loading of Ehrlich ascites tumor cells (normally devoid of creatine) with creatine phosphate or cyclocreatine phosphate has been suggested to provide these highly proliferating and undifferentiated cells with the homeostatic control mechanism found in nondividing muscle and nerve cells (3). In a more recent paper growth rate of transplantation tumors into rats and nude mice was significantly reduced by 1% creatine or cyclocreatine in the diet (65). The tumors used were rat mammary tumors, rat sarcoma, and two human neuroblastoma cell lines. Creatine kinase, therefore, seems to be a new target for antitumor chemotherapy (66).

Recently a lipid-lowering effect of creatine has been established (37). In the study, 32- to 70-year-old men and women were fed for 5 days with 20 g of creatine daily and thereafter with 10 g per day for 51 consecutive days. There was a reduction in low-density lipoprotein (LDL) cholesterol and triglycerides of 22 and 23%, respectively.

In an ex vivo trial creatine was shown to prevent anoxic damage of brain slices (67), indicating that it may have neuroprotective activities.

X. CONCLUSIONS

Creatine is useful as a ergogenic aid in the sprint disciplines of running, cycling, and swimming after short-term supplementation. During continuous exercise of long duration, potential beneficial effects warrant further investigation, particularly whether higher training intensity can be achieved. In team ball games and racket sports (e.g., soccer, tennis, basketball) with periods of high-intensity exercise, creatine supplementation may be of some advantage, but this has not yet been proven. Body builders may also benefit from creatine feeding by increasing their lean body mass.

Long-term effects of creatine use on performance and safety still need to be elucidated. Potential new indications (e.g., ischemia injury, muscle weakness, movement disorders, tumors, hyperlipidemia, metabolic myopathy) should be pursued.

ACKNOWLEDGMENTS

We thank Dr. P. P. Hoppe for his comments on the manuscript. Thanks are also extended to U. Oberfrank for the skillful preparation of the figures.

REFERENCES

1. Applegate EA, Grivetti LE. Search for the competitive edge: a history of dietary fads and supplements. J Nutr 1997; 127:869S–873S.
2. Lykken GI, Robert AJ, Munoz JM, Sandstead HH. A mathematical model of creatine metabolism in normal males—comparison between theory and experiment. Am J Clin Nutr 1980; 33:2674–2685.
3. Walker JB. Creatine: biosynthesis, regulation and function. Adv Enzymol Relat Areas Mol Biol 1979; 50:177–242.
4. Harris RC, Söderlund K, Hultman E. Elevation of creatine in resting and exercised muscle of normal subjects by creatine supplementation. Clin Sci 1992; 83:367–374.
5. Balsom PB, Söderlund K, Ekblom B. Creatine in humans with special reference to creatine supplementation. Sports Med 1994; 18:268–280.

6. Wallimann T, Wyss M, Brdiczka D, Nicolay K, Eppenberger HM. Intracellular compartmentation, structure and function of creatine kinase isoenzymes in tissues with high and fluctuating energy demands: the ''phosphocreatine circuit'' for cellular energy homeostasis. Biochem J 1992; 281:21–40.
7. Löffler G, Petrides PE. Biochemie und Pathobiochemie, 5th ed. Berlin: Springer-Verlag, 1997.
8. Delanghe J, De Slypere JP, De Buyzere M, Robbrecht J, Wieme R, Vermeulen A. Normal reference values for creatine, creatinine, and carnitine are lower in vegetarians. Clin Chem 1989; 35:1802–1803.
9. Greenhaff PL, Bodin K, Soderlund K, Hultman E. Effect of oral creatine supplementation on skeletal muscle phosphocreatine resynthesis. Am J Physiol 1994; 266: E725–E730.
10. Balsom PD, Söderlund K, Sjödin B, Ekblom B. Skeletal muscle metabolism during short duration high-intensity exercise: influence of creatine supplementation. Acta Phys Scand 1995; 154:303–310.
11. Green AL, Simpson EJ, Littlewood JJ, Macdonald IA, Greenhaff PL. Carbohydrate ingestion augments creatine retention during creatine feeding in humans. Acta Phys Scand 1996; 158:195–202.
12. Green AL, Hultman EM, Macdonald IA, Sewell DA, Greenhaff PL. Carbohydrate ingestion augments skeletal muscle creatine accumulation during creatine supplementation in humans. Am J Physiol 1996; 271:E821–E826.
13. Haughland RB, Chang DT. Insulin effects on creatine transport in skeletal muscle. Proc Soc Exp Biol Med 1975; 148:1–4.
14. Greenhaff PL, Casey A, Short AH, Harris R, Soderlund K, Hultman E. Influence of oral creatine supplementation of muscle torque during repeated bouts of maximal voluntary exercise in man. Clin Sci 1993; 84:565–571.
15. Balsom PD, Ekblom B, Söderlund K, Sjödin B, Hultman E. Creatine supplementation and dynamic high-intensity intermittent exercise. Scand J Med Sci Sports 1993; 3:143–149.
16. Birch R, Noble D, Greenhaff PL. The influence of dietary creatine supplementation on performance during repeated bouts of maximal isokinetic cycling in man. Eur J Appl Physiol Occup Physiol 1994; 69:268–270.
17. Earnest CP, Snell PG, Rodriguez R, Almada AL, Mitchell TL. The effect of creatine monohydrate ingestion on anaerobic power indices, muscular strength and body composition. Acta Phys Scand 1995; 153:207–209.
18. Grindstaff P, Kreider R, Weiss L, Fry A, Wood L, Bullen D, Miyaji M, Ramsey L, Li Y, Almada A. Effects of ingesting a supplement containing creatine monohydrate of 7 days on isokinetic performance (abstr). Med Sci Sports Exercise 1995; 27:S146.
19. Almada A, Kreidner R, Weiss L, Fry A, Wood L, Bullen D, Miyaji M, Grindstaff P, Ramsey L, Li Y. Effects of ingesting a supplement containing creatine monohydrate for 28 days on isokinetic performance (abstr). Med Sci Sports Exercise 1995; 27:S146.
20. Bosco C, Tihanyi J, Pucspk J, Kovacs I, Gabossy A, Colli R, Pulvirenti G, Tranquilli C, Foti C, Viru M, Viru A. Effect of oral creatine supplementation on jumping and running performance. Int J Sports Med 1997; 18:369–372.
21. Balsom PB, Harridge S, Söderlund K, Sjödin B, Ekblom B. Creatine supplementa-

tion per se does not enhance endurance exercise performance. Acta Phys Scand 1993; 14:521–523.
22. Stroud MA, Holliman D, Bell D, Green AL, Macdonald IA, Greenhaff PL. Effect of oral creatine supplementation on respiratory gas exchange and blood lactate accumulation during steady-state incremental treadmill exercise and recovery in man. Clin Sci 1994; 87:707–710.
23. Febbraio MA, Flanagan TR, Snow RJ, Zhao S, Carey MF. Effect of creatine supplementation on intramuscular TCr, metabolism and performance during intermittent, supramaximal exercise in humans. Acta Phys Scand 1995; 155:387–395.
24. Terrillion KA, Kolkhorst FW, Dolgener FA, Joslyn SJ. The effect of creatine supplementation on two 700-m maximal running bouts. Int J Sports Nutr 1997; 7:138–143.
25. Rossiter HB, Cannel ER, Jakeman PM. The effect of oral creatine supplementation on the 1000-m performance of competitive rowers. J Sports Sci 1996; 14:175–179.
26. Jacobs I, Bleue S, Goodman J. Creatine ingestion increases anaerobic capacity and maximum accumulated oxygen deficit. Can J Appl Physiol 1997; 22:231–243.
27. Greenhaff PL, Casey A, Green A. Kreatin-Supplementierung neu unter der Lupe. Insider 4(3):1996.
28. Casey A, Constantin-Teodosiu D, Howell S, Hultman E, Greenhaff PL. Creatine ingestion favorably affects performance and muscle metabolism during maximal exercise in humans. Am J Physiol 1996; 271:E31–E37.
29. Maughan RJ. Creatine supplementation and exercise performance. Int J Sport Nutr 1995; 5:94–101.
30. Bogdanis GC, Nevill ME, Boobis LH, Lakomy HKA. Contribution of phosphocreatine and aerobic metabolism to energy supply during repeated sprint exercise. J Appl Physiol 1996; 80:876–884.
31. Sipilä I, Rapola J, Simell O, Vannas A. Supplementary creatine as a treatment of gyrate atrophy of the choroid and retina. N Engl J Med 1981; 304:867–870.
32. British Olympic Commitee. Ergogenic aids—creatine. Sports Sci Update 1, 1995.
33. Greenhaff PL. Kreatin: seine Rolle in Bezug auf die körperliche Leistungsfähigkeit sowie Ermüdung; seine Anwendung als ein Sporternährungs-Supplement. Insider 4(1):1995.
34. Hultman E, Soderlund K, Timmons JA, Cederblad G, Greenhaff PL. Muscle creatine loading in men. J Appl Physiol 1996; 81:232–237.
35. Vandenberghe K, Gillis N, Van Leemputte M, Van Hecke P, Vanstapel F, Hespel P. Caffeine counteracts in ergogenic action of muscle creatine loading. J Appl Physiol 1996; 80:452–457.
36. Sanders LR. Exercise-induced acute renal failure associated with ibuprofen, hydrochlorothiazide, and triamteren. J Am Soc Nephrol 1995; 5:2020–2023.
37. Earnest CP, Almada AL, Mitchell TL. High-performance capillary electrophoresis—pure creatine monohydrate reduces blood lipids in men and women. Clin Sci 1996; 91:113–118.
38. Stöckler S, Holzbach U, Hanefeld F, Marquardt I, Helms G, Requart M, Hänicke W, Frahm J. Creatine deficiency in the brain: a new, treatable inborn error of metabolism. Pediatr Res 1994; 36:409–413.
39. Nathan I, Hensel R, Dvilonsky A, Shainkin-Kestenbaum R. Effects of uremic tox-

ins—guanidino compounds and creatinine—on proliferation of HL60 and K562 cell lines. Nephron 1989; 52:251–252.
40. Seki S, Yuyama N, Hiramatsu M. Effect of guanidino compounds on hen egg development. Adv Exp Med Biol 1982; 153:465–470.
41. Brönnimann M. Kreatin in der (Sport-)Medizin. DIA-GM 1997; 18:127–130.
42. Mikami H, Orita Y, Ando A, Fujii M, Kikuchi T, Yoshihara K, Okada A, Abe H. Metabolic pathway of guanidino compounds in chronic renal failure. Adv Exp Med Biol 1982; 153:449–458.
43. Gonella M, Barsotti G, Lupetti S, Giovanetti S. Metabolic production of methyl guanidine. Clin Sci Mol Med 1975; 48:341–347.
44. Yokozawa T, Fujitsuka N, Oura H, Ienaga K, Nakamura K. Comparison of methylguanidine production from creatinine and creatol in vivo. Nephron 1991; 58:125–126.
45. Yokozawa T, Mo ZL, Oura H. Comparison of toxic effects of methylguanidine, guanidinosuccinic acid and creatinine in rats with adenine-induced chronic renal failure. Nephron 1989; 51:388–392.
46. D'Hooge R, Rei YQ, Marescau B, De Deyn PP. Convulsive action and toxicity of uremic guanidino compounds: behavioural assessment and relation to brain concentration in adult mice. J Neurol Sci 1992; 112:96–105.
47. Sato T, Ota M, Matsuo M, Tasaki H, Miyazaki S. Recurrent reversible rhabdomyolysis asociated with hyperthermia and status epilepticus. Acta Paediatr 1995; 84: 1083–1085.
48. Warren DJ, Leitch AG, Legett RJE. Hyperuricaemic acute renal failure after epileptic seizures. Lancet 1975; 2:385–387.
49. Conger JD. Acute uric acid nephropathy. Med Clin North Am 1990; 74:859–871.
50. Knochel JP, Dotin LN, Hamburger RJ. Heatstress, exercise, and muscle injury: effects on urate metabolism and renal function. Ann Intern Med 1974; 81:312–328.
51. Mac Searraigh ETM, Kallmeyer JC, Schiff HB. Acute renal failure in marathon runners. Nephron 1979; 24:236–240.
52. Aizawa H, Morita K, Minami H, Sasaki N, Tobise K. Exertional rhabdomyolysis as a result of sterous military training. J Neurol Sci 1995; 132:239–240.
53. Hageloch W, Apell HJ, Weickerer H. Rhabdomyolyse bei Bodybuilder unter Anabolika-Einnahme. Sportverletzung Sportschäden 1988; 2:122–125.
54. Kuipers H. Exercise-induced muscle damage. Int J Sports Med 1994; 15:132–135.
55. Penn AS. Myoglobinuria. In: Engel AG, Banker BG, eds. Myology. New York: McGraw-Hill, 1985:1785–1805.
56. Ogilvie I, Pourfarzam M, Jackson S, Stockdale C, Bartlett K, Turnbull DM. Very long-chain acyl coenzyme A dehydrogenase deficiency presenting with exercise-induced myoglobinuria. Neurology 1994; 44:467–473.
57. Lochmüller H, Reimers CD, Fischer P, Heuss B, Müller-Höcker J, Pongratz DE. Exercise-induced myalgia in hypothyroidism. Clin Invest 1993; 71:999–1001.
58. Toler SM. Creatine is an ergogen for anaerobic exercise. Nutr Rev 1997; 55:21–25.
59. Laastuen LE, Todd WR. Rat liver glycogen-lowering activity of fed creatine—a retraction. J Nutr 1969; 99:446–448.
60. Mirvish SS, Cairnes DA, Hermes NH, Raha CR. Creatinine: a food component that

is nitrosated—denitrosated to yield methyl urea. J Agric Food Chem 1982; 30:824–828.

61. Khanna NK, Madan BR. Studies on the anti-inflammatory activity of creatine. Arch Int Pharmacodyn Ther 1978; 231:340–350.
62. Stöckler S, Hanefeld F, Frahm J. Creatine replacement therapy in guanidinoacetate methyltransferase deficiency, a novel inborn error of metabolism. Lancet 1996; 348: 789–790.
63. Ferraro S, Maddalena G, Fazio S, Santomauro M, Lo Storto M, Codella C, D'Agosto V, Sacca L. Acute and short-term efficacy of high doses of creatine phosphate in the treatment of cardiac failure. Curr Ther Res 1990; 47:917–923.
64. Gordon A, Hultman E, Kaijser L, Kristjansson S, Rolf CJ, Nyquist O, Sylvén C. Creatine supplementation in chronic heart failure increases skeletal muscle creatine phosphate and muscle performance. Cardiovasc Res 1995; 30:413–418.
65. Miller EE, Evans AE, Cohn M. Inhibition of rate of tumor growth by creatine and cyclocreatine. PNAS USA 1993; 90:3304–3308.
66. Bergnes G, Yuan W, Khandekar VS, O'Keefe MM, Martin KJ, Teicher BA, Kaddurah-Daouk R. Creatine and phosphocreatine analogs: anticancer activity and enzymatic analysis. Oncol Res 1996; 8:121–130.
67. Carter AJ, Mueller RE, Pschorn U, Stransky W. Preincubation with creatine enhances levels of creatine phosphate and prevents anoxic damage of rat hippocampal slices. J Neurochem 1995; 64:2691–2699.

11

Plant Phenols and Cardiovascular Disease: Antioxidants and Modulators of Cell Response

Fabio Virgili and Cristina Scaccini
National Institute for Food and Nutrition Research, Rome, Italy

Peter-Paul Hoppe
BASF, Offenbach/Queich, Germany

Klaus Krämer
BASF Aktiengesellschaft, Ludwigshafen, Germany

Lester Packer
University of Southern California School of Pharmacy, Los Angeles, California

I. INTRODUCTION

All cells that constitute the human body rely on the vascular system for their supply of oxygen and nutrients, without which either anoxic necrosis or dysfunction can occur. By far the most frequent causes of vascular stenosis, occlusion, or rupture are atherosclerosis and hypertension, acting alone or in concert.

Atherosclerosis is a chronic, progressive disease of large- and medium-sized arteries that slowly alters and thickens the arterial walls. It can either promote an occlusive thrombosis in the altered artery or produce a gradual but relentless stenosis of the arterial lumen. In the first case, an infarction of the organ supplied by the afflicted vessel occurs, such as in a heart attack (when a coronary artery is affected) and in a thrombotic stroke (when a cerebral artery is suddenly blocked). In the second case, stenosis of the vessel leads to a progressive and gradual destruction of the affected organ part.

Hypertension, on the other hand, is a disease that mainly affects small arteries, causing either a stenosis, with subsequent disappearance and fibrous replacement of the dependent organ part, or the rupture of the altered wall leading to hemorrhage.

Together with these dramatic outcomes, which occur at the tissue level, a number of subtle dysfunctions occurs at the cellular and molecular levels in the early stages of disease progression, which leads to the loss of homeostatic functions. These events include the modification of the pattern of gene expression, cell proliferation, and apoptosis.

The blood vessel is composed of a monolayer of endothelial cells, which is in contact with a layer of smooth muscle cells and encircled by a layer of connective tissue. The endothelial cell layer behaves as the interface between the circulating blood and the vessel itself and has the role of both sensor and signal transducer within the microenvironment. Endothelial cells play a central role in vessel homeostasis by releasing factors regulating vessel tone, coagulation state, cell growth, cell death, and leukocyte trafficking. Vascular smooth muscle cells maintain the tone of blood vessels in response to vasoactive substances and, in turn, release cytokines and other regulatory factors. The pathogenesis of atherosclerosis involves a series of critical events, including endothelial dysfunction, infiltration of inflammatory cells into the vessel wall, alteration in vascular cell phenotype, and vascular remodeling.

Endothelial cell dysfunction is characterized by impairment in vasorelaxation and increased adhesiveness of the endothelial cell layer. Several lines of evidence suggest that endothelial cell dysfunction is associated with alterations in the cell redox state, while many of the risk factors associated with atherosclerotic vascular disease, such as diabetes, hyperlipidemia, and hypertension, are characterized by the presence of an oxidative insult.

Evidence supports the hypothesis that the oxidative modification of low-density lipoprotein (LDL) is a critical step in the pathogenesis of atherosclerosis (1). Oxidation of LDL in vitro leads to its enhanced uptake by a scavenger receptor on the surface of macrophages and subsequent foam cell formation (2,3).

Several immunocytochemical studies have indicated that oxidized LDL is generated in vivo. Proteins with physical, chemical, and immunological properties of oxidized LDL have been demonstrated to be present in atherosclerotic lesions of human and rabbit aorta (4). Furthermore, human and rabbit serum contain autoantibodies against oxidized LDL, and atherosclerotic lesions contain IgG specific for oxidized LDL (5). Moreover, an oxidatively modified LDL subfraction has been found in human subjects (6).

The proposed role of oxidized LDL in atherogenesis, based on studies in vitro, is shown in Figure 1. LDL, modified by oxidation, glycation, and aggregation, is considered a major cause of injury to the endothelium and underlying smooth muscle LDL, entrapped in the subendothelial space, can undergo progressive oxidation (minimally modified LDL, mm-LDL) and then can activate the

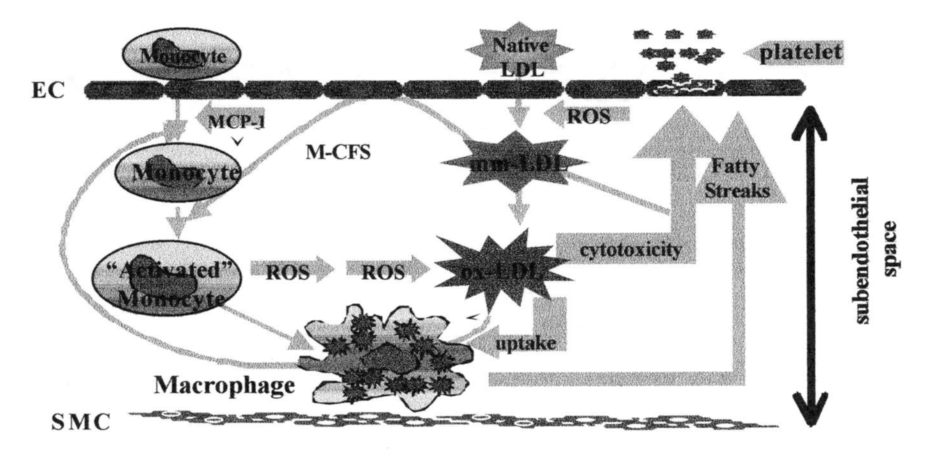

Figure 1 Sequence of events in atherogenesis and role of low-density lipoprotein. Native LDL, in the subendothelial space, undergoes progressive oxidation (minimally modified LDL, mm-LDL) and activates the expression of monocyte chemotactic protein (MCP-1) and monocyte colony-stimulating factor (M-CSF) in the endothelium (EC). MCP-1 and M-CSF promote the entry and maturation of monocytes to macrophages, which further oxidize LDL (ox-LDL). Ox-LDL is specifically recognized by the scavenger receptor of macrophages and, once internalized, formation of foam cells occurs. Both mm-LDL and ox-LDL induce endothelial dysfunction associated with changes of the adhesiveness to leukocytes or platelets and to wall permeability.

expression of molecules entitled for the recruitment of monocytes and for the stimulation the formation of monocyte colonies (monocyte chemotactic protein, MCP-1; monocyte colony-stimulating factor M-CSF) in the endothelium. These molecules promote the entry and maturation of monocytes to macrophages, which further oxidize LDL (ox-LDL). Modified LDL is also able to induce endothelial dysfunction, which is associated with changes of the adhesiveness to leukocytes or platelets and the wall permeability. Dysfunctioning endothelium also displays procoagulant properties and the expression of a variety of vasoactive molecules, cytokines, and growth factors.

LDL, oxidized in vitro by several cell systems or by cell-free systems (metal ions or azo initiators), is recognized by the scavenger receptor of macrophages (7). The increasing LDL affinity for the scavenger receptor is associated with changes in structural and biochemical properties of LDL, such as the formation of lipid hydroperoxides, oxidative modification, and fragmentation of apoprotein B-100 and an increase in negative charge (8).

The exact mechanism of LDL oxidation in vivo is still unknown, but transition metal ions, myeloperoxidase, lipoxygenase, and nitric oxide are thought to be involved (1).

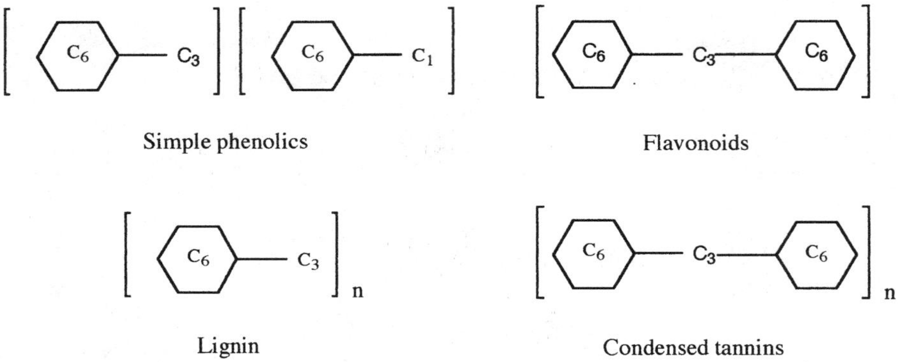

[C_6—C_3] [C_6—C_1]

Simple phenolics

[C_6—C_3—C_6]

Flavonoids

[C_6—C_3]$_n$

Lignin

[C_6—C_3—C_6]$_n$

Condensed tannins

Figure 2 Basic arrangement of carbon skeleton of plant phenols. (From Ref. 107.)

Several epidemiological studies have shown that increased dietary intake of natural phenolic antioxidants correlates with reduced coronary heart disease (9,10). Food antioxidants exert a twofold action: they prolong the shelf life of the product, protect its constituents during processing, and prevent the formation of toxic compounds. These foods also supply antioxidants to the human body, thus contributing to the antioxidant defense system.

Plants produce a large variety of secondary products containing a phenol group, i.e., a hydroxyl group on an aromatic ring. These compounds are a chemically heterogeneous group that includes simple phenols, flavonoids, lignin, and condensed tannins. The basic structures of the principal classes of plant phenols are schematized in Figure 2. Each phenolic class contains a number of compounds that are widely distributed in plants. The daily intake of flavonoids in Western countries has been estimated to be about 23 mg/d (11). No analogous calculation has been done for phenolic acids.

The growing interest in these compounds principally involves their antioxidant activity and their inhibitory effect on certain enzyme systems. In this chapter, the capacity of single purified compounds or plant/food phenolic components to modulate LDL susceptibility to oxidative modification will be reviewed, together with their activity in metabolic pathways other than in an antioxidant capacity.

II. IN VITRO AND EX VIVO MODULATION OF LDL OXIDATION BY PLANT PHENOLS

As described above, the susceptibility of LDL to oxidative modification is considered a key (even if still unclear) element in the atherosclerotic process. Since

LDL fatty acid composition and circulating level of antioxidants are the principal modulators of LDL oxidization (8), in the last decade a number of natural antioxidants have been tested to define their capacity to strengthen the resistance of LDL to oxidation both in vitro and ex vivo. In the in vitro studies, human LDL are oxidized by activated cells or by cell-free systems (metal ions or azo initiators) in the presence of antioxidants at micromolar concentration. In the ex vivo studies, the oxidation of the LDL is done after supplementation of subjects (humans or animals) with the test compound(s). It is evident that the ex vivo test gives a much more physiological and complete representation of the activity in vivo, taking into account bioavailability, metabolism, incorporation in LDL, and synergism with other compounds of the molecule(s) under study. As a consequence, the antioxidant effect ex vivo is often less dramatic than the effect observed in vitro. An example is given in Figure 3, showing (a) the in vitro inhibition of Cu(II)-catalyzed oxidation of human LDL by increasing concentrations of caffeic acid (21) and (b) the ex vivo inhibition of Cu(II)-catalyzed oxidation of rat LDL after 4-week supplementation with two caffeic acid–containing diets (31).

From these short considerations, it is possible to acknowledge that the in vitro activity in the LDL system can only be utilized to screen antioxidants and define their mechanism of action against oxidant species, while ex vivo studies can offer information of the likely activity in vivo.

The in vitro antioxidant capacity of phenols is generally ascribed to their reaction with oxidants to form resonance-stabilized phenoxyl radicals (12,13). In general, the antioxidant activity of a molecule is strengthened by the presence of a second hydroxyl group through the formation of an intramolecular hydrogen bond. Moreover, in the case of metal-catalyzed oxidation, the presence of the two hydroxyl groups in the *ortho* position produces the formation of the M^{+n}–phenolic acid complex, resulting in chelation of the metal anion (14).

A. Phenolic Acids

Phenolic acids (Fig. 4) are ubiquitous in plant food (i.e., fruits, vegetables, coffee) (15) either in the free form or glycosylated or esterified with quinic acid and organic acids.

The absorption of specific phenolic acids has been demonstrated in both rats and humans, and specific metabolites have been identified in human and rat urine (16,17). A Na^+-dependent, carrier-mediated transport across the brush border membrane of rat jejunum has been proposed (18).

The antioxidant activity of some of these small monomeric phenols has been studied in various model systems. Several phenolic derivatives of cinnamic and benzoic acids were studied for their capacity to reduce ferrylmyoglobin (19) and to inhibit oxidative modification of LDL induced by azoinitiators and by metal catalysts (20,21) or by ferrylmyoglobin and metmyoglobin (22,23). Me-

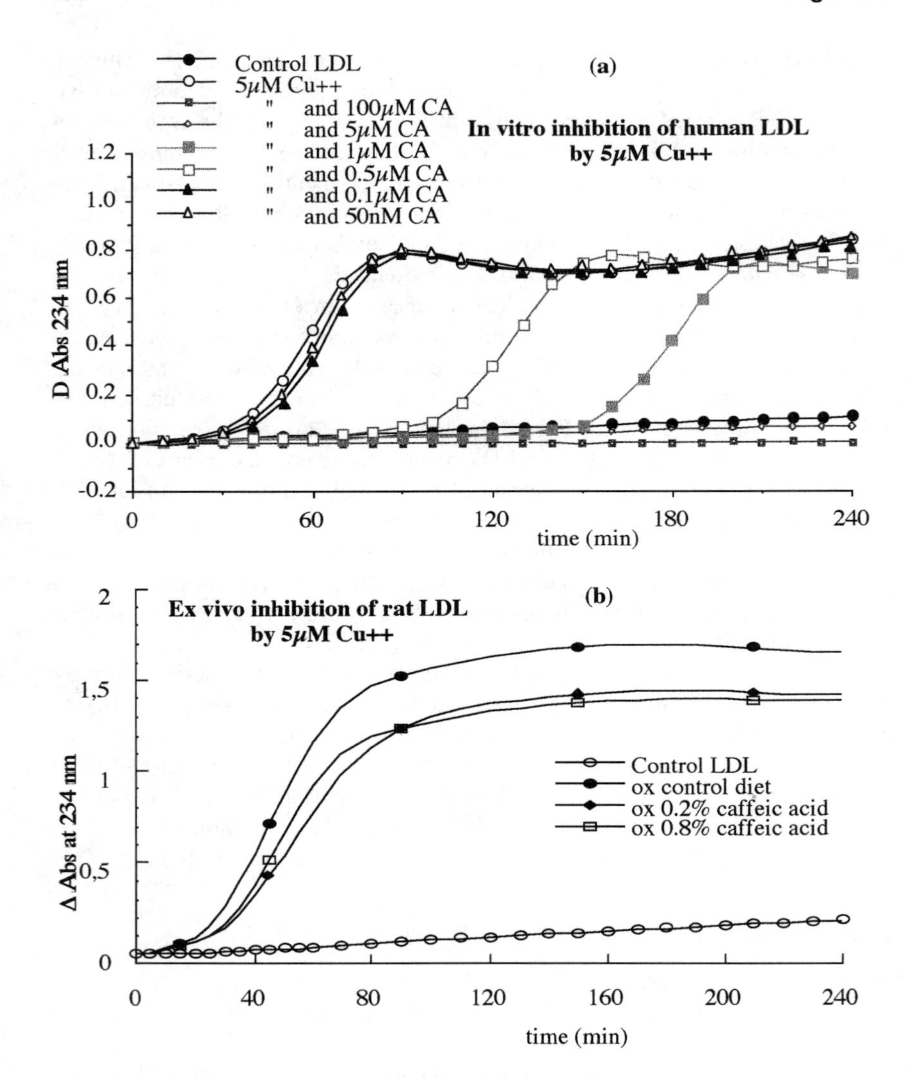

Figure 3 In vitro and ex vivo antioxidant effect of caffeic acid. (a) In vitro inhibition of human LDL by 5 μM Cu^{2+}. (b) Ex vivo inhibition of rat LDL by 5 μM Cu^{2+}.

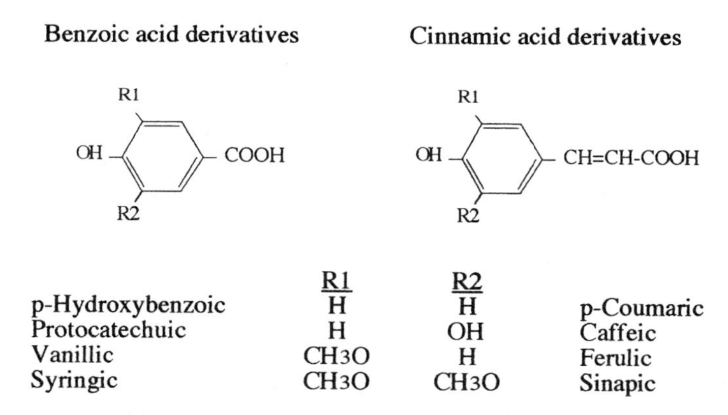

Figure 4 Chemical structure of the major phenolic acids.

thodical studies on a number of phenolic acids reported their ability to inhibit methyl linoleate (24) and lard oxidation (25) under strong oxidation conditions and their relative ability to scavenge the radical cation ABTS$^{\cdot}$ in the aqueous phase (26).

These studies indicate that the antioxidant activity in vitro of phenolic acids is related to their structure, namely the substitutions on the aromatic ring and structure of the side chain (27). In particular:

The antioxidant activity of the aromatic ring is enhanced by the presence of the propenoic side group (as in the case of the hydroxycinnamic acid derivatives), instead of the carboxylic group of benzoic acid derivatives, the conjugated double bond in the side chain having a stabilizing resonance effect on the phenoxyl radical.

The stability of the phenoxyl radical is further enhanced by the two methoxy groups, which increase the steric hindrance in the region of the radical, and the second hydroxyl group, which forms an intramolecular hydrogen bond.

The results of these studies point to the derivatives of cinnamic acid (mainly ferulic and caffeic acids) as being the most active phenolic acids, and several papers report the antioxidant capacity of these compounds in different model systems. Vieira et al. (28) found that caffeic and *p*-coumaric acids at micromolar concentrations synergistically interact in vitro with ascorbate in protecting LDL from oxidation promoted by ferrylmyoglobin. The same authors recently proposed that five naturally occurring phenolic acids (ferulic, protocatechuic, ellagic, *p*-coumaric, and caffeic) can prevent apoptosis of endothelial cells induced by coincubation with oxidized LDL. Among the compounds tested, caffeic acid was again the most protective. The antiapoptotic effect of caffeic acid results from (1) indirect antioxidant action, which prevents LDL oxidation and toxicity and (2) a direct cytoprotective effect, which blocks the intense and sustained cytosolic [Ca^{2+}] rise elicited by oxidized LDL (29). The ability of caffeic acid to affect the cellular response to *t*-butyl hydroperoxide–induced oxidative stress was studied in U937 human monocytic cells. Caffeic acid was incorporated into cells without any cytotoxic effect, and caffeic acid–treated cells showed an increased resistance to oxidative challenge, as revealed by a higher percent of survival and the maintenance of a higher proliferative capacity compared to control cells. This effect is probably due to the ability of caffeic acid to reduce glutathione depletion and to inhibit lipid peroxidation (30).

In addition, caffeic acid was found to have a role in vivo in antioxidant defenses of rats (31). Dietary supplementation of caffeic acid in rats resulted in a statistically significant increase of α-tocopherol in both plasma and lipoprotein. Moreover, caffeic acid was found to be present in postprandial plasma at micromolar concentrations, doubling the plasma antioxidant capacity. Lipoproteins from caffeic acid fed rats were more resistant to oxidation ex vivo than controls.

B. Flavonoids

The flavonoids, ubiquitous in plants, constitute a large class of compounds that contain a number of phenolic hydroxyl groups attached to a ring structure, conferring antioxidant activity. The differences among the compounds result from the variation in the number and arrangement of the hydroxyl groups as well as from the nature and extent of alkylation and/or glycosylation of these groups. The chemical skeleton of the main subclasses is shown in Figure 5.

Many studies have been undertaken to establish the structural criteria for the activity of polyhydroxy flavonoids in enhancing the stability of fatty acid dispersions, lipids, oils, and LDL (26,32). As for phenolic acids, the inhibition of oxidation by flavonoids is related to the chelation of metal ions via the *ortho*-dihydroxy phenolic structure, the scavenging of alkoxyl and peroxyl radicals, and the regeneration of α-tocopherol through reduction of the tocopheryl radical.

About 4000 plant substances belong to the flavonoid class, about 900 of which are present in the human diet. For this reason, the choice of the molecules to be studied for their capacity to exert an antioxidant action in vitro and ex vivo has been governed by three criteria: (1) general nutritional significance, i.e., occurrence in foods and beverages, as for catechins (flavanols), and quercetin (flavonol); (2) specific interest, i.e., occurrence in particular foodstuffs, such as licorice (glabridin); and (3) possible therapeutic significance, such as phenolics in traditional herbal medicine.

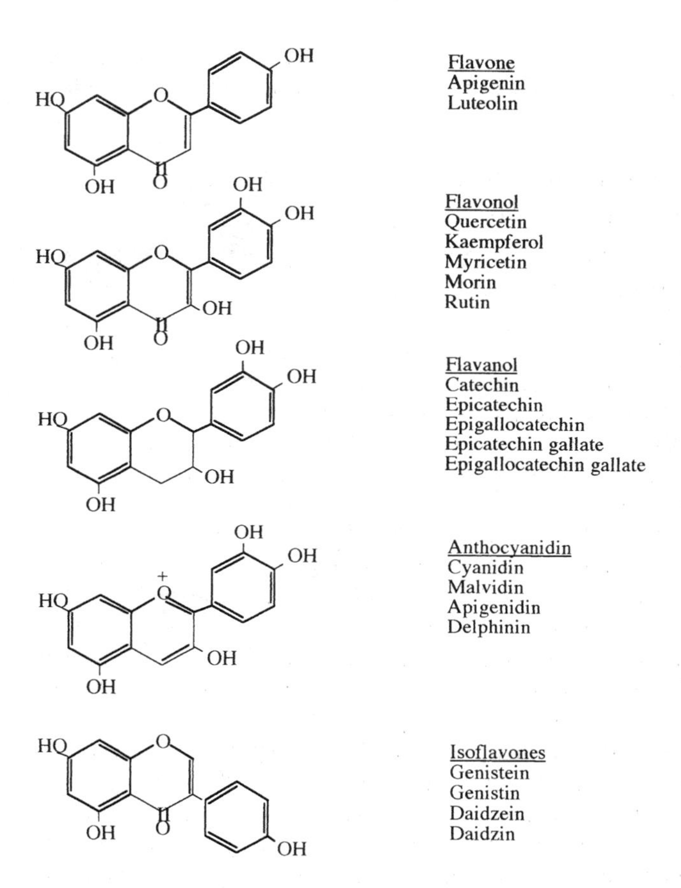

Figure 5 Carbon skeletons of major flavonoid types. (From Ref. 107.)

A number of studies have examined single flavonoids. These studies are useful in defining the relationship between structure and mechanism of action of the molecule. However, these studies may overestimate the importance of compounds with high antioxidant activity but with poor dietary impact, and they may underestimate the possible synergism between molecules. Finally, it is important to be aware that unknown "minor" components may modulate the biological activity.

On the basis of these considerations, the papers reporting the antioxidant activity of the phenolic component of (1) foods and beverages that are extensively used and studied, as in the case of tea, wine, and soybean and (2) plants with pharmacological interest (liquorice and sage) and plant extracts such as the extract from the bark of the French pine, *Pinus marittima* (Pycnogenol®) will be reviewed.

1. Tea (Catechin, Epicatechin, Epigallocatechin, Epicatechin Gallate, Epigallocatechin Gallate)

Green tea is a rich source of flavonoids, namely catechins and flavonols. In black tea, due to the fermentation process, catechins are converted to complex condensation products.

Tea flavonoids have been shown to act as antioxidants, according to the mechanism described above. With regard to in vitro LDL oxidation, gallate esters were found to be more efficient than the respective free forms in inhibiting oxidation catalyzed by Cu(II): epigallocatechin gallate > epicatechin gallate > catechin > epicatechin (33,34). In a metal-free system, all the compounds were effective as chain-breaking antioxidants except for epigallocatechin (35). Catechin and quercetin inhibited LDL oxidation induced by human monocyte–derived macrophages, lymphoid and endothelial cells, and protected lymphoid cells against cytotoxic effects of oxidized LDL. Catechin also inhibited the uptake and degradation of oxidized LDL by macrophages (36).

Recently, Lotito and Fraga demonstrated that the addition of (+)-catechin to human plasma prevents or delays its oxidation through the sparing of the endogenous antioxidants β-carotene and α-tocopherol (37).

The effect ex vivo of tea flavonoids on LDL susceptibility to oxidation depends on their absorption and partitioning into LDL and/or the subendothelial space. The data available are conflicting. In one case (38), consumption of six cups of green or black tea (900 mL/d for 6 weeks) had no significant effect on LDL resistance to copper-catalyzed oxidation. In another study, Ishikawa et al. (39) showed a small but significant increase in the lag time of LDL oxidation after 4 weeks of black tea consumption (600 mL/d).

These findings indicate that tea flavonoids act as strong inhibitors of LDL oxidation in vitro, while the assessment of activity either in vivo or ex vivo still needs further investigation. For an extensive review of tea flavonoids and cardiovascular diseases, see Ref. 40.

2. Wine (Phenolic Acids, Quercetin, Catechins, Anthocyanidins)

Wine, especially red wine, contains a wide range of polyphenols that have desirable biological properties. These include the phenolic acids (*p*-coumaric, cinnamic, caffeic, gentisic, ferulic, and vanillic), trihydroxy stilbenes (resveratrol and polydatin), and flavonoids (catechin, epicatechin, and quercetin). Polyphenols in grape vine are synthesized through a common pathway from phenylalanine involving polyketide condensation reactions. Metabolic regulation is provided by competition between resveratrol synthase and chalcone synthase for a common precursor pool of acyl-CoA derivatives. Polymeric aggregation in turn gives rise to the viniferins (potent antifungal agents) and procyanidins (strong antioxidants that also inhibit platelet aggregation).

The quantity and distribution of polyphenols into the different chemical classes vary with cultivar, area of production, agronomic techniques, vinification processes, vintage, age, etc.

The positive effect of red wine phenolics on the modulation of human LDL resistance against oxidative modification has been demonstrated in vitro (41). The antioxidant activity of wines in protecting LDL from oxidation is distributed widely among the principal phenolic classes, including catechin oligomers, procyanidin dimers and trimers, and the monomers catechin, epicatechin, and myricetin (42). Using liquid/liquid extraction Ghiselli et al. (43) obtained three fractions from an Italian red wine containing single polyphenolic subfractions: (1) phenolic acids and quercetin-3-glucuronide, (2) catechins and quercetin-3-glucoside, and (3) anthocyanins. The antioxidant activity of these fractions was compared with that of the original red wine before and after dealcoholization. The anthocyanin fraction was the most effective both in scavenging reactive oxygen species and in inhibiting lipoprotein oxidation. This higher activity was explained by both its high concentration in red wine and its antioxidant efficiency, which, at least for peroxyl radical scavenging, was three times as high as that of the other two fractions.

Another study (44) reports that in the presence of red wine or grape juice, LDL is significantly more resistant to oxidation in vitro than control LDL. Flavonoids, but not ethanol or nonflavonoid phenolic compounds, were reported to contribute to the antioxidant properties of red wine and grape juice.

While the activity of wine phenols in vitro is well known, data ex vivo after consumption of wine are controversial, probably due to variable experimental conditions. Fuhrman et al. (45) found that chronic red wine consumption (400 mL/d) reduced the susceptibility of LDL to lipid peroxidation catalyzed by copper. In contrast, consumption of 200 mL per day of red wine (46) or 550 mL per day of partially dealcoholized (3.5%) red wine (47) was not associated with protection from oxidation. A significant antioxidant activity was confirmed by Miyagi et al. (44) in LDL from humans after drinking red wine but not grape juice, suggesting that flavonoids in red wine may be absorbed more efficiently than those from grape juice. The discrepancies could be accounted for by a decreased intestinal absorption of polyphenols in the absence of alcohol or by the different quantities of wine consumed. Moreover, different oxidative conditions were utilized in different studies.

In a recent study, Carbonneau et al. (48) demonstrated that the supplementation of human volunteers with a phenolic extract from red wine led to a significant increase of plasma antioxidant capacity and of LDL vitamin E. This increase was not accompanied by any modification of LDL susceptibility to oxidation, suggesting that phenolic compounds localize in the aqueous phase of plasma and at the surface of lipoproteins.

3. Soybean (Genistein, Genistin, Daidzein)

Recently, soy isoflavones (12 different isomers including genistein, genistin, daidzein, daidzin, glycitein, glycitin, in free form and as glycosides) have been proposed to be responsible for the protective effect of a soy diet against chronic vascular diseases and early atherogenetic events.

In a study in vitro, genistein inhibited the oxidation of LDL by metal anion, superoxide/nitric oxide, and endothelial cells. Moreover, genistein protected endothelial cells from damage by oxidized lipoproteins, probably by blocking the upregulation of two tyrosine-phosphorylated proteins (49).

The feeding of a soy protein high-fat diet (isoflavones 21 g/100 g protein) to C57BL/6 mice (50) resulted in (1) reduction of plasma cholesterol levels, (2) increased resistance of LDL against oxidation, and (3) decrease of the atherosclerotic lesion area. The same effects were not observed in LDL receptor–deficient mice, suggesting that soy isoflavones might lower cholesterol levels by increasing LDL receptor activity.

The effect of soybean isoflavones on LDL oxidation resistance has been studied in human volunteers receiving three soy bars (containing 12 mg genistein and 7 mg daidzein) daily for 2 weeks (51). Plasma isoflavone level increased after supplementation, but less than 1% of the plasma isoflavones were associated with LDL. In spite of this, the resistance of LDL to copper-catalyzed oxidation was increased, suggesting that circulating isoflavones may promote the formation of ''modified'' LDL in vivo.

4. Other Phenolic Extracts (*Glycyrrhiza glabra*, *Salvia miltiorrhiza*, and *Pinus marittima*—Pycnogenol®)

Some recent papers demonstrate the use of phenolic extracts from plants (licorice, sage and pine bark) as antioxidants in studies in vitro and ex vivo.

Isoflavans isolated from licorice root (*Glycyrrhiza glabra*) protect LDL from oxidation. Glabridin (the major flavonoid constituent) inhibits LDL oxidation in vitro by inhibiting lipid peroxide and oxysterol formation and by protecting endogenous antioxidants in LDL (52,53). Experiments ex vivo (humans and apo E–deficient mice) showed that the feeding of licorice extract or glabridin rendered LDL more resistant to oxidation than controls. In addition, the consumption of licorice by apo E–deficient mice resulted in a reduction of the incidence and extent of atherosclerotic lesions in the aortic arch (54).

Sage (*Salvia miltiorrhiza*) is used in China and Japan in the treatment of cardiovascular diseases. The aqueous extract of sage contains phenolic compounds with antioxidant activity in biological systems (55). Feeding an atherogenic diet (high cholesterol) to NZW rabbits in the presence of the water-soluble extract of sage (5%) (1) reduced plasma cholesterol, (2) increased the α-tocopherol content of LDL and its resistance to oxidation, and (3) reduced endothelial damage and the extent of atherosclerotic lesions in the abdominal aorta, as compared to the control group (high cholesterol) (56).

Pine bark extract (Pycnogenol® PBE) has been reported to be an efficient scavenger of both the superoxide anion radical (57–59) and hydroxyl radical (55). The superoxide anion–scavenging activity of PBE studied by Virgili et al. (57) was reported as hundreds of units of SOD equivalents per mg. In the same investigation, the specific scavenging activity of PBE toward the hydroxyl radical, generated by the iron/ascorbate redox system was reported to be in the order of micromoles EPC-K1 (a water-soluble synthetic reference antioxidant) per milligram in solution. Both $OH^{\bullet}$ and $O_2^{-\bullet}$ scavenging activity were maintained after treatment with ascorbate oxidase, indicating that ascorbate, possibly present in the mixture, was not responsible for the antioxidant activity. On the other hand, $O_2^{-\bullet}$ scavenging activity was in part affected by ultrafiltration, implying that high molecular weight compounds present in the mixture contributed to the antioxidant activity. When compared to other phytochemicals and plant extracts, PBE was the highest ranking oxygen free radical scavenger (60). Another interesting possibility is that PBE flavonoids, as a result of their intermediate potential, may exert their activity within the cellular antioxidant network. Studies conducted on different cell lines (macrophages, endothelium) showed that incubation with PBE is associated with higher tocopherol levels both in normal conditions and following oxidative stress induced by reactive nitrogen species (61). These observations were confirmed in intact cells and in other ESR studies by Cossins and coworkers (62), indicating that PBE may prolong the ascorbyl radical lifetime. Nelson and collaborators have studied the capacity of PBE to protect LDL from copper-induced oxidation and have reported a dose-dependent decrease in lipid peroxide generation, starting at concentrations as low as 2 μg/mL (63). Nitric oxide (NO), a molecule that is attracting increasing interest as a free radical, becomes potentially harmful once its concentration overwhelms its neurotransmitter and second messenger functions. A study conducted in our laboratory has demonstrated that PBE significantly decreased, in a dose-dependent fashion, the accumulation of nitrite after the spontaneous decomposition of sodium nitroprusside, acting as a nitric oxide radical scavenger (57). PBE is composed of flavonoids, mainly procyanidins, like that of the grape seed extract, and it is therefore likely that these two mixtures display a similar spectrum of biological activities.

III. POLYPHENOLS AS MODULATORS OF CELLULAR RESPONSE

The contribution of flavonoids and phenolic acids to the prevention and possibly to the therapy of cardiovascular disease (CVD) can also be found on metabolic pathways other than antioxidation. As previously mentioned, CVD and atherosclerosis are characterized by early cellular events and by the dysregulation of normal cellular homeostasis (64). Molecular mechanisms by which polyphenols may play a role either in the etiopathology or in the pathophysiology of CVD will be discussed here, especially modulation of gene expression regulated by NF-κB activation and induction of either apoptotic or proliferative responses.

A. NF-κB and CVD

The transcription factors of the nuclear factor-κB/Rel family control the expression of a wide spectrum of different genes involved in inflammatory and proliferation responses. The typical NF-κB dimer is composed of the subunits p50 and p65, and it is present as its inactive form in the cytosol bound to the inhibitory proteins IκB. Following activation by various stimuli, including inflammatory or hyperproliferative cytokines, ROS and bacterial wall components, the phosphorylation and proteolytic removal of IκB from the complex occurs. The activated NF-κB immediately enters the nucleus, where it interacts with regulatory κB elements in the promoter and enhancer regions, thereby controlling the transcription of inducible genes (65,68).

NF-κB is a rapid pathway for transcriptional activation of various genes encoding cytokines, growth factors, adhesion molecules, and chemoattractant factors. Dysregulation of NF-κB control of gene expression has recently been reported in the pathogenesis of atherosclerosis (61,64,65). Oxidized LDL, a major component of the early and advanced atherosclerotic lesion (68), can modulate NF-κB activation. Incubation with minimally or more extensively oxidized forms of LDL activates NF-κB in endothelial cells and in macrophages (69,70). Oxidative stress and antioxidants have been reported to modulate the NF-κB system (65,71,72). Recently it has been proposed that H_2O_2 is a sort of second messenger molecule that can induce NF-κB activation (65).

Data reporting an effect of LDL, either native or oxidatively modified, on NF-κB activation and the role of this important regulatory pathway in the formation of the atheroma are still conflicting (see Ref. 73 for review). However, it is accepted that NF-κB is activated in monocyte-macrophages, in endothelial cells, and in smooth muscle cells in the early stages of the formation of an atherosclerotic lesion by stimuli such as IL-1, TNF-α, or modified LDL. Chronic exposure to oxidized LDL may be associated with inhibition of the NF-κB transcriptional system, leading to a dysregulation of gene expression.

B. Regulation of Gene Expression by NF-κB in CVD

A wide spectrum of different genes expressed in atherosclerosis have been shown to be regulated by NF-κB, including the genes encoding TNF-α, IL-1, the macrophage or granulocyte colony-stimulating factor (M/G-CSF), MCP-1, c-myc, and the adhesion molecules VCAM-1 and ICAM-1 (73). In the early stages of the atherosclerotic lesion, different types of cells (macrophages, smooth muscle cells, and endothelial cells) interplay, and when a shift from the normal homeostasis occurs, a vicious circle may be triggered, exacerbating dysfunction.

1. NF-κB in Macrophages

The material accumulated in the vessel wall during the formation of the lesion is removed by the phagocytic activity of macrophages (68). Macrophages are the principal inflammatory cell type in the atheroma microenvironment, where they interact with endothelial cells, smooth muscle cells, and T cells expressing a variety of genes such as those encoding TNF-α, IL-1, and ICAM-1, that are known to be regulated by NF-κB.

2. NF-κB in Smooth Muscle Cells

During lesion formation, smooth muscle cells change from a contractile to a synthetic phenotype, displaying fibroblast-like features and expressing several potential NF-κB target genes, such as those encoding M-CSF and MCP-1 (74).

3. NF-κB in Endothelial Cells

The expression of several adhesion molecules involved in the interaction of blood cells with the endothelium, such as ICAM-1, VCAM-1, or ELAM-1, has been shown to be regulated by NF-κB in cultured endothelial cells (65,75). Thus in vivo, dysfunction of the NF-κB system in regulating gene expression in endothelial cells may play an important role in the pathogenesis of atherosclerosis, especially in the early stages of the disease (68,75). Activated NF-κB may also modulate the endothelial cell production of chemoattractant substances, such as MCP-1, that attract macrophages to the lesion (75).

C. Flavonoids and Phenolic Acids and NF-κB Regulated Gene Expression

Even though no studies are yet available directly addressing the relationship between NF-κB activation in CVD and flavonoids or phenolic acids, some tentative conclusions can be inferred from experiments on the modulation of gene expression performed both in vivo and on cultured cells. In the scenario described above, polyphenols may play an important role either by directly affecting key steps in the activation pathway of NF-κB or by modulating the intracellular redox status, which is in turn one of the major determinants of NF-κB activation (75,77). Both complex mixtures of polyphenols (such as those extracted from the bark of the *Pinus marittima* or from *Ginkgo biloba* leaves) and purified molecules have been reported to affect gene expression in different cellular types. Preincubation with either the procyanidin-containing extract from the bark of the pine tree *Pinus marittima*, or Egb761, the extract from *Ginkgo biloba* leaves, has been reported to inhibit expression of the inducible form of the enzyme nitric oxide synthase in mouse macrophages activated by INF-γ and LPS (57,78). In both cases, no effect was observed on the activation of NF-κB, which is the main factor regulating the expression of this enzyme, suggesting that these complex mixtures of polyphenols possibly act at a post-transcriptional level on mRNA expression. Other purified polyphenols have been reported to affect the expression of adhesion molecules such as ICAM-1 in endothelial cells, and significantly decrease the adhesion of activated lymphocytes to endothelial cells (79–81). Figure 6 illustrates the regulation of NF-κB activation by oxidants/antioxidants. Some of major genes involved in the pathogenesis of CVD are also listed.

D. Other Aspects of Polyphenols as Modulators of Signal Transduction

Several studies have demonstrated that, depending on their structure, flavonoids may be inhibitors of several kinases involved in signal transduction, mainly protein kinase C (PKC) and tyrosine kinases (82–85). Agullo and collaborators (86) tested 14 flavonoids of different chemical classes and reported that myricetin, luteolin, and apigenin were efficient inhibitors of phosphatidylinositol 3-kinase, PKC, and tyrosine kinase activity. A structure-function study indicated that the position, number, and substitution of hydroxyl groups on the B ring and the saturation of C2-C3 bonds affect flavonoid activity on different kinases (86). Wolle and collaborators (79) examined the effect of flavonoids on endothelial cell expression of adhesion molecules. A synthetic flavonoid, 2-(3-amino-phenyl)-8-methoxy-chromene-4-one, an analog to apigenin, markedly inhibited TNF-α–induced VCAM-1 cell surface expression in a concentration-dependent fashion but had no effect on ICAM-1 expression. The inhibition correlated with decreases in steady-state mRNA levels, resulting in a reduction in the rate of gene transcription rather than changes in mRNA stability. No effects on NF-κB activation were observed either by mobility shift assay or by reporter gene assay, indicating that the modulation of VCAM-1 gene expression is due to a NF-κB–independent mechanism (79). Taken together, these studies opened an important issue in the ability of polyphenols to modulate the expression of genes responsible for pro-

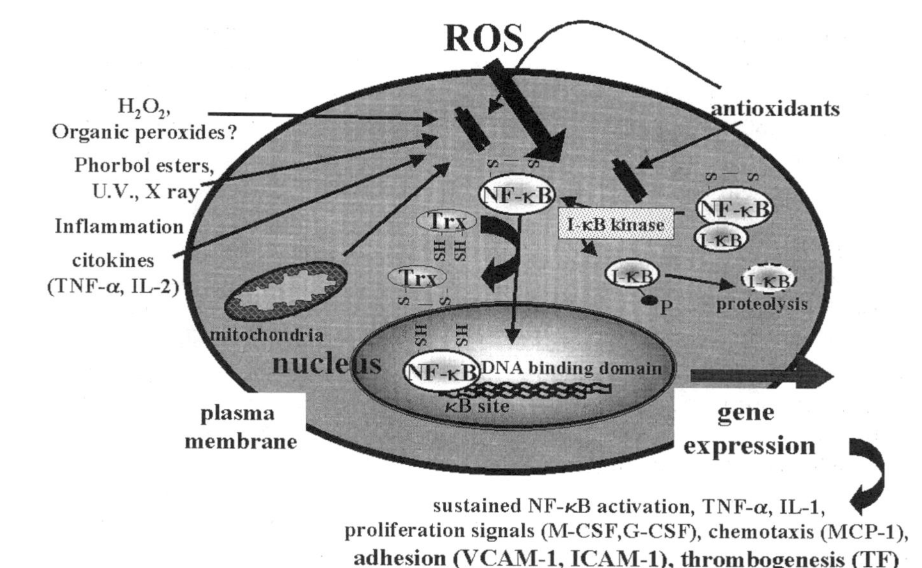

Figure 6 Simplified scheme of oxidant/antioxidant regulation of NF-κB activation. Different stimuli, leading to an increase of ROS generation inside the cell, activate the phosphorylation of IκB inhibitory protein and the subsequent proteolysis. Thioredoxin (Trx) may reduce activated NF-κB proteins, facilitating nuclear translocation. Once released from IκB, the NF-κB complex translocates into the nucleus and binds to DNA domain in the promoters and enhancers of genes such as TNF-α, IL-1, proliferation and chemotactic factors, adhesion molecule. Some of these genes, in turn, may further induce NF-κB activation, leading to a vicious circle if the regulatory cellular system escapes from control.

atherogenic processes with or without altering the activity of NF-κB, which can be considered fundamental for other cellular functions.

Hu et al. (87) reported that oncogene expression (c-myc, c-raf, and c-H-ras) in vivo, induced by nitrosamine treatment, is inhibited in mouse lung by tea drinking. The same authors also reported that topical pretreatment with the tea flavonoid (−)-epigallocatechin gallate significantly inhibits oncogene expression induced by PMA in mouse skin (87). Similarly, c-fos expression, cell growth, and PKC activity induced by PMA in NIH3T3 cells were inhibited by the natural flavonoid apigenin, as reported by Huang et al. (88). Green tea polyphenol extract stimulates the expression of detoxifying enzymes through antioxidant-responsive element in the cultured human hepatoma cell line HepG2 (89). This activity seems to be mediated by potentiation of the mitogen-activated protein kinases (MAPKs) signaling pathway, suggesting an indirect activity of polyphenols in the regulation of cellular responses to oxidative injury. Lin and coworkers (90) reported that both curcumin and apigenin inhibit PKC activity induced by PMA treatment in mouse skin. The same inhibitory effect can be observed in mouse isolated fibroblasts pretreated with curcumin. Also, apigenin, kaempferol, and genistein revert the transformation of the morphology of the v-H-ras transformed NIH3T3 line, and the authors suggest that both PKC activity and oncogene expression may be the mechanism by which polyphenols exert their antitumor activity (90). The flavonoid silymarin inhibits the expression of TNF-α mRNA induced by either 7,12 dimethylbenz(a)anthracene or okadaic acid (OA) in the SENCAR mouse skin model (91). This inhibitory activity, which is associated with a complete protection of mouse epidermis from tumor promotion by OA and results in a significant reduction (up to 85%) of tumor incidence induced by 7,12-dimethylbenz(a)anthracene (92), may also be relevant in the pathogenesis of CVD, since TNF-α plays a central role in the vicious circle of macrophage-endothelial cell dysfunction (73).

A review of the effects of flavonoids on immune and inflammatory cell functions, including macrophages, has been published by Middleton and Kandaswami (92), covering the matter from flavonoid activity, usually inhibitory, on secretory processes, mitogenesis, and cell-to-cell interaction. The same review included data on gene expression and cytokine effects. The authors point out that different cell types are not significantly affected by flavonoids while resting but become highly sensitive once activated. In other words, phenolics seem to have the ability to alter the outcome of the activation process either by interacting with molecules generated after the stimulus or by interfering with activation pathways (92).

The cell-to-cell interaction following the expression of adhesion molecules (ICAM-1, VCAM-1, and selectin) in endothelial cells induced by cytokine treatment has been reported to be blocked by hydroflavones and flavanols (93). Apigenin, the most potent flavone tested in this study, inhibited the expression of adhesion molecules, the expression of both interleukin-6 and interleukin-8 induced by TNF-α, and interleukin-1–induced prostaglandin synthesis. Apigenin was found to have no effect on the nuclear translocation of NF-κB, but it significantly inhibited the expression of the reporter gene β-galactosidase driven by NF-κB elements in SW480 cells induced by TNF-α, suggesting that NF-κB transcriptional activation was affected (93). Also the adhesion of cytokine-treated lymphocytes to endothelial cells was blocked by pretreatment of endothelial cells with apigenin (93). Finally, the same study reports apigenin to have a strong anti-inflammatory activity in vivo on carrageenin-induced rat paw edema and on delayed-type hypersensitivity in the mouse. Taken together, these data suggest that both flavonoids and phenolic acids may have important effects in diseases involving leukocyte adhesion and trafficking and oxidant-induced gene expression.

E. Polyphenols, Cell Proliferation, and Apoptosis

The effect of flavonoids on cell proliferation has been studied by Carrero et al. (94), who demonstrated that pure quercetin and a grape-derived beverage decreased the apoptotic response of lymphocytes in the presence of minimally oxidized LDL (mm-LDL) and restore both the utilization of cholesterol and the proliferating activity. As described earlier, Vieira and coworkers (29) reported that natural phenolic molecules, such as caffeic and ferulic acids, significantly inhibit apoptosis of human cultured endothelial cells induced by treatment with mildly oxidized LDL. The ability of phenolic acids in preventing LDL-induced apoptosis results from two different activities: an indirect protective effect due to the protection of LDL from oxidation and a direct cytoprotective activity.

Conversely, other authors demonstrated a pro-apoptotic activity of other flavonoids. A downregulation of c-myc and Ki-ras expression and a rapid reduction of the cellular concentration of inositol-1,4,5-triphosphate, associated with the activation of both apoptosis and differentiation programs, were reported by Csokay et al. (95) after a single treatment with micromolar concentrations of quercetin activate in K562 human leukemia cells. Plaumann and collaborators (96) reported that apigenin, luteolin, and quercetin induced the accumulation of p53 and apoptosis in the nontumor cell line C3H10T1/2CL8. The activity of baicalein, a flavonoid contained in the herbal medicine sho-saiko-to, has been tested by Matsuzaki et al. (97) in three different cell lines of human hepatocellular carcinoma. Treatment with baicalein strongly inhibited topoisomerase II activity and suppressed cell proliferation. Baicalein induced apoptosis in one cell line, while it was cytotoxic in the other two lines. Treatment with the naturally occurring citrus flavone tangeretin elicits differential response in tumor and normal cell lines. Tangeretin was reported to induce apoptosis in human promyelocytic leukemia HL-60 cells, while no cytotoxicity was observed when tested on normal human peripheral blood mononuclear cells (98). Similarly, catechin compounds (catechin, epigallocatechin, and epigallocatechin gallate) have been reported to induce programmed cell death in human lymphoid leukemia cells (99). These observations, though not all directly addressed to CVD, indicate that phenolic molecules can modulate uncontrolled cellular proliferation.

F. Indirect Evidence for Polyphenol Activity in CVD

An indirect effect of flavonoids and phenolic acids on NF-κB activation, and therefore on NF-κB–driven gene expression, may be inferred from two kinds of study: ones addressing the modulation of NF-κB activity by other antioxidant molecules (α-tocopherol, thiolic antioxidants such as *N*-acetylcysteine, lipoic acid, pyrrolidinedithiocarbamate), and others addressing the role of flavonoids and phenolic acids in the antioxidant network. α-Tocopherol and lipoic acid inhibit NF-κB in different cellular models (71,72,100), and several studies describe the ability of flavonoids and phenolic acids to exert a significant tocopherol and glutathione sparing effect either under basal homeostatic conditions or following oxidative challenge.

Roy and coworkers demonstrated that the adhesion of lymphocyte to endothelial cells is regulated by the thiolic antioxidant α-lipoic acid and by α-tocopherol (101). Similarly, an enhancement of the endogenous levels and a protective effect on α-tocopherol after peroxynitrite treatment by the procyanidin-containing extract from pine bark PBE was reported by Virgili et al. (61). The same complex mixture of procyanidins has been reported to enhance the activity of the enzymatic machinery, which regulates the GSH redox status in endothelial cells (102,103). In fact, a significant increase in GSH levels, an increased activity of the GSH redox enzymes (GSH reductase and GSH peroxidases), and an increase in the enzymatic activity of both SOD and catalase have been reported and proposed by Wei and collaborators to be mediated by an increase in protein synthesis (102).

Purified flavonoids and phenolic acids (quercetin, kaempherol, catechin, caffeic acid, and others) may enhance the cellular thiol content either under basal conditions or during oxidative stress, both in endothelial cells and in lymphocytes (Nardini et al., personal communications). This important role in the antioxidant network usually results in a greater resistance to pro-oxidant cytotoxicity and, in general, leads to a greater resistance of cells to dysfunction (64).

Proliferation of vascular smooth muscle cells is one of the most important features of atherosclerosis (74). Vascular smooth muscle cells display a unique susceptibility to antioxidants, which indicates that they respond differently than other types to changes in the redox status. In fact, hydrogen peroxide has been demonstrated to stimulate the proliferation of vascular smooth muscle cells while inhibiting the proliferation of vascular endothelial cells (104). However, the effect of antioxidants on smooth muscle cell proliferation is still unclear. α-Tocopherol inhibits the proliferation of smooth muscle cells by preventing the activation of PKC (105). Two structurally different thiol-containing compounds, NAC and PDTC, have been reported to induce apoptosis in cultured vascular smooth muscle cells in a dose- and time-dependent fashion (106). The overexpression of the proto-oncogene bcl-2 blocked PDTC- and NAC-induced apoptosis, suggesting that the thiol oxidation status within the cell plays an important role in switching on the apoptotic program.

IV. CONCLUSIONS

Nutrition can be a major determinant of human health. Recent findings on polyphenols support the philosophical concept that ''man is what he eats'' by demonstrating the ability of different nutritional components to significantly contribute to the maintenance of health and affect the pathophysiology of different diseases. Dietary consumption of polyphenols has been known for decades to be significantly associated with a lower risk of degenerative diseases. In particular, protection of serum lipids from oxidation, which is a major step in the development of atherosclerosis, has been demonstrated. Data reviewed here strongly suggest that polyphenols may significantly contribute to LDL protection from oxidation in vitro. The effect obtained from experiments performed ex vivo, i.e., the protection from oxidative damage of LDL isolated after dietary supplementation with polyphenols, appears much less dramatic. However, on a long-term basis (we could say on a lifelong term), this slight though significant effect is likely to result in a better preservation of the chemical and physical characteristics of lipoproteins, which in turn may result in a better regulation of vessel homeostasis and integrity. Even though the real significance of the oxidative modification of LDL fraction is not totally clear, a wide consensus has been reached in identifying the oxidative modification of lipoproteins as one of the earliest and major features in the pathogenesis of arteriosclerosis. Moreover, so far the protection of LDL from oxidative injury exerted by polyphenols has confirmed in vivo the hypothesis that the beneficial effect of certain dietary regimens, such as the so-called Mediterranean diet, is due, at least in part, to antioxidant activity.

New avenues have been more recently explored involving the capacity of polyphenols to interact with the expression of the human genetic potential. The present challenge for researchers is to fully understand the interaction between this heterogeneous class of compounds and cellular responses, due to their ability to affect the cellular antioxidant network or to directly affect gene expression. Some directions can be suggested to optimize the research, in consideration of the complexity of the phenolic components in plant foods and considering the major role played by nutrition.

Thus, the study of individual phenolic molecules, although useful in describing the structure-activity relationship defined above, has some problems: (1) overestimation of compounds with high antioxidant activity but poor dietary impact; (2) underestimation of synergism between molecules; and (3) lack of awareness of the action of "still unknown" compounds. For these reasons, investigations of the biological effects of complex mixtures of polyphenols from natural sources are warranted.

The main outcomes to be investigated would be the effect of plant extracts on:

- Antioxidant activity in vitro utilizing different model systems.
- The inhibitory/activating effect on key enzymes involved in the pathogenesis of atherosclerosis. In particular, enzymes regulating signal transduction and involved in phosphorylation of proteins such as PKC

and tyrosine protein kinase seem to be somehow modulated by different polyphenols.

- The ability to modulate redox-sensitive pathways of cellular response in endothelial cells, lymphocytes, and smooth muscle cells, such as NF-κB, AP-1, and other transcription factors sensitive to the cellular redox status in response to modified lipoproteins. Some data are already available on oxidatively modified LDL, while the cellular response to lipoproteins modified by the exposure to reactive nitrogen species is largely unknown.
- Regulation of gene expression by identifying target genes involved in the pathogenesis of CVD. Cytokines and adhesion molecules appear to be among the most important genes expressed during the pro-inflammatory situation that precedes the formation of the atheroma and have also been reported to be affected, at least in part, by phenolics.

These investigations should be paralleled by studies addressing the bioavailability of the extract of interest and eventually by the attempt to identify, through appropriate fractionation of the extract itself, the most active component(s) of the mixture. Such identification could open the avenue for the utilization of selected molecules at a pharmaceutical level, rather than for nutritional utilization.

ACKNOWLEDGMENTS

The authors thank S. Loukianoff and Eric Witt for help in editing the manuscript.

REFERENCES

1. Berliner JA, Heinecke JW. The role of oxidized lipoproteins in atherosclerosis. Free Rad Biol Med 1996; 20:707–727.
2. Witztum JL, Steinberg D. Role of oxidized low-density lipoprotein in atherogenesis. J Clin Invest 1991; 88:1785–1792.
3. Steinbrecher UP, Zhang HML. Role of oxidatively modified LDL in atherosclerosis. Free Rad Biol Med 1990; 9:155–168.
4. Palinski W, Yla-Herttuala S, Rosenfeld ME, Butler SW, Socher SA, Parthasarathy S, Curtiss LK. Antisera and monoclonal antibodies specific for epitopes generated during oxidative modification of LDL. Arteriosclerosis 1990; 10:325–335.
5. Yla-Herttuala S, Lipton BA, Rosenfeld ME, Sarkioja T, Yoshimura T, Leonard EJ, Witztum JL, Steinberg D. Macrophages express monocyte chemotactic protein (MCP-1) in human and rabbit atherosclerotic lesions. Proc Natl Acad Sci USA 1991; 88:5252–5256.
6. Avogaro P, Bittolo-Bon G, Cazzolato G. Presence of a modified low density lipoprotein in human. Arteriosclerosis 1998; 8:78–87.

7. Brown MS, Goldstein JL. Scavenging for receptors. Nature 1990; 343:508–509.
8. Esterbauer H, Gebiki J, Puhl H, Jurgens G. The role of lipid peroxidation and antioxidants in oxidative modification of LDL. Free Rad Biol Med 1992; 13:341–390.
9. Hertog MGL, Fesrens EJM, Hollman PCK, Katan MB, Kromhout D. Dietary antioxidant flavonoids and risk of coronary heart disease: the Zutphen elderly study. Lancet 1993; 342:1007–1011.
10. Stampfer MJ, Hennekens CH, Manson JE, Colditz GA, Rosner B, Willet WC. Vitamin E consumption and the risk of coronary disease in women. N Engl J Med 1993; 328:1444–1449.
11. Hertog MG, Hollman PH, Katan MB, Kromhout D. Intake of potentially anticarcinogenic flavonoids and their determinants in adults in the Netherlands. Nutr Cancer 1993; 20:315–347.
12. Baum BO, Perun AL. Antioxidant efficiency versus structure. Soc Plast Engrs Trans 1962; 2:250–257.
13. Stryer L. Biochemistry. San Francisco: Freeman, 1975.
14. Gordon MH. The mechanism of antioxidant action in vitro. In: Hudson BJF, ed. Food Antioxidant. London: Elsevier, 1990:1–18.
15. Herrmann K. Occurrence and content of hydroxycinnamic and hydroxybenzoic acid compounds in foods. Crit Rev Food Sci Nutrition 1989; 28:315–347.
16. Jacobson EA, Newmark H, Baptista J, Bruce WR. A preliminary investigation of the metabolism of dietary phenolics in human. Nutr Rep 1983; 28:1409–1417.
17. Booth AN, Emerson O, Jones FT, De Eds F. Urinary metabolites of caffeic and chlorogenic acids. J Biol Chem 1957; 229:51–59.
18. Wolffram S, Weber T, Grenacher B, Scharrer E. A Na^+-dependent mechanism in involved in mucosal uptake of cinnamic acid across the jejunal brush border in rats. J Nutr 1995; 125:1300–1308.
19. Laranjinha J, Almeida LM, Madeira VMC. Reduction of ferrylmyoglobin by dietary phenolic acids derivatives of cinnamic acid. Free Rad Biol Med 1995; 19: 329–337.
20. Laranjinha J, Almeida LM, Madeira VMC. Reactivity of dietary phenolic acids with peroxyl radicals: antioxidant activity upon low density lipoprotein peroxidation. Bochem Pharmacol 1994; 48:487–494.
21. Nardini MD, Aquino M, Tomassi G, Di Felice M, Scaccini C. Inhibition of human low-density lipoprotein oxidation by caffeic acid and other hydroxycinnamic acid derivatives. Free Rad Biol Med 1995; 19:541–552.
22. Laranjinha J, Vieira O, Madeira VMC, Almeida LM. Two related phenolic antioxidants with opposite effects on vitamin E content in low density lipoproteins oxidized by ferrylmyoglobin: consumption vs regeneration. Arch Biochem Biophys 1995; 323:373–381.
23. Castelluccio C, Paganga G, Melikian N, Bolwell GP, Pridham J, Sampson J, Rice-Evans C. Antioxidant potential of intermediates in phenylpropanoid metabolism in higher plants. FEBS Lett 1995; 368:188–192.
24. Cuvelier ME, Richard H, Berset C. Comparison of the antioxidant activity of some acid-phenols: structure-activity relationship. Biosci Biotech Biochem 1992; 56: 324–325.
25. Marinova EM, Yanishlieva NV. Inhibited oxidation of lipid II: comparison of the

antioxidative properties of some hydroxy derivatives of benzoic and cinnamic acids. Fat Sci Technol 1992; 11:428–432.

26. Rice-Evans CA, Miller NJ, Pananga G. Structure-antioxidant activity relationship of flavonoids and phenolic acids. Free Radic Biol Med 1996; 20:933–956.
27. Shahidi F, Wanasundara PKJ. Phenolic antioxidants. Crit Rev Food Sci Nutr 1992; 32:67–103.
28. Vieira O, Laranjinha J, Madeira V, Almeida L. Cholesteryl ester hydroperoxide formation in myoglobin-catalyzed low density lipoprotein oxidation: concerted antioxidant activity of caffeic and p-coumaric acids with ascorbate. Biochem Pharmacol 1998; 55:333–340.
29. Vieira O, Escargueil-Blanc I, Meilhac O, Basile JP, Laranjinha J, Almeida L, Salvayre R, Negre-Salvayre A. Effect of dietary phenolic compounds on apoptosis of human cultured endothelial cells induced by oxidized LDL. Br J Pharmacol 1998; 123:565–573.
30. Nardini M, Pisu P, Gentili V, Natella F, Di Felice M, Piccolella E, Scaccini C. Effect of caffeic acid on tert-butyl hydroperoxide induced oxidative stress in U937. Free Rad Biol Med 1998; 25:1098–1105.
31. Nardini M, Natella F, Gentili V, Di Felice M, Scaccini C. Effect of caffeic acid dietary supplementation on the antioxidant defense system in rat: an in vivo study. Arch Biochem Biophys 1997; 342:157–160.
32. Bors W, Heller W, Michel C, Saran M. Flavonoids as antioxidants: determination of radical-scavenging efficiency. Meth Enzymol 1990; 186:343–355.
33. Miura S, Watanabe J, Sano M, Tomita T, Osawa T, Hara Y, Tomita I. Inhibitory effects of tea polyphenols (flavan-3-ol derivatives) on Cu^{++}-mediated oxidative modification of low density lipoprotein. Biol Pharm Bull 1994; 17:1567–1572.
34. Vinson JA, Dabbagh YA, Serry MM, Jang J. Plant flavonoids, especially tea flavonoids, are powerful antioxidants using an in vitro model for heart disease. J Agric Food Chem 1995; 43:2800–2802.
35. Salah N, Miller NJ, Paganga G, Tijburg L, Bolwell GP, Rice-Evans C. Polyphenolic flavonoids as scavenger of aqueous phase radicals and as chain-breaking antioxidants. Arch Biochem Biophys 1995; 322:339–346.
36. Mangiapane H, Thompson J, Salter A, Brown S, Bell D, White DA. The inhibition of the oxidation of low-density lipoprotein by (+)catechin, a naturally occurring flavonoid. Biochem Pharmacol 1992; 43:445–450.
37. Lotito S, Fraga CG. (+)-Catechin prevents human plasma oxidation. Free Rad Biol Med 1998; 24:435–441.
38. Van het Hof KH, de Boer HS, Wiseman SA, Weststrate JA, Tijburg LBM. Consumption of green tea or black tea does not increase the resistance of LDL to oxidation in humans. Am J Clin Nutr 1997; 66:1125–1132.
39. Ishikawa T, Suzukawa M, Toshimitsu I, Yoshida H, Ayaori M, Nishiwaki M, Yonemura A, Hara Y, Nakamura H. Effect of tea flavonoid supplementation on the susceptibility of low-density lipoprotein to oxidative modification. Am J Clin Nutr 1997; 66:261–266.
40. Tijburg LBM, Mattern T, Folts JD, Weisgerber UM, Katan MB. Tea flavonoids and cardiovascular diseases: a review. Crit Rev Food Sci Nutr 1997; 37:771–785.

41. Frankel EN, Kanner J, German JB, Parks E, Kinsella JE. Inhibition of human LDL oxidation by phenolic substances in red wine. Lancet 1993; 341:454–457.
42. Frankel EN, Waterhouse AL, Teissedre PL. Principal phenolic phytochemicals in selected California wines and their antioxidant activity in inhibiting oxidation of human low density lipoproteins. J Agric Food Chem 1995; 43:890–894.
43. Ghiselli A, Nardini M, Baldi A, Scaccini C. Antioxidant activity of different phenolic fractions separated from an Italian red wine. J Agric Food Chem 1998; 46:361–367.
44. Miyagi Y, Miwa K, Inoue H. Inhibition of human low-density lipoprotein oxidation by flavonoids in red wine and grape juice. Am J Cardiol 1997; 80:1627–1631.
45. Fuhrman B, Lavy A, Aviram M. Consumption of red wine with meals reduces the susceptibility of human plasma and low density lipoprotein to lipid peroxidation. Am J Clin Nutr 1995; 61:549–554.
46. Sharpe PC, McGrath L, McClean E, Young IS, Archbold GP. Effect of red wine consumption on lipoprotein (a) and other risk factors for atherosclerosis. Q J M 1995; 82:101–108.
47. de Rijke YB, Demacker PNM, Assen NA, Sloots LM, Katan MB, Stalenhoef AFH. Red wine consumption does not affect oxidizability of low-density lipoproteins in volunteers. Am J Clin Nutr 1995; 63:329–334.
48. Carbonneau MA, Leger CL, Monnier L, Bonnet C, Michel F, Fouret G, Dediue F, Descomps B. Supplementation with wine phenolic compounds increases the antioxidant capacity of plasma and vitamin E of low-density lipoprotein without changing the lipoprotein Cu(II) oxidizability: possible explanation by phenolic location. Eur J Clin Nutr 1997; 51:682–690.
49. Kapiotis S, Hermann M, Held I, Seelos C, Ehringer H, Gmeiner BM. Genistein, the dietary-derived angiogenesis inhibitor, prevents LDL oxidation and protects endothelial cells from damage by atherogenic LDL. Arterioscler Thromb Vasc Biol 1997; 17:2868–2874.
50. Kirk EA, Sutherland P, Wang SA, Chait A, LeBoeuf RC. Dietary isoflavones reduce plasma cholesterol and atherosclerosis in C57BL/6 mice but not LDL receptor-deficient mice. J Nutr 1998; 128:954–959.
51. Tikkanen MJ, Wahala K, Ojala S, Vihma V, Adlercreutz H. Effect of soybean phytoestrogen intake on low density lipoprotein oxidation resistance. Proc Natl Acad Sci USA 1998; 95:3106–3110.
52. Vaya J, Belinky P, Aviram M. Antioxidant constituents from licorice roots: isolation, structure elucidation and antioxidative capacity toward LDL oxidation. Free Radic Biol Med 1997; 23:302–313.
53. Belinky P, Aviram M, Fuhrman B, Rosenblat M, Vaya J. The antioxidative effects of the isoflavan glabridin on endogenous constituents of LDL during its oxidation. Atherosclerosis 1998; 137:49–61.
54. Fuhrman B, Buch S, Vaya J, Belinky P, Coleman R, Hayek T, Aviram M. Licorice extract and its major polyphenol glabridin protect low-density lipoprotein against lipid peroxidation: in vitro and ex vivo studies in humans and in atherosclerotic apolipoprotein E-deficient mice. Am J Clin Nutr 1997; 66:267–275.
55. Liu GT, Zhang TM, Wang BE, Wang YW. Protective action of seven natural phe-

nolic compounds against peroxidative damage to biomembranes. Biochem Pharmacol 1992; 43:147–152.

56. Wu YJ, Hong CH, Lin SJ, Wu P.; Shiao MS. Increase of vitamin E content in LDL and reduction of atherosclerosis in cholesterol-fed rabbits by a water-soluble antioxidant-rich fraction of *Salvia miltiorrhiza*. Arterioscler Thromb Vasc Biol 1998; 18:481–486.
57. Virgili F, Kobuchi H, Packer L. Procyanidins extracted from *Pinus maritima* (Pycnogenol®): scavengers of free radical species and modulators of nitrogen monoxide metabolism in activated murine RAW 264.7 macrophages. Free Rad Biol Med 1998; 24:1120–1129.
58. Blazso G, Gabor M, Sibbel R, Rohdewald P. Antiinflammatory and superoxide radical scavenging activities of procyanidins containing extract from the bark of *Pinus pinaster* Sol. and its fractions. Pharm Pharmacol 1994; 3:217–220.
59. Elstner EF, Kleber E. Radical scavenger properties of leucocyanidine. In: Das NP, ed. Flavonoids in Biology and Medicine III: Current Issues in Flavonoids Research. Singapore: National University of Singapore Press, 1990:227–235.
60. Noda Y, Anzai K, Mori A, Kohno M, Shinmei M, Packer L. Hydroxyl and superoxide anion radical scavenging activities of natural source of antioxidants using the computerized JES-FR30 ESR spectrometer system. Biochem Mol Biol Int 1997; 42:35–44.
61. Virgili F, Kim D, Packer L. Procyanidins extracted from pine bark protect α-tocopherol in ECV 304 endothelial cells challenged by activated RAW 264.7 macrophages: role of nitric oxide and peroxynitrite. FEBS Lett 1998; 431:315–318.
62. Cossins E, Lee R, Packer L. ESR studies of vitamin C regeneration, order of reactivity of natural source phytochemical preparations. Biochem Mol Biol Int 1998; 45: 583–598.
63. Nelson AB, Lau BHS, Ide N, Rong Y. Pycnogenol inhibits macrophage oxidative burst, lipoprotein oxidation and hydroxil radical induced DNA damage. Drug Dev Indust Med 1998; 24:1–6.
64. Gibbons GH, Dzau VJ. Molecular therapies for vascular disease. Science 1996; 272:689–693.
65. Baeuerle PA, Henkel T. Function and activation of NF-κB in the immune system. Ann Rev Immunol 1994; 12:141–179.
66. Baldwin ASJ. The NF-κB and IκB proteins: new discoveries and insights. Ann Rev Immunol 1996; 14:649–681.
67. Brand K, Page S, Rogler G, Bartsch A, Brandl R, Knuechel R, Page M, Kaltschmidt C, Baeuerle PA, Neumeier D. Activated transcription factor NF-κB is present in the atherosclerotic lesion. J Clin Invest 1996; 97:1715–1722.
68. Berliner JA, Navab M, Fogelman AM, Frank JS, Demer LL, Edwards PA, Watson AD, Lusis AJ. Atherosclerosis: basic mechanisms—oxidation, inflammation and genetics. Circulation 1995; 91:2488–2496.
69. Rajavashisth TB, Yamada H, Mishra NK. Transcriptional activation of macrophage stimulating factor gene by minimally modified LDL. Atherioscler Thromb Vasc Biol 1995; 15:1591–1598.
70. Peng HP, Rajavashisth TB, Libby P, Liao JK. Nitric oxide inhibits macrophage

stimulating colony factor gene transcription in vascular endothelial cells. J Biol Chem 1995; 270:17050–17055.
71. Suzuki YJ, Packer L. Inhibition of NF-κB activation by vitamin E derivatives. Biochem Biophys Res Commun 1993; 193:277–283.
72. Suzuki YJ, Aggarwal BB, Packer L. Alpha-lipoic acid is a potent inhibitor of NF-κB activation in human T cells. Biochem Biophys Res Commun 1992; 189:1709–1715.
73. Brand K, Page S, Walli AK, Neumaier D, Baeuerle PA. Role of nuclear factor κB in atherogenesis. Exp Physiol 1997; 82:297–304.
74. Ross R. The pathogenesis of atherosclerosis: a perspective for the 90s. Nature 1993; 362:529–532.
75. Collins T. Endothelial nuclear factor κB and the initiation of the atherosclerotic lesion. Lab Invest 1993; 68:499–508.
76. Sen CK, Packer L. Antioxidant and redox regulation of gene expression. FASEB J 1996; 10:709–720.
77. Suzuki YJ, Forman HJ, Sevanian A. Oxidants as stimulators of signal transduction. Free Rad Biol Med 1997; 22:269–285.
78. Kobuchi H, Droy-Lefaix MT, Christen Y, Packer L. *Ginkgo biloba* extract (EGb761): inhibitory effect on nitric oxide production in the macrophage cell line RAW 264.7. Biochem Pharmacol 1997; 53:897–903.
79. Wolle J, Hill RR, Ferguson E, Devall LJ, Trivedi BK, Newton RS, Saxena U. Selective inhibition of tumor necrosis factor-induced vascular cell adhesion molecule-1 gene expression by a novel flavonoid. Lack of effect on transcriptional factor NF-κB. Arterioscler Thromb Vasc Biol 1996; 16:1501–1508.
80. Panes J, Gerritsen ME, Anderson DC, Miyasaka M, Granger DN. Apigenin inhibits TNF-induced intercellular adhesion molecule-1 upregulation in vivo. Microcirculation 1996; 3:279–286.
81. Gerritsen ME, Carley WW, Ranges GE, Shen CP, Phan SA, Ligon GF, Perry CA. Flavonoids inhibit cytokine induced endothelial cell adhesion protein gene expression. Am J Pathol 1995; 147:278–292.
82. Middleton EJ, Kandashwami C. The impact of plant flavonoids on mammalian biology: implications for immunity, inflammation and cancer. In: Harborne JH, Liss AR, eds. The Flavonoids: Advances in Research Since 1986. New York: 1993: 619–652.
83. Ferriola PC, Cody V, Middleton E. Protein kinase C inhibition by plant flavonoids. Kinetic mechanisms and structure activity relationship. Biochem Pharmacol 1989; 38:1617–1624.
84. Cushman M, Nagarathman D, Burg DL, Geahlen RL. Synthesis and protein-tyrosine kinase inhibitory activity of flavonoid analogues. J Meed Chem 1991; 34:798–806.
85. Hagiwara M, Inoue S, Tanaka T, Nunoki K, Ito M, Hidaka H. Differential effects of flavonoids as inhibitors of tyrosine protein kinases and serine/threonin protein kinases. Biochem Pharmacol 1988; 37:2987–2992.
86. Agullo G, Gamet-payrastre L, Manenti S, Viala C, Remesy C, Chap H, Payrastre B. Relationship between flavonoid structure and inhibition of phosphatidylinositol

3-kinase: a comparison with tyrosine kinase and protein kinase C inhibition. Biochem Pharmacol 1997; 53:1649–1657.
87. Hu G, Han C, Chen J. Inhibition of oncogene expression by green tea and (−)-epigallocatechin gallate in mice. Nutr Cancer 1995; 24:203–209.
88. Huang YT, Kuo ML, Liu JY, Huang SY, Lin JK. Inhibition of protein kinase C and proto-oncogene expression in NIH 3T3 cells by apigenin. Eur J Cancer 1996; 32A:146–151.
89. Yu R, Jiao JJ, Duh JL, Gudehithlu K, Tan TH, Kong AN. Activation of mitogen-activated protein kinases by green tea polyphenols: potential signaling pathways in the regulation of antioxidant responsive elements-mediated phase II enzyme gene expression. Carcinogenesis 1997; 18:451–456.
90. Lin JK, Chen YC, Huang YT, Lin-Shiau SY. Suppression of protein kinase C and nuclear oncogene expression as possible molecular mechanisms of cancer chemoprevention by apigenin and curcumin. J Cell Biochem Suppl 1997; 28–29:39–48.
91. Zi X, Mukhtar H, Agarval R. Novel cancer chemopreventive effects of a flavonoid antioxidant silymarin: inhibition of mRNA expression of an endogenous tumor promoter TNF alpha. Biochem Biophys Res Comm 1997; 239:334–339.
92. Middleton EJ, Kandashwami C. Effects of flavonoids on immune and inflammatory cell functions. Biochem Pharmacol 1992; 43:1167–1179.
93. Gerritsen ME, Carley WW, Ranges GE, Shen CP, Phan SA, Ligon GF, Perry CA. Flavonoids inhibit cytokine-induced endothelial cell adhesion protein gene expression. Am J Pathol 1995; 147:278–292.
94. Carrero P, Ortega H, Martinez-Botas J, Gomez-Coronado D, Lasuncion MA. Flavonoid-induced ability of minimally modified low-density lipoproteins to support lymphocyte proliferation. Biochem Pharmacol 1998; 55:1125–1129.
95. Csokay B, Prajda N, Weber G, Olah E. Molecular mechanisms in the antiproliferative action of quercetin. Life Sci 1997; 60:2157–2163.
96. Plaumann B, Fritsche M, Rimpler H, Brandner G, Hess RD. Flavonoids activate wild-type p53. Oncogene 1996; 13:1605–1614.
97. Matsuzaki Y, Kurokawa N, Terai S, Matsumura Y, Kobayashi N, Okita K. Cell death induced by baicalein in human hepatocellular carcinoma cell lines. Jpn J Cancer Res 1996; 87:170–177.
98. Hirano T, Abe K, Gotoh M, Oka K. Citrus flavone tangeretin inhibits leukaemic HL-60 cell growth partially through induction of apoptosis with less cytotoxicity on normal lymphocytes. Br J Cancer 1995; 72:1380–1388.
99. Hisabami H, Achiwa Y, Fujikawa T, Komiya T. Induction of programmed cell death (apoptosis) in human lymphoid leukemia cells by catechin compounds. Anticancer Res 1996; 16:1943–1946.
100. Adcock IM, Brown CR, Kwon O, Barnes PJ. Oxidative stress induces NF-κB DNA binding and inducible NOS mRNA in human epithelial cells. Biochem Biophys Res Comm 1994; 199:1518–1524.
101. Roy S, Sen CK, Kobuchi H, Packer L. Antioxidant regulation of phorbol ester-induced adhesion of human Jurkat T-cells to endothelial cells. Free Rad Biol Med 1998; 25:229–241.
102. Wei Z, Peng Q, Lau BHS. Pycnogenol enhances endothelial cell antioxidant defences. Redox Rep 1997; 3:147–155.

103. Rimbach G, Virgili F, Packer L. Effect of reactive nitrogen species on GSH levels in endothelial cells: role of kinetic mode of generation and protection by flavonoids. Redox Rep 1999; 4:171–177.
104. Rao GN, Berk BC. Active oxygen species stimulate vascular smooth muscle cell growth and proto-oncogene expression. Circ Res 1992; 70:593–599.
105. Tasinato AD, Boiscoboinik D, Bartoli GM, Maroni P, Azzi A. d-α-tocopherol inhibition of vascular smooth muscle cell proliferation occurs at physiological concentrations, correlates with protein kinase C inhibition, and is independent of its antioxidant properties. Proc Natl Acad Sci 1995; 92:12190–12194.
106. Tsai J-C, Jain M, Hsieh C-M, Lee W-S, Yoshizumi M, Patterson C, Perrella MA, Cooke C, Wang H, Haber E, Schlegel R, Lee M-E. Induction of apoptosis by pyrrolidinedithiocarbamate and N-acetylcysteine in vascular smooth muscle cells. J Biol Chem 1996; 271:3667–3670.
107. Taiz L, Zeiger E. Plant Physiology. Redwood City, CA: The Benjamin/Cummings Publishing Co. Inc., 1991.

12

L(−)-Carnitine and Its Precursor, γ-Butyrobetaine

Hermann Seim
Institute of Clinical Chemistry and Pathobiochemistry, University of Leipzig, Leipzig, Germany

Knut Eichler
BASF Aktiengesellschaft, Ludwigshafen, Germany

Hans-Peter Kleber
Institute of Biochemistry, University of Leipzig, Leipzig, Germany

I. INTRODUCTION

L(−)-Carnitine, a name derived from the Latin *carnis* (flesh), is a hygroscopic and extremely water-soluble compound ubiquitous in nature. The history of L(−)-carnitine research has extended over this century (Table 1). L(−)-Carnitine was first isolated from meat extracts in 1905 (1), and soon after, its chemical formula ($C_7H_{15}NO_3$) was proposed. In spite of many studies on the biological effects of L(−)-carnitine, its function remained unclear for half a century. Because of the vitamin-like properties of L(−)-carnitine in the mealworm *Tenebrio molitor*, the name vitamin B_T was created (3), but soon after it was found that microorganisms and higher animals are also able to synthesize L(−)-carnitine by themselves (7,8,17). Hence, the assumption upon which L(−)-carnitine was included among the vitamins failed. Further investigations demonstrated a function for L(−)-carnitine in the β-oxidation of fatty acids (18). It was shown that this quaternary ammonium compound is essential for the transport of long-chain fatty acids through the inner mitochondrial membrane of mammals. In 1962 the configuration of the physiological enantiomer was determined (9) and in 1997 confirmed as L(−)- or R(−)-3-hydroxy-4-*N*,*N*,*N*-trimethylaminobutyrate (19). The discov-

Table 1 History of Carnitine Research

1905	Isolation of carnitine from muscle (1)
1927	Elucidation of structure of carnitine (2)
1952	Carnitine was shown to be a vitamin (B_T) for mealworm (*Tenebrio molitor*) (3,4)
1955	Discovery of reversible enzymatic acetylation of carnitine by the carnitine acetyltransferase in liver (5): Acetyl-CoA + L(−)-carnitine → acetyl-L(−)-carnitine + CoA L(−)-Carnitine was shown to stimulate long-chain fatty acid oxidation in liver homogenates (6)
1961	Evidence of γ-butyrobetaine as precursor of L(−)-carnitine (7,8)
1962	Determination of configuration of the physiological enantiomer L(−)-carnitine (9)
1962–1963	Fatty acid esters of carnitine were shown to be intermediates in fatty acid oxidation; discovery of carnitine palmitoyltransferase (CPT), which catalyzes the reaction: Palmitoyl-CoA + L(−)-carnitine → palmitoyl-L(−)-carnitine + CoA and the postulate of its role in fatty acid oxidation (10–13)
1966	Evidence of localization of CPT (inner mitochondrial membrane) and acyl-CoA synthetase (outer mitochondrial membrane) (14,15)
1970	Detection of formation of branched chain acylcarnitines (16)
1971	Role of lysine in carnitine biosynthesis in *Neurospora crassa* was elucidated (17)
1973	Inborn errors in carnitine metabolism were found (20,21)
1975	Report on the existence of the carnitine carrier, the carnitine acylcarnitine translocase (22,23)
1977	Evidence of malonyl-CoA as inhibitor of CPT I (24)
1981	Purification of γ-butyrobetaine hydroxylase, the last enzyme in the biosynthetic pathway of L(−)-carnitine (25)
1987	CPT I was shown to be localized in the outer membrane of the mitochondria (26)
1988–1998	Cloning and sequencing of genes of carnitine acyltransferases (28–32)
1995	Evidence for the function of L(−)-carnitine in the transfer of acyl groups from the peroxisomes to the mitochondria (33)

ery that L(−)-carnitine is ultimately derived from the essential amino acid lysine (17,27) and the description of human carnitine deficiency syndromes of apparent genetic origin (20), were the impetus for extensive investigation into its metabolism, function, and applications. These studies led not only to a series of clinical applications of L(−)-carnitine but also to the idea of its use as a nutraceutical.

Cheap, racemic D,L(−)-carnitine can no longer be applied because the D-enantiomer is not as harmless as was assumed in the past (34). Thus, D(+)-

carnitine is bound and transported by the active L(−)-carnitine transport system of cell membranes, thereby diminishing L(−)-carnitine within the cells and inhibiting L(−)-carnitine–specific reactions.

The growing demand for L(−)-carnitine, particularly in medicine and as a nutraceutical, has caused a worldwide search for ways of synthesizing this betaine in an optically pure form. Therefore, besides chemical synthesis, microbiological and enzymatic procedures have also been developed in the last years for the production of enantiomerically pure L(−)-carnitine (35).

II. PHYSIOLOGY AND BIOCHEMISTRY

A. Biosynthesis

Although the ability to synthesize L(−)-carnitine seems to be nearly as ubiquitous as L(−)-carnitine itself, the pathway has been studied most extensively in the rat. The first clues to the mechanism of carnitine biosynthesis were obtained in 1961 (Table 1), when it was shown that γ-butyrobetaine is converted to L(−)-carnitine (7,8,36). The precursors of L(−)-carnitine are the two essential amino acids lysine and methionine (37) (Fig. 1). In *Neurospora crassa* free lysine is methylated with S-adenosylmethionine as the methyl donor (38,39). In animals, however, 6-*N*-trimethyllysine is formed by the methylation of lysine residues in proteins such as myosin, actin, histones, cytochrome *c*, and calmodulin (40,41). 6-*N*-Trimethyllysine is hydrolyzed from the proteins in the lysosome (42) and transported to the cytosol, where it is hydroxylated at carbon 3 by 6-*N*-trimethyllysine-3-hydroxylase (43). The product 3-hydroxy-6-*N*-trimethyllysine is converted to γ-trimethylaminobutyraldehyde by the 3-hydroxy-6-*N*-trimethyllysine aldolase, a pyridoxal phosphate-dependent enzyme (44). This enzyme apparently is identical to serine hydroxymethyltransferase (43). The resulting aldehyde is then oxidized by one of several NAD^+-linked cytosolic aldehyde dehydrogenases (including one apparently specific for this substrate) to form γ-butyrobetaine (44,45) (Fig. 1). The latter is hydroxylated at carbon 3 by γ-butyrobetaine hydroxylase [4-trimethylaminobutyrate, 2-oxoglutarate: oxygen oxidoreductase (3-hydroxylating)]. This enzyme belongs to a class of nonheme ferrous iron dioxygenases in which the hydroxylation of the substrate is linked to the oxidative decarboxylation of 2-oxoglutarate. These enzymes require Fe^{2+} and a reducing cofactor, e.g., ascorbate, and are stimulated by catalase. The trimethyllysine-3-hydroxylase is also a member of this class of enzymes.

All enzymes in the pathway of L(−)-carnitine biosynthesis are ubiquitous in mammalian tissues except γ-butyrobetaine hydroxylase. This enzyme is present only in a few tissues, and it also shows species variations in tissue distribution. In all species it is found in the liver (18). In the rat it is also found to a small extent in the testis, but it is absent from all other tissues (46–48). In humans

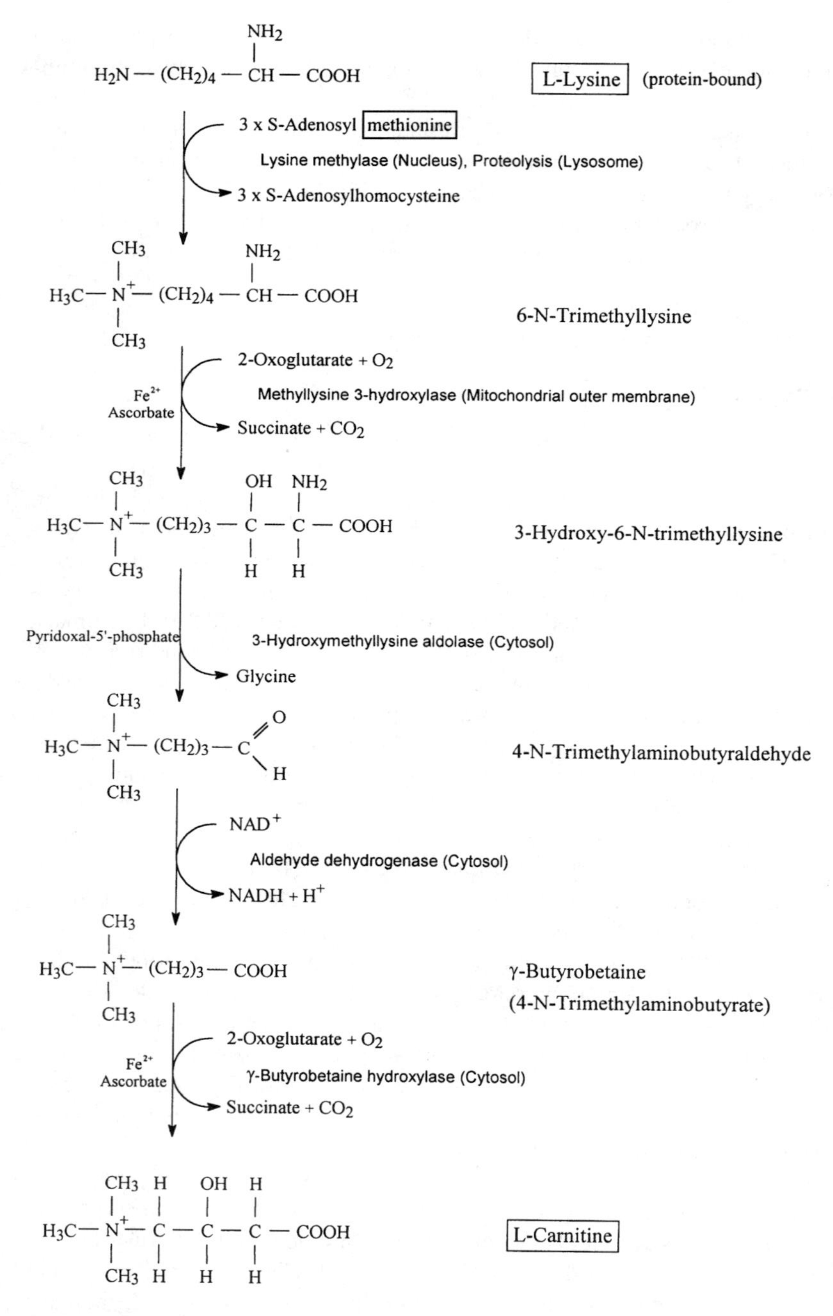

Figure 1 Biosynthesis of L(−)-carnitine.

γ-butyrobetaine hydroxylase is present in liver, kidney, and brain but not in skeletal muscle or heart (41,44,49). Most of the carnitine is found in skeletal muscle [about 1 mM in rat (50), 3 mM in humans (51)], with the highest concentration in epididymis [up to 80 mM, varying with species (52)], yet it is formed mainly in the liver. Therefore, it is evident that an exensive transport and redistribution of carnitine takes place.

The normal rate of L(−)-carnitine biosynthesis in humans is approximately 1.2 μmol/kg body weight/day (53). This rate is sufficient to meet normal requirements. Deficient synthesis may occur by lack of substrates, cofactors, or activators, e.g., in deficiency of lysine (54,55), methionine, Fe^{2+}, ascorbate (56), or vitamin B_6.

L(−)-Carnitine biosynthesis in mammals is apparently regulated by the availability of 6-*N*-trimethyllysine and its ability to penetrate the membrane to the intramitochondrial site of 6-*N*-trimethyllysine hydroxylase. In humans, 30–50% of total 6-*N*-trimethyllysine (from diet and endogenous synthesis) is converted to L(−)-carnitine, and the remainder is excreted in urine (58). The availability of γ-butyrobetaine in liver seems to be a regulatory factor for L(−)-carnitine biosynthesis in rats (58,59). Until now, no other regulation of its biosynthesis has been found. Its absorption in the gut is slow and is influenced by the L(−)-carnitine content of the diet.

B. Absorption

In addition to endogenous biosynthesis, dietary intake of L(−)-carnitine serves to maintain tissue L(−)-carnitine stores. L(−)-Carnitine is found in a variety of sources. However, foods of animal origin and dairy products are much richer in this compound than plant-derived food (see Sec. V.A). The contribution of dietary and endogenous carnitine to the tissue stores has not been established, but it has been suggested that about 50% of L(−)-carnitine normally originates in food (60). In humans and rats between 20 and 85% of the dietary L(−)-carnitine is absorbed. The remainder is excreted as metabolites (see Sec. II.D) in urine and feces following bacterial degradation in the large intestine (61–65). Less than 1–2% of dietary L(−)-carnitine have been found in human feces but a high percentage of γ-butyrobetaine was measured (66,67).

Absorption and transport of L(−)-carnitine have been studied in intestinal preparations from humans and various animals (e.g., rats, pigs, guinea pigs). The studies demonstrated relatively rapid transport of L(−)-carnitine from the lumen into small intestinal mucosa of rats, acetylation of up to 50% of the L(−)-carnitine taken up from the lumen, and slower release of free and acetylcarnitine into the circulation (68–70). The results obtained concerning the mechanism by which L(−)-carnitine is absorbed in the small intestine are partly contradictory, because different techniques and preparations were used and possible inherent differences between species studied exist. Using everted rat intestinal rings and sacs, active transport of L(−)-carnitine into the duodenum and the jejunum but not the ileum was observed (71). The transport of L(−)-carnitine was diminished by D(+)-carnitine and acetyl-L(−)-carnitine, which suggests that these compounds utilize the same transport system. From the results of in vitro studies of L(−)-carnitine transport across the proximal small intestinal mucosa of humans, it was also concluded that an active uptake mechanism that depended on sodium cotransport exists (72,73). For the absorption of large doses of L(−)-carnitine, a passive diffusion of this quaternary ammonium compound was also identified. These results are similar to those reported by other groups using live rats and isolated perfused intestine (68–70,74). Recently, the mechanism of L(−)-carnitine uptake was studied using a human-derived intestinal epithelial cell line (Caco-2) (75). McLoud et al. (75) demonstrated an energy-dependent saturable uptake of L(−)-carnitine. The uptake process was Na^+ dependent and was inhibited by D(+)-carnitine and γ-butyrobetaine. In this context it should be mentioned that γ-butyrobetaine, 6-*N*-trimethyllysine, and 3-hydroxy-6-*N*-trimethyllysine are also absorbed (76). In contrast to these studies, only passive diffusion could be demonstrated using jejunal brush border membrane vesicles from rats (77) and enterocytes isolated from guinea pigs (78). Gross et al. (79) postulated that L(−)-carnitine is taken up from the enterocytes by facilitated diffusion. They suggested the existence of a specific carrier for L(−)-carnitine in the mucosal membrane (68).

C. Distribution, Tissue Uptake, and Turnover Time

L(−)-Carnitine is available from dietary sources and from endogenous biosynthesis, as discussed above. L(−)-Carnitine homeostasis in mammals is maintained by a combination of these two sources with a highly efficient reabsorption of L(−)-carnitine (see Sec. II.D). The body distribution of L(−)-carnitine is determined by the L(−)-carnitine transport into cells against a concentration gradient, an independent efflux process, and exchange mechanisms, which are tissue-specific.

The total body pool of L(−)-carnitine in a normal 70 kg human adult is approximately 100 mmol (80). Of this quantity, 98% is found in muscle and only about 1.5% in liver and kidney and 0.6% in extracellular fluids (81,82). L(−)-Carnitine concentration in the brain is relatively low (0.5–1.0 μmol/g wet weight), though brain is one of the few tissues capable of endogenous biosynthesis. Several factors, especially hormones (e.g., sex hormones and the glucagon-to-insulin ratio), may impact on L(−)-carnitine distribution and levels in tissues (81,82). Plasma total L(−)-carnitine levels in normal adults ranged from 30 to 89 μM, but females have lower levels than males (80,83). Under physiological conditions, the plasma L(−)-carnitine concentration is maintained within a narrow range. It should be emphasized that the concentration of L(−)-carnitine in skeletal muscle is approximately 70 times higher than in plasma. Similar differences exist also between other tissues and extracelluar fluid.

L(−)-Carnitine in tissues and extracellular fluids is present as either free (nonesterified) L(−)-carnitine or L(−)-carnitine esters (acylcarnitines) (81,82). Normally the short-chain acyl-L(−)-carnitine ester pool consists primarily of acetyl-L(−)-carnitine. Remarkably, the proportion of acylcarnitine may vary greatly with nutritional conditions, exercise, and disease status.

For L(−)-carnitine to carry out its principal function in mitochondrial fatty acid oxidation, the molecule must enter the cell. Most cell types possess a stereospecific mechanism for transporting L(−)-carnitine across the cell membrane, with a resulting 10- to 100-fold gradient between extracellular and intracellular concentrations (18,81). Liver plays a unique role in L(−)-carnitine homeostasis. This organ is the major site of γ-butyrobetaine hydroxylation, and the corresponding transport system shows a higher affinity for γ-butyrobetaine ($K_m \sim 0.5$ mM) (84) than for L(−)-carnitine ($K_m \sim 5.0$ mM) (84,85). Additionally, adsorbed L(−)-carnitine appears primarily in portal circulation and is extracted by the liver prior to systemic distribution. A movement of L(−)-carnitine into bile has been observed, but the total L(−)-carnitine concentrations found in bile are highly variable and related to different metabolic conditions (86).

The uptake system has been studied in isolated hepatocytes (84) and perfused liver (87–89). It is energy- and sodium-dependent as well as saturable, consistent with a carrier-mediated process. The transporter postulated shows low stereospecificity. For the efflux of L(−)-carnitine a separate system, which is saturable and energy independent, has been demonstrated (87,88). It has been postulated that acyl carnitines are transported out of hepatocytes faster than L(−)-carnitine. Other tissues studied, e.g., heart (91,92), skeletal muscle (92,93), and kidney (68,94), have a temperature- and sodium-dependent saturable uptake system. In contrast to the liver, it is of a high-affinity type. In contrast to the skeletal muscle the high-affinity carnitine uptake system in the heart and in the kidney is not energy dependent. Until now the apparent differences have not been clarified (95).

Using the technique of kinetic compartmental analysis (66) and a two-compartment model following intravenous administration of labeled L(−)-carnitine (96), respectively, turnover times have been estimated. The different turnover times of L(−)-carnitine in different organs in the rat (between 0.39 hour in spleen and 903 hours in the "slow" compartment of liver) (50), but also in other animals (86), presumably reflect the variable relationship of cellular uptake and release mechanisms in these locations. Turnover time for L(−)-carnitine in extracellular fluid was approximately 1 hour and for the whole body about 65 days (50).

D. Degradation and Excretion

L(−)-Carnitine is a nontoxic substance with a LD_{50} of 8.9 (97) and 9.1 g L(−)-carnitine/kg (98), respectively, approximately equivalent to those of amino acids. For the D-enantiomer a LD_{50} of 10.3 g/kg has been determined (97,99). Carnitine esters with long-chain acyls are more toxic; e.g., palmitoylcarnitine is 23-fold more toxic than free L(−)-carnitine (100).

There are no degradation pathways of L(−)-carnitine in the mammalian body except degradation of dietary L(−)-carnitine by intestinal bacteria. Using oral administration of pharmacological doses or radiolabeled forms of L(−)-carnitine ([methyl-^{14}C] or [methyl-^{3}H]), it has been shown that L(−)-carnitine is primarily degraded in mammals to γ-butyrobetaine and trimethylamine (61–65). After absorption and oxidation in the liver, trimethylamine is excreted as trimethylamine oxide in urine. γ-Butyrobetaine has been found primarily in feces (67). In humans, trimethylamine oxide in urine accounted for 8–39% and γ-butyrobetaine in feces accounted for 0.1–8% of total dietary L(−)-carnitine (61). The fecal loss of L(−)-carnitine accounts for less than 1–2% of the total (79). Studies comparing catabolism of orally administered L(−)-carnitine in germ-free and conventional rats led to the conclusion that bacteria in the gastrointestinal tract were entirely responsible for metabolite formation (62,63). Bacteria are able to metabolize L(−)-carnitine and other trimethylammonium compounds in different ways (101). *Acinetobacter* species degrade only the carbon backbone with formation of trimethylamine (102–104). Various members of the Enterobacteriaceae, such as *Escherichia coli*, *Salmonella typhimurium*, and *Proteus vulgaris*, are able to convert L(−)-carnitine, via crotonobetaine, to γ-butyrobetaine in the presence of carbon and nitrogen sources under anaerobic conditions (105–107).

The only two known routes for removing body L(−)-carnitine are via excretion in the urine or by bile in the gut (67,70,108,109). The kidneys play an important role in maintenance of L(−)-carnitine homeostasis in mammals. The kidneys are involved not only in highly efficient L(−)-carnitine reabsorption but also participate in the synthesis (not in all mammals) and secretion of L(−)-carnitine and acyl-L(−)-carnitines (86). The daily urinary excretion of L(−)-carnitine averages approximately 0.1–0.3% of the total body store in healthy individuals (18,110). In humans with normal plasma L(−)-carnitine concentrations, 90–98% of filtered L(−)-carnitine is reabsorbed by the kidney (95,111,112). In rats, a clearance of about 40 mL of plasma per day could be calculated (113). In normal humans clearance of short-chain acyl-L(−)-carnitine esters is greater than that for nonesterified, free L(−)-carnitine, in spite of the lower concentration of acyl-L(−)-carnitine esters, compared to L(−)-carnitine in the circulation (114). The rate of L(−)-carnitine excretion is influenced by physiological factors, e.g., a diet high in fat and low in carbohydrate increases the rate of L(−)-carnitine excretion by increasing the filtered load of L(−)-carnitine (115). Consumption of a diet rich in protein also increases the rate of L(−)-carnitine excretion (115). Reabsorption of more than 95% was found with γ-butyrobetaine and D(+)-carnitine, showing that the reabsorption mechanisms have a relatively low specificity (113).

III. FUNCTION

L(−)-Carnitine is an essential factor for the β-oxidation of long-chain fatty acids in mitochondria. This L(−)-carnitine function has been studied since the 1950s and has become well known in the meantime (see Table 1). The function results from the fact that long-chain fatty acids are activated by the acyl-CoA synthetase at the outer mitochondrial membrane and that fatty acid acyl-CoA esters are not able to penetrate the inner mitochondrial membrane. If there is a carnitine deficiency or a defect in L(−)-carnitine–specific enzymes, no energy can be produced from the main energy source of the body, i.e., from fat. The involved carnitine system consists of three enzymes and is demonstrated in the upper part of Figure 2.

Carnitine palmitoyltransferase I (CPT I) is located in the outer membrane of mitochondria and forms acylcarnitine from acyl-CoA. By means of carnitine-acylcarnitine translocase acylcarnitine is transported through the inner mitochondrial membrane in strict stoichiometric exchange with intramitochondrial L(−)-carnitine (22,23). In the matrix, the site of β-oxidation, acylcarnitine has to be transformed back in acyl-CoA to enter the pathway of β-oxidation. This last step is realized by the CPT II located at the matrix side of the inner mitochondrial membrane. This is the physiological flow of substrates to the fatty acid oxidation, but in principle the reactions of the three enzymes are also reversible.

The regulation of the substrate flux takes place on the level of the CPT I reaction. This enzyme is metabolically inhibited by malonyl-CoA, the substrate for the de novo biosynthesis of fatty acids. So the CPT I is regulated by the hormonal conditions, phosphorylation, and on the level of m-RNA transcription (24,26,30,116–121).

The CPTs are not restricted to mitochondria. They also exist in peroxisomes, microsomes (endoplasmic reticulum), cell membranes, and even in nuclear membranes. Their functions in these cell organelles are not quite clear; influences on membrane fluidity and transport processes have been discussed (116).

Other carnitine functions are demonstrated in the lower part of Figure 2. They are carried out on the level of the carnitine acetyltransferase and connected with the reaction of the carnitine-acylcarnitine translocase, i.e., with the transport of short-, medium-, or branched-chain activated acids through the mitochondrial inner membrane.

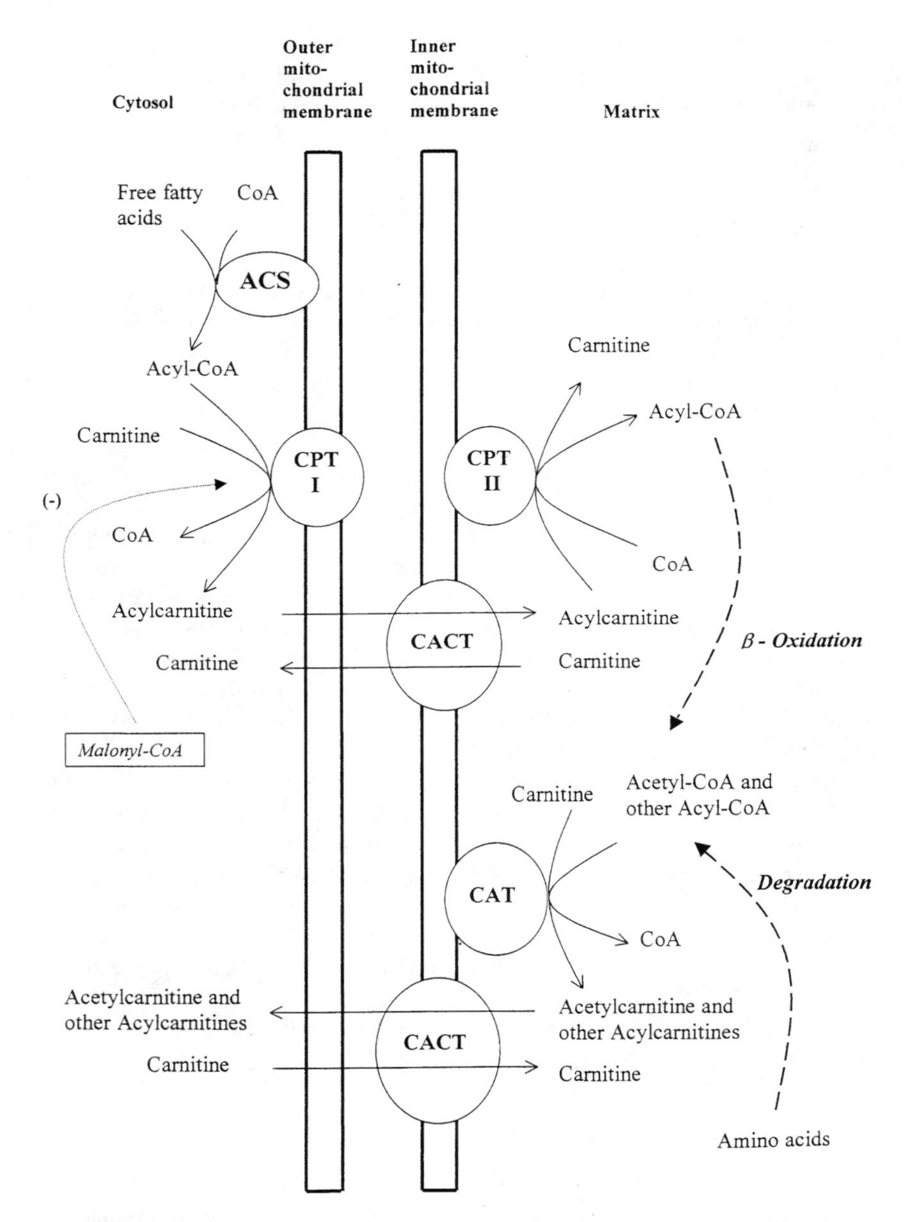

Figure 2 The mitochondrial carnitine system. ACS = Acylcoenzyme A synthetase; CPT I = carnitine palmitoyltransferase I; CPT II = carnitine palmitoyltransferase II; CACT = carnitine-acylcarnitine translocase; CAT = carnitine acetyltransferase.

The carnitine acetyltransferase is able to transform activated acetyl groups from acetyl-CoA to L(−)-carnitine, liberating CoA. Free CoA is required for a variety of processes in intermediary metabolism, e.g., for β-oxidation, amino acid degradation, detoxification of organic acids and xenobiotics, dehydrogenation and decarboxylation of pyruvate (PDH-complex), and of α-ketoglutarate influencing the citric acid cycle, ketogenesis, and glycolysis. Activated organic acids are transported out of the mitochondria, out of the cell, and out of the body by the kidneys in the form of acylcarnitines. The urinary elimination of specific acylcarnitines is relevant for the diagnosis and therapy of several inborn errors of amino acid and fatty acid degradation. Thus the carnitine-CoA relationship is pivotal for the energy production in the cells.

Acetyl groups and medium-chain acyl groups are transported from the peroxisomes to the mitochondria as acylcarnitines by the so-called L(−)-carnitine shuttle (28,33,122). Apart from carnitine acetyltransferase, a carnitine octanoyltransferase exists in peroxisomes for this purpose (32). Acetylcarnitine itself is an energy substrate, which can be transported through the whole body by the blood and utilized in the mitochondria of different blood cells and tissues.

Many of the pleiotropic effects of L(−)-carnitine administered can be explained by the relationship between L(−)-carnitine and CoA on the level of carnitine acetyltransferase.

IV. DEFECTS OF THE CARNITINE SYSTEM

Disturbances of the carnitine system can be caused by a deficiency of substrates or by significantly decreased or missing activity of the involved enzymes. A classification scheme is shown in Figure 3.

A. Carnitine Deficiency Syndromes

As a new syndrome in humans, L(−)-carnitine deficiency was first described in 1973 (20). In most cases the carnitine concentration has to fall to less than 10–20% of the normal range before metabolic effects can be seen in patients. Carnitine deficiency syndromes commonly are classified according to the etiopathogenesis and the organ involvement. Primary deficiency is caused by disturbances in the carnitine system itself; secondary deficiencies may occur as a result of other, defined genetic or acquired defects or may be associated with complex diseases (123–125).

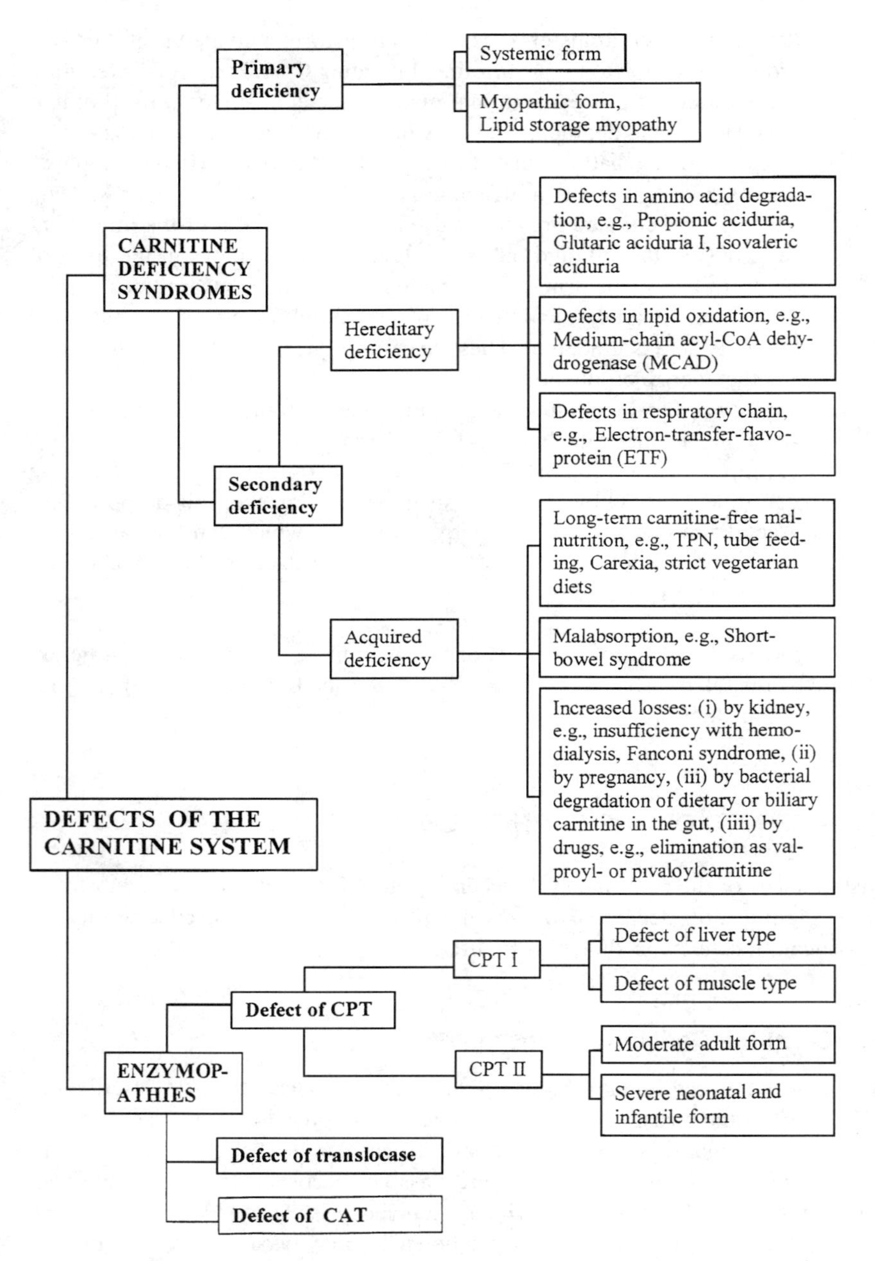

Figure 3 Classification of defects in the carnitine system. CPT = Carnitine palmitoyltransferase; CAT = carnitine acetyltransferase.

Primary carnitine deficiency syndromes are defined according to the following criteria (126):

1. The disorder is caused directly by inadequate carnitine levels in plasma or tissues or both.
2. Patients have impaired fatty acid oxidation.
3. The metabolic abnormalities are corrected when carnitine concentrations are restored to the normal values.
4. Primary defects of intramitochondrial β-oxidation have been ruled out.

Among the primary deficiency syndromes, at least two different entities have been described: systemic carnitine deficiency and muscle carnitine deficiency.

Systemic primary carnitine deficiency is readily detectable by the low serum L(−)-carnitine concentration. Further organ involvement is present including the liver as well as the cardiac and skeletal muscles (127–129). Clinical manifestations vary depending on the organ more heavily affected, correspondingly leading to hepatic encephalopathy with hepatomegaly or progressive congestive cardiomyopathy. During periods of fasting, reduced ketogenesis and hypoglycemia can be determined.

The underlying cause for primary systemic carnitine deficiency is obviously a defect in the carnitine transport system of the cell membranes (carnitine-carrier$_{in}$ deficiency) normally accumulating carnitine inside the cells against the concentration gradient. As a result, absorption from the intestine is inhibited and renal involvement leads to a reduction of L(−)-carnitine reabsorption from the glomerular filtrate, i.e., a depletion of L(−)-carnitine with urine.

Family studies with fibroblasts revealed an autosomal-recessive inheritance. In heterozygous individuals, carnitine carriers with decreased affinity have been described. Primary systemic carnitine deficiency manifests itself during infancy or early childhood, and, if left untreated, it is characterized by a severe, life-threatening clinical course.

Myopathic carnitine deficiency is restricted to muscles (skeletal muscle and myocard); serum level and liver concentration are within the reference range with no signs of renal carnitine losses (20,126,128). Clinical symptoms include episodes of progressive muscle weakness and myalgias. Compensatory ketogenesis occurs during periods of fasting or during intake of a high-fat diet. Histochemically, a form of lipid storage myopathy is present, showing fat droplets stored within type I muscle fibers. A study in cultured myoplasts from a patient suffering from myogenous carnitine deficiency demonstrated normal carnitine uptake but increased carnitine efflux, suggesting a possible carnitine-carrier$_{out}$ deficiency (128,130). The myopathic form is inherited via an autosomal-recessive mode or acquired. The onset of symptoms is observed during childhood up to adulthood; the clinical course is less progressive than that seen in the systemic form of the disease.

Secondary carnitine deficiencies are associated with a wide variety of hereditary or acquired diseases (Fig. 3) (126,128,129). They are characterized by decreased availability of free L(−)-carnitine in serum and tissues. Secondary deficiencies are considered as consequences of L(−)-carnitine losses, impaired intake, or increased acylcarnitine formation. In cases of functional carnitine deficiency, total carnitine levels may still be within the reference range, but free carnitine is significantly reduced because of the excessively increased portion of acylcarnitines (the acylcarnitine/carnitine ratio is pathologically high = carnitine insufficiency) (131,132). Thus, carnitine is unable to be a transfer recipient of acyl groups from acyl-CoA and cannot liberate CoA.

Whereas primary carnitine deficiencies are considered to be rare, clinical occurrence of secondary deficiencies are observed more frequently.

B. Enzymopathies

Among the enzyme defects demonstrated in Figure 3, the moderate adult muscle form of the CPT II deficiency is by far the most frequent. The CPT I activity of these patients is in the normal range. CPT II deficiency is the most common disorder of lipid metabolism affecting skeletal muscle. This defect has also been described as one of the most common biochemically defined causes of myoglobinuria (rhabdomyolysis) in adults (the disease develops in young adulthood). The muscle form of CPT II deficiency manifests itself especially following strenuous physical activity, but periods of fasting, exposure to cold, recurrent infections, and high-fat intake can also precipitate the symptoms.

CPT II protein is the product of a single gene localized at chromosome 1p32 (133). The enzyme can be isolated from patients or expressed in vitro in its catalytic active form. In the meantime several mutations with more or less decreased enzyme activities have been described (128,134–136). One of the most common mutations of CPT II is the Ser113Leu substitution, in which the catalytic activity of the mutant enzyme is drastically diminished (137). But the reduction of CPT II activity alone cannot account for the clinical heterogeneity of the disease. In cases of the adult muscle form or in the early onset hepatic form of CPT II deficiency, the reduction of the CPT II activity was the same, but the clinical outcome and the underlying mutations were very different (reviewed in Refs. 128, 135).

The CPT II deficiency of neonates and infants has a significantly poorer prognosis. Besides hepatic involvement, cardiac defects are predominant, and increased long-chain acylcarnitine content of plasma and tissues with lipid accumulation have been described (135,138).

In humans and a variety of mammals CPT I is expressed in two isoforms (reviewed in Refs. 128, 139). For the liver-specific isoenzyme (L-CPT I) and the muscle specific isoenzyme (M-CPT I), two different mRNAs were isolated and the cDNAs expressed (140,141). The predicted primary structures of both enzymes showed 62.6% homology. The calculated molecular masses were 88,150 (773 amino acids) and 88,227 (772 amino acids) for the liver and skeletal muscle isoforms, respectively. The genes for human liver CPT I (CPT I alpha) or skeletal muscle (CPT I beta) have been designed to chromosome 11q13 (142) and 22q13.3 (142,143). In rats the L-CPT I is the dominant isoform not only in liver but also in kidney, lung, ovary, spleen, brain, intestine, and pancreatic islets, whereas M-CPT I predominates in skeletal muscle, heart, white and brown adipose tissue, and testis (144).

The expression of L- or M-CPT I in organs depends on the state of differentiation (145). When neonatal rat heart myocytes are subjected to electrical stimulation, there is a marked proliferation of mitochondria accompanied by an approximate 50% decrease in the mRNA level of L-CPT I and about a 2.5-fold increase in the mRNA level of M-CPT I. The mRNA changes were reflected in the activity of the isoenzymes (146). The same changes take place in the differentiation of adipocytes in vitro. Undifferentiated rat or human preadipocytes expressed solely L-CPT I, but significant levels of M-CPT I emerged after 3 days of differentiation, while the M-CPT I form predominated in mature adipocytes (144). Multiple mature mRNAs in rat heart derived from alternative splicing of CPT Ibeta transcript were also described (147). The fact that human fibroblasts express solely the liver-type isoenzyme is relevant for diagnostic studies (148).

CPT I deficiency is relatively rare. L-CPT I deficiency manifests itself by hypoketotic hypoglycemia, especially triggered by fasting (149,150). No myopathic or cardiomyopathic involvement was seen, a consequence of an intact M-CPT I (151,152).

The clinical manifestation of M-CPT I deficiency is recurrent rhabdomyolysis with a normal ketogenic response to fasting (153). In skeletal muscle homogenate palmitate or palmitoyl-CoA was not oxidized, unlike palmitoylcarnitine.

Carnitine translocase deficiency is one of the most severe disorders of fatty acid oxidation with a very early onset and usually lethal outcome in the perinatal or early infantile period of life (128,154). Fewer than 10 patients have been reported in the literature. A characteristic feature of the disease is a significant increase in plasma long-chain acylcarnitines with very low free carnitine (functional carnitine deficiency). CPT II was not affected. The human genome contains a single gene for the expression of the carnitine-acylcarnitine translocase (155). In two cases of translocase deficiency, the accompanying mutations have been identified (154).

From the nutritional point of view it should be mentioned that frequent feedings, nighttime snacks, and avoidance of fasting and high-fat diets can reduce the development of clinical symptoms in the CPT deficiencies.

V. L-(−)-CARNITINE AS NUTRIENT AND DIETARY SUPPLEMENT

A. Dietary Sources

L(−)-Carnitine is widely distributed in nature. Food of animal origin, primarily red meat and dairy products, contain much more L(−)-carnitine than food of plant origin. The carnitine content of selected food is listed in Table 2 (reviewed in Refs. 157, 158).

L(−)-Carnitine exists in food either free or in acylated form, bound to long-chain, middle-chain, or short-chain fatty acids, including acetic acid (= acetylcarnitine). The rate of acylcarnitine amounts for about 5–30% of total carnitine. L(−)-Carnitine content in food has to be determined after hydrolysis of all acylcarnitines to get the total L(−)-carnitine.

In general, a diet rich in meat is considered to supply a large amount of L(−)-carnitine, while a vegetable-based diet supplies only traces. Consequently, strict vegetarians have a high risk to be deficient in L(−)-carnitine. It should be mentioned that L(−)-carnitine is a water-soluble small molecule. Any cooking with water naturally causes losses of L(−)-carnitine, when the water phase is

Table 2 Carnitine Contents of Various Foods (fresh weight)

Animal origin of food	Total carnitine (mg/100 g)	Plant origin of food	Total carnitine (mg/100 g)
Sheep muscle	209.3	Apple puree	3.1
Lamb muscle	78.0	Tomatoes	2.9
Beef rump steak	61.6	Pears	2.7
Sheep heart	59.0	Rice	1.8[a]
Pork muscle	30.0	Apple juice	1.3
Rabbit muscle	21.0	Asparagus	1.3
Beef heart	19.3	Avocado	1.3
Chicken muscle	4.5–9.7	Peas	1.2
Pork liver	4.9	Pineapple	1.1
Cow's milk	0.5–3.9	Wheat seeds	0.35–1.22[a]
Sheep liver	2.2	Bread	0.81
Beef kidney	1.8	Cauliflower	0.13
Chicken liver	0.6	Carrots, spinach, potatoes, cabbage, corn kernels	0

[a] mg/100 g dry weight.
Source: Refs. 157, 158.

not further used. During cooking the L(−)-carnitine molecule is stable, and no decomposition takes place.

B. Bioavailability

Concerning the absorption of L(−)-carnitine after oral application and the increase in blood (including in the interstitial fluid) and in organs, a remarkable result has to be discussed. The higher the applied dosages, starting with the physiological L(−)-carnitine content of food to high pharmacological doses, the less the percentage of absorbed carnitine in blood and tissues (from 100% to 4%). Degradation of L(−)-carnitine and elimination by kidneys were described in Secs. II.B and II.C.

L-Carnitine is absorbed in the duodenum and, to a lesser extent, in jejunum (see Sec. II.B). The active saturable transport process allows small amounts of L-carnitine to be almost entirely absorbed. This can occur with dietary intake. Higher amounts of L(−)-carnitine, for instance pharmacological doses of 1–6 g per day, are absorbed mainly by diffusion, with the active process being saturated (67,159–161).

Absorption, bioavailability, and urinary elimination of carnitine in men were studied with a single high oral dose of L(−)-carnitine, 6 g/subject or 100 mg/kg body weight, and compared with a single lower oral dose, 2 g/subject or 30 mg/kg (162–164). During the first 24 hours after application, the urinary recovery of L(−)-carnitine was only 8% and 4% for the 2 g and 6 g doses in six healthy subjects on a low-carnitine diet. Oral bioavailability of the low carnitine dose ranged from 9 to 25%, whereas that of the high dose was only 4 to 10% (162).

Plasma levels were increased up to about 90 μmol/L (basal values had been subtracted from the concentration measured) with oral application of 100 mg/kg, while plasma concentration was increased only by about 25 μmol/L with application of 30 mg/kg. The maximal blood concentration was reached 3–6 hours after application (163,164).

The urinary recovery of L(−)-carnitine is much higher after intravenous administration, as it is also the case with the maximal blood concentration. Healthy subjects given an intravenous dose of 40 mg/kg demonstrated a peak serum L(−)-carnitine level of 1612.3 μmol/L, a value 36 times higher than the baseline concentration (165). The urine recovery in 24 hours was 77.2–95.4%. In another study 2 intravenous dosages (30 mg/kg or 100 mg/kg) were compared (164). The highest mean plasma concentrations measured were 1444.8 ± 157.9 and 2913.9 ± 320.4 μmol/L, respectively. The urinary elimination was more than 80% of the dose.

The bioavailability of three different oral dosage forms of L(−)-carnitine were tested in 15 healthy subjects. Based on the free or total L(−)-carnitine plasma concentrations, the mean absolute bioavailability of tablets, oral solutions, and chewable tablets relative to an i.v. dose was approximately 18% for all three oral formulations (166).

The administration of L(−)-carnitine encapsulated in liposomes and the direct intravenous administration of the drug were tested in rats (167). The retention in the blood system of L(−)-carnitine in liposomes was up to 300% higher. L(−)-Carnitine in the novel dosage form accumulated to a higher extent in liver (156%), while the concentration in heart (55%) and skeletal muscle (54%) decreased markedly compared to the standard injection.

Brass reviewed pharmacokinetic studies for therapeutic use of carnitine in hemodialysis patients (168). He concluded that intravenous carnitine may have theoretical advantages in initiating treatment when high peak concentrations are required to facilitate L(−)-carnitine reaching nonhepatic tissue sites or when oral therapy is not feasible due to poor tolerance or compliance. Orally administered L(−)-carnitine was reported to have clinical efficacy in hemodialysis patients in doses of 2–4 g/day and can be used for long-term maintenance therapy.

C. Carnitine Requirement in Pregnancy and Infancy

At parturition neonates have to adapt to fat as a major metabolic fuel. Immediately at birth a rapid elevation of blood free fatty acid levels occurs due to lipolysis from adipose tissue. Later the high free fatty acid concentration in serum depends on absorption of dietary fat. Human milk contains more than 40% of total calories as lipid. Thus, L(−)-carnitine becomes an essential factor for energy production from fatty acids in neonates.

During pregnancy the fetus gets L(−)-carnitine from the mother. L(−)-Carnitine stores are low in the fetus early in gestation (169), and premature infants have a higher risk of developing carnitine deficiency if exogenous L(−)-carnitine is not provided by nutrition (170).

At delivery plasma L(−)-carnitine levels of pregnant women are decreased to about half the concentrations seen in nonpregnant women (171–174). During the twelfth week of gestation total L(−)-carnitine concentration was found to be at a significantly lower level of 21 ± 3.4 μmol/L in plasma (nonpregnant controls 40 ± 14.3 μmol/L) and was further reduced to 15 ± 6.0 μmol/L at delivery. The free L(−)-carnitine level fell to 10 ± 4.6 μmol/L at this time. The causes for this deficiency were found in the transport of L(−)-carnitine through the placenta and a higher clearance of the kidneys for acylcarnitines (173). During the prenatal and perinatal period the L(−)-carnitine amount in the fetuses seems to be involved in fetal lung maturation influencing respiratory distress syndrome (175).

In a study with 353 metabolically healthy children, Schmidt-Sommerfeld et al. (176) found a high concentration of both free and acylcarnitine in plasma on the first day of life (36.4 ± 10.8 μmol/L for total carnitine), while from the second to seventh days the value was decreased to 25.2 ± 4.1 μmol/L. They discussed this phenomenon considering a mobilization from tissue stores during the immediately postnatal metabolic adaptation. A high ratio of acylcarnitine to free L(−)-carnitine was determined during this period. After the first week, total L(−)-carnitine plasma concentrations progressively increased and adult values were reached after the first year (176).

Human milk contains 28–95 μmol/L total L(−)-carnitine (177,178). Sandor et al. found that total L(−)-carnitine in breast milk remained at a constant level during the first 21 days postpartum, then fell significantly until the fiftieth day (178). In the colostrum of mothers who delivered premature or full-term newborns, total carnitine concentration was the same (75 μmol/L). About 50% of total L(−)-carnitine occurred in the form of acetyl and short-chain acyl L(−)-carnitines (179).

When neonates were fed orally or parenterally with carnitine-free formulas, many studies evidenced that the L(−)-carnitine level was decreased in serum to a level of secondary carnitine deficiency (reviewed in Refs. 180–182). When the L(−)-carnitine amount in tissues was determined, this level was also found to be reduced (170). L(−)-Carnitine application normalized the blood level in all cases and could influence the lipid metabolism positively (183,184). Therefore, one can recommend that a L(−)-carnitine level for neonates be obtained at least on the physiological level of breast-fed babies to ensure a proper energy production from fat.

D. Carnitine-Deficient Nutrition

Because food of plant origin generally contains very little L(−)-carnitine (see Table 2), vegetarians take in limited amounts of this conditionally essential substance. Consequently, it is not surprising that vegetarians have a significantly lower level of free or total L(−)-carnitine in serum compared with omnivores on mixed diet (112,185–187). Dietary L(−)-carnitine provides more than half the total L(−)-carnitine available in omnivores, whereas in strict vegetarians less than 15% comes from food (53).

The serum L(−)-carnitine level of vegetarians is lower but usually not dramatically decreased to a severe carnitine deficiency state because endogenous L(−)-carnitine is efficiently conserved by the kidneys (112). Plasma carnitine concentrations often remain in the lower borderline of "normal" range. A study with 49 healthy probands on a mixed diet and 46 lacto-ovo-vegetarians demonstrated that the well-known lower L(−)-carnitine serum concentration in women also manifests itself with a vegetarian diet: total serum L(−)-carnitine in men on a normal mixed diet accounts for 46.1 ± 9.2 μmol/L, while in vegetarian men the concentration was significantly lower at 37.3 ± 8.6 μmol/L. In women the corresponding values were 39.4 ± 9.1 and 31.5 ± 10.0 μmol/L (187). Whether the lower L(−)-carnitine level of vegetarian men in the range of healthy nonvegetarian women caused adequate physical performance was not examined. Strict vegetarians and ovo-vegetarians have the highest risk of receiving too little L(−)-carnitine from food, while as a rule milk-containing food delivers enough L(−)-carnitine for an intact metabolism. There are some cases of extremely restrictive vegetarian diets being responsible for various deficiency disorders (188,189).

While the vegetarian lifestyle is a voluntary decision made by healthy adults, nutritionists and physicians recommend the food ingredients for carnitine-free nutrition of tube-fed or parenterally fed patients. In patients fed L(−)-carnitine–free diets, the serum carnitine concentration fell into the pathological range depending on the duration of carnitine-free nutrition and the age of patients. Neonates react with low L(−)-carnitine levels after less than one week (190,191). Adult patients can maintain plasma levels of L(−)-carnitine much longer, but after about 4 weeks of carnitine-free nutrition, patients showed a significant decrease in serum-free and total L(−)-carnitine (192,193). Only some of the patients receiving home parenteral nutrition for 1–80 months had very low serum-free L(−)-carnitine concentrations, between 10 and 15 μmol/L (194). In another group of patients with severe malabsorption on long-term total parenteral nutrition (96 ± 11 month), mean plasma L(−)-carnitine was significantly below the mean value normal for females and borderline low for males. Patients with normal levels had elevated serum creatinine, indicating lower glomerular filtration (195).

Sixteen children (average 6.2 years) suffering from severe neurological symptoms received a balanced carnitine-free tube diet for at least 2.3 month. All children showed a pathologically low free and total L(−)-carnitine level in serum (9.5 ± 3.2 and 10.2 ± 3.6 μmol/L). After substitution with 1 g L(−)-carnitine per day the carnitine values in serum rose significantly and did not differ from the normal values (196). The oxidation of ^{13}C-labeled trioleine to $^{13}CO_2$ was examined by means of a breath test before and after L(−)-carnitine application in these children. With this test the stimulation of fatty acid oxidation by L(−)-carnitine supplementation was proved in vivo (197,198). Other groups of patients that benefit from L(−)-carnitine application were reviewed in 1998 (199).

E. Sports

During the last decade L(−)-carnitine has increasingly gained attention in the nutrition of athletes. This application is based on its proven function in fatty acid metabolism. In particular, L(−)-carnitine appears to be promising dietary supplement for endurance training. At the end of the 1960s, L(−)-carnitine in combination with vitamin B_6 and potassium aspartate (Aminox) was being used to prevent fatigue (200,201). Numerous studies have tried to prove the effects of L(−)-carnitine supplementation on athletic performance. The results were not always consistent, but in the majority of cases beneficial effects of L(−)-carnitine were found in athletes (for reviews see, e.g., Refs. 110, 202–207).

Today L(−)-carnitine supplementation in extreme sport is an established part of the diet. It is mostly used by endurance athletes on a regular basis to prevent relative L(−)-carnitine deficiency (208). Various reasons for an induced relative L(−)-carnitine deficiency for top-level athletes have been reported in the literature. As already mentioned (Sec. II. A) L(−)-carnitine biosynthesis requires niacin, vitamin B_6, vitamin C, and iron. Biosynthesis starts with protein-bound L-lysine and uses methionine supplied as S-adenosyl methionine. An insufficient supply of these molecules leads to a decrease in L(−)-carnitine synthesis and raises the need for supplementation. Nutritional studies have demonstrated that about 20% of endurance athletes suffer a shortage of vitamin B_6 (209). A significant number of elite athletes prefer a vegetarian diet and often show iron deficiencies in addition to a low exogenous L(−)-carnitine and lysine supply. A change to a normal mixed diet or L(−)-carnitine supplementation led to significantly improved performance (210). It was shown that endurance training increased muscular L(−)-carnitine consumption. In addition, the excretion of acetyl-L(−)-carnitine by sprinters was reduced after administration of 1 g of L(−)-carnitine per day (211).

L(−)-Carnitine is involved in several physiological effects, which, from a theoretical biochemical point of view, suggests a contribution to enhance muscular performance:

1. Excess of L(−)-carnitine reducing the acetyl-CoA /CoA ratio: During physical exercise the fraction of acyl- L(−)-carnitine in plasma increases by a factor of 2–3. Of this fraction, 90% consists of acetyl-L(−)-carnitine (212–214). Several studies revealed a shift from free L(−)-carnitine to acyl-L(−)-carnitine in the muscle during exercise. The total amount of L(−)-carnitine (free and acylesters) did not change significantly. The amount of free L(−)-carnitine drops from 80–90% to 30–40% when shifting from resting to active status (215–217). The ratio of acetylcarnitine to CoA is regulated by CAT. Free intramitochondrial CoA is indispensable for β-oxidation and the citric acid cycle. Therefore, a high acetyl-CoA/CoA ratio inhibits the pyruvate dehydrogenase complex. As a consequence, pyruvate cannot be decarboxylated and used in the citric acid cycle for aerobic energy production (218). Campos et al. defined the term "carnitine insufficiency" when more than 20% of total blood L(−)-carnitine is acetylated (129). Application of 50–200 mg/kg/day of L(−)-carnitine significantly reduced muscle insufficiency in 19 of 20 patients.

   During intensive exercise, L(−)-carnitine supplementation modulates the acetyl-CoA/CoA ratio. Acetyl residues are transferred to

L(−)-carnitine by CAT, making CoA available for other intramitochondrial reactions. This mechanism has been proven in patients. The first studies with sprinters revealed an increase of free L(−)-carnitine levels (219) and a reduced excretion of short-chain acyl-L(−)-carnitine esters after L(−)-carnitine supplementation (211).

2. Increase of mitochondrial fatty acid oxidation: β-oxidation is strongly dependent on the transport of fatty acids into the mitochondrial matrix. As discussed above, this transport relies on acyl-L(−)-carnitine esters as intermediates. An augmentation of L(−)-carnitine levels could therefore lead to stimulation of β-oxidation, reduced glycogen consumption, and a delayed fatigue. Physical exercise increases the uptake and oxidation of fatty acids by contracting muscles (220). CPT I was suggested to be responsible for a specific regulation (118). Animal experiments have shown that CPT I activity doubled after physical exercise in red and white muscles (221). A CPT I K_m value of 480 μmol/L was determined in human skeletal muscle (117). The total L(−)-carnitine concentration of human muscle was estimated at 3–4 mmol/L (203). Taking into account the fact that only 30% of total muscular L(−)-carnitine is available as free L(−)-carnitine allows enough room for an activity increase of CPT I by L(−)-carnitine application. It should also be mentioned that the regulation of CPT I is a rather complex area since various isoenzymes have been found whose regulation may differ between tissues. Certainly more work is needed in this field. Führenbach et al. demonstrated that 30 mg L(−)-carnitine/kg body weight of elite athletes applied for 6 weeks significantly changed fatty acid metabolism in vivo (210). Very low-density lipoprotein cholesterol decreased by 20%, free fatty acids by 16%, and body fat by 10%.
3. Modulation of erythrocyte properties and numbers by L(−)-carnitine: L(−)-carnitine and acyl-L(−)-carnitine are able to modify the properties of erythrocyte membranes and improve the rheological quality of the blood. In contrast to choline or β-methylcholine, L(−)-carnitine inhibits the aggregation of erythrocytes caused by fibrinogen (222). Activated fatty acids are incorporated directly into the phospholipids of erythrocyte membranes via O-acyl-L(−)-carnitine independently of ATP (223). In addition, short-chain acyl-L(−)-carnitines, such as acetyl- and propionyl-L(−)-carnitine, change the molecule of phospholipid groups in the erythrocyte membrane (224). In erythrocytes the total L(−)-carnitine concentration is 240 μmol/L compared with 60 μmol in plasma. Furthermore, the content of acyl-L(−)-carnitine is enhanced 2.5 times relative to plasma levels (225). The authors propose a putative function in the modulation of membrane lipids and a stimula-

tion of Na^+/K^+-ATPase activity. An improved oxygen release by modified membrane properties could explain the augmentation of VO_2max after L(−)-carnitine application (213,226).

F. Geriatric Nutrition

Only a few authors have reported on L(−)-carnitine and its requirements during the life cycle (53). The published data on blood L(−)-carnitine levels of elderly people are contradictory. Women older than 40 displayed increased L(−)-carnitine levels. No differences were found in the blood of men of different ages (227). In contrast, a decrease in men of L(−)-carnitine concentration in blood with age was observed (228). The activity of the citric acid cycle and β-oxidation enzymes as well as the L(−)-carnitine muscle content decreased with increasing age (229). Based on these results, an influence on heart metabolism, sperm maturation and mobility, as well as cognitive behavior of elderly people was suggested. Furthermore, it was postulated that L(−)-carnitine biosynthesis in liver, kidney, and brain declined with age, creating a secondary lack of L(−)-carnitine (230). Additional studies to demonstrate clinical conditions of secondary L(−)-carnitine deficiency are still needed. On the other hand, L(−)-carnitine and its short-chain acyl esters were recommended for the treatment of chronic degenerative disease. It has been clinically demonstrated that acetyl-L(−)-carnitine slowed down the progression of Alzheimer's disease (231–233). The neuroprotective effects of L(−)-carnitine seem to have more to do with its steric resemblance to acetylcholine than to be related to nonspecific membrane interactions (234). Other studies using acetyl-L(−)-carnitine have reported on the slowing down of aging processes and forms of dementia (235–240). Mitochondrial decay may be one of the principal underlying causes of cellular decline in the aging process. Recently it was shown in old rats that acetyl-L(−)-carnitine and lipoic acid administered for a few weeks restored mitochondrial function, lowered oxidants to the levels of young rats, and increased ambulatory activity. Thus, these two metabolites were considered to be necessary for health in old age and were therefore proposed as conditional micronutrients (241,242).

VI. APPLICATION OF γ-BUTYROBETAINE

γ-Butyrobetaine is the direct precursor of L(−)-carnitine in many organisms, including humans (see Fig. 1). The last step of its biosynthesis is carried out in the liver, kidney, testis, and brain by γ-butyrobetaine hydroxylase (18,44,243). The hydroxylation of the substrate is linked to the oxidative decarboxylation of α-ketoglutarate (see Fig. 1). The reaction requires cofactors (see Sec. II.A) and can be stimulated by catalase (244). L(−)- and D(+)-Carnitine are inhibitors of the enzyme (245). Kidney tissue displays the highest γ-butyrobetaine hydroxylase activity in humans (44). In other species the main activity is differently distributed, e.g., in rat the last step is almost exclusively located in the liver (59). In contrast to other enzymes of L(−)-carnitine biosynthesis, the activity of γ-butyrobetaine hydroxylase increases with age. In infants the enzyme activity is only about 10% that of adults (44).

γ-Butyrobetaine and other L(−)-carnitine precursors (6-*N*-trimethyllysine, 3-hydroxy-6-*N*-trimethyllysine) are absorbed like L(−)-carnitine (see Sec. II.B) (76). A large amount of dietary L(−)-carnitine is degraded via crotonobetaine to γ-butyrobetaine by Enterobacteriaceae in the human intestine under anaerobic conditions (101,105). It seems likely that part of the formed γ-butyrobetaine is taken up and transformed to L(−)-carnitine by the body.

Based on the above given explanations it should theoretically be possible to stimulate L(−)-carnitine synthesis by γ-butyrobetaine supplementation. Rebouche et al. (58) tested the utilization of dietary precursors for L(−)-carnitine synthesis in human adults. Excess amounts of the L(−)-carnitine precursors lysine plus methionine, 6-*N*-trimethyllysine, and γ-butyrobetaine were fed as supplements to a low L(−)-carnitine diet for 10 days. Dietary γ-butyrobetaine dramatically increased L(−)-carnitine production, 6-*N*-trimethyllysine had a somewhat smaller effect, and lysine plus methionine had even less effect on L(−)-carnitine synthesis (58). Comparable studies were carried out with rats (246,247) and a clear increase in L(−)-carnitine levels in plasma, kidney, and liver were found. The effect of γ-butyrobetaine is dependent on its concentration. Like L(−)-carnitine, in vivo γ-butyrobetaine reduces de novo L(−)-carnitine synthesis from 6-*N*-trimethyllysine (246). Sandor proposed γ-butyrobetaine as a potential L(−)-carnitine replacement (247). Supporting this suggestion is the fact that γ-butyrobetaine hydroxylase is not rate limiting for L(−)-carnitine synthesis (248). It was argued that γ-butyrobetaine uptake by tissues involved in L(−)-carnitine synthesis could restrict its transformation to L(−)-carnitine (58), but recently Berardi et al. demonstrated that γ-butyrobetaine transport is not rate limiting for L(−)-carnitine synthesis in liver (249).

γ-Butyrobetaine could replace L(−)-carnitine as a supplement. The advantage to the consumer would be a lower price for the same physiological effect because γ-butyrobetaine is an achiral molecule and its synthesis would be easier as well as less expensive than the production of the chiral L(−)-carnitine. As a prerequisite for such a recommendation, additional studies are required. The equivalence of γ-butyrobetaine and L(−)-carnitine must be demonstrated over a wide concentration range. Levels of free and total L(−)-carnitine and γ-butyrobetaine should be measured in plasma and relevant organs (e.g., kidney, liver, muscle, brain). In addition, experiments using γ-butyrobetaine with established L(−)-

carnitine deficiency should be carried out before γ-butyrobetaine is used as a supplement and L(−)-carnitine substitute in humans.

VII. CONCLUDING REMARKS

L(−)-Carnitine plays an important role in fatty acid metabolism, transporting activated fatty acids from the cytosol into the mitochondrial matrix. In addition, L(−)-carnitine is involved in other biochemical pathways, e.g., modulation of acyl-CoA/CoA ratio. The molecular basis of genetic disorders of the carnitine system is under research. The liver and muscle isoforms of CPT 1 cDNAs and more or less active mutations of the CPT II were described and brought about a better understanding of the carnitine system and its disturbances.

The human body is able to synthesize L(−)-carnitine from protein-bound L-lysine and methionine. Its biosynthesis requires several cofactors: niacin, vitamin B_6, vitamin C, and iron. Furthermore, intake of L(−)-carnitine serves to maintain tissue L(−)-carnitine stores. Two uptake mechanisms have been described in the human intestine: active transport and passive diffusion. Meat is the preferred nutritional source for L(−)-carnitine, therefore strict vegetarians have a relatively high risk of receiving too little L(−)-carnitine from food. When tube-fed or parenterally fed patients receive L(−)-carnitine-free food, neonates react with carnitine deficiency in serum and tissues after one week, adults only after months. L(−)-Carnitine application is a helpful tool for stabilization of fatty acid oxidation in humans.

The systemic primary carnitine deficiency syndrome manifests itself either as hepatic encephalopathy or as progressive cardiomyopathy; the underlying cause is obviously a defect in the carnitine transport system of cell membranes accumulating L(−)-carnitine inside the cell against the concentration gradient. Secondary carnitine deficiencies are associated with a wide variety of hereditary or acquired diseases.

Several studies have shown that L(−)-carnitine is an interesting nutritional supplement for athletes supporting energy production. An excess of L(−)-carnitine reduces the acetyl-CoA/CoA ratio and liberates CoA for other metabolic functions. Finally, the modulation of erythrocyte properties and number by L(−)-carnitine was demonstrated.

A positive influence of L(−)-carnitine on heart metabolism, sperm maturation, and mobility as well as cognitive behavior of elderly people has been suggested. Acetyl-L(−)-carnitine and lipoic acid administered for a few weeks restored mitochondrial function during aging.

γ-Butyrobetaine, the direct precursor of L(−)-carnitine, could also be an interesting and cheap nutritional supplement replacing L(−)-carnitine.

REFERENCES

1. Gulewitsch W, Krimberg R. Zur Kenntnis der Extraktivstoffe der Muskeln. II. Mitteilung. Über das Carnitin. Hoppe Seyler's Z Physiol Chem 1905; 45:326–330.
2. Tomita M, Sendju Y. Über die Oxyaminoverbindungen, welche die Biuretreaktion zeigen. III. Spaltung der γ-Amino-β-oxybuttersäure in die optisch-aktiven Komponenten. Hoppe-Seyler's Z Physiol Chem 1927; 169:263–277.
3. Carter HE, Bhattacharrya PK, Weidman KR, Fraenkel G. Chemical studies on vitamin B_T isolation and characterization as carnitine. Arch Biochem Biophys 1952; 38:405–416.
4. Fraenkel G, Blewett M, Coles M. B_T, a new vitamin of the B-group and its relation to the folic acid group and other anti-anaemia factors. Nature 1948; 161:981–983.
5. Friedman S, Fraenkel G. Reversible enzymatic acetylation of carnitine. Arch Biochem Biophys 1955; 59:491–501.
6. Fritz IB. The effects of muscle extracts on the oxidation on palmitic acid by liver slices and homogenates. Acta Physiol Scand 1955; 34:367–385.
7. Lindstedt G, Lindstedt S. On the biosynthesis and degradation of carnitine. Biochem Biophys Res Commun 1961; 6:319–323.
8. Bremer J. Carnitine precursors in the rat. Biochim Biophys Acta 1962; 57:327–335.
9. Kaneko T, Yoshida R. On the absolute configuration of L-carnitine (vitamin B_T). Bull Chem Soc Jpn 1962; 35:1153–1155.
10. Bremer J. Carnitine in intermediary metabolism. Reversible acetylation of carnitine by mitochondria. J Biol Chem 1962; 237:2228–2231.
11. Bremer J. Carnitine in intermediary metabolism. The metabolism of fatty acid esters of carnitine by mitochondria. J Biol Chem 1962; 237:3628–3632.
12. Fritz IB, Yue KTN. Long-chain carnitine acyltransferase and the role of acylcarnitine derivatives in the catalytic increase of fatty acid oxidation induced by carnitine. J Lipid Res 1963; 4:279–288.
13. Bremer J. Carnitine in intermediary metabolism. The biosynthesis of palmitoylcarnitine by cell subfractions. J Biol Chem 1963; 238:2774–2779.
14. Norum KR, Farstad M, Bremer J. The submitochondrial distribution of acid: CoA ligase (AMP) and palmityl-CoA: carnitine palmityltransferase in rat liver mitochondria. Biochem Biophys Res Commun 1966; 24:797–804.
15. Yates DW, Shepherd D, Garland PB. Organization of fatty-acid activation in rat liver mitochondria. Nature 1966; 209:1213–1215.
16. Solberg HE, Bremer J. Formation of branched chain acylcarnitines in mitochondria. Biochim Biophys Acta 1970; 222:372–380.
17. Horne DW, Tanphaichitr V, Broquist HP. Role of lysine in carnitine biosynthesis in *Neurospora crassa*. J Biol Chem 1971; 246:4373–4375.
18. Bremer J. Carnitine—metabolism and functions. Physiol Rev 1983; 63:1420–1480.
19. Bau R, Schreiber A, Metzenthin T, Lu RS, Lutz F, Klooster WT, Koetzle TF, Seim

H, Kleber H-P, Brewer F, Englard S. Neutron diffraction structure of (2R, 3R)-L-(−)-[2-D] carnitine tetrachloroaurate $[(CH_3)_3N\text{-}CH_2\text{-}CHOH\text{-}CHD\text{-}COOH]^+$ $[AuCl_4^-]$: determination of the absolute stereochemistry of the crotonobetaine-to-carnitine transformation catalyzed by L-carnitine dehydratase from *Escherichia coli*. J Am Chem Soc 1997; 119:12055–12060.
20. Engel AG, Angelini C. Carnitine deficiency of human muscle with associated lipid storage myopathy: a new syndrome. Science 1973; 179:899–902.
21. DiMauro S, DiMauro PM. Muscle carnitine palmityltransferase deficiency and myoglobinuria. Science 1973; 182:929–931.
22. Ramsay RR, Tubbs PK. The mechanism of fatty acid uptake by heart mitochondria: an acylcarnitine-carnitine exchange. FEBS Lett 1975; 54:21–25.
23. Pande SV. A mitochondrial carnitine acylcarnitine translocase system. Proc Natl Acad Sci USA 1975; 72:883–887.
24. McGarry JD, Leatherman GF, Foster DW. Carnitine palmitoyltransferase I. The site of inhibition of hepatic fatty acid oxidation by malonyl-CoA. J Biol Chem 1978; 253:4128–4136.
25. Kondo A, Blanchard JS, Englard S. Purification of calf liver gamma-butyrobetaine hydroxylase. Arch Biochem Biophys 1981; 212:338–346.
26. Murthy MSR, Pande SV. Malonyl-CoA binding site and the overt carnitine palmitoyltransferase activity reside on the opposite sides of the outer mitochondrial membrane. Proc Natl Acad Sci USA 1987; 84:378–382.
27. Tanphaichitr V, Horne DW, Broquist HP. Lysine, a precursor of carnitine in the rat. J Biol Chem 1971; 246:6364–6366.
28. Chatterjee B, Song CS, Kim JM, Roy AK. Cloning, sequencing, and regulation of rat liver carnitine octanoyltransferase: transcriptional stimulation of the enzyme during peroxisome proliferation. Biochemistry 1988; 27:9000–9006.
29. Woeltje KF, Esser V, Weis BC, Sen A, Cox WF, McPhaul MJ, Staughter CA, Foster DW, McGarry JD. Cloning, sequencing, and expression of a cDNA encoding rat liver mitochondrial carnitine palmitoyl transferase II. J Biol Chem 1990; 265: 10720–10725.
30. Esser V, Britton CH, Weis BC, Foster DW, McGarry JD. Cloning, sequencing, and expression of a cDNA encoding rat liver carnitine palmitoyltransferase I. Direct evidence that a single polypeptide is involved in inhibitor interaction and catalytic function. J Biol Chem 1993; 268:5817–5822.
31. Johnson TM, Kocher HP, Anderson RC, Nemecek GM. Cloning, sequencing and heterologous expression of a cDNA encoding pigeon liver carnitine acyltransferase. Biochem J 1995; 305(Pt 2):439–444.
32. Caudevilla C, Serra D, Miliar A, Codony C, Asins G, Bach M, Hegardt FG. Natural trans-splicing in carnitine octanoyltransferase pre-mRNAs in rat liver. Proc Natl Acad Sci USA 1998; 95:12185–12190.
33. Jacobs BS, Wanders RJA. Fatty acid oxidation in peroxisomes and mitochondria: the first unequivocal evidence for the involvement of carnitine in shuttling propionyl-CoA from peroxisomes to mitochondria. Biochem Biophys Res Commun 1995; 213:1035–1041.
34. Meier PJ. D-Carnitin, harmlos? In: Gitzelmann R, Baerlocher K, Steinmann B, eds. Carnitin in der Medizin. Stuttgart: Schattauer, 1987:101–104.

35. Jung H, Jung K, Kleber H-P. Synthesis of L-carnitine by microorganisms and isolated enzymes. Adv Biochem Engin Biotechnol 1993; 50:22–44.
36. Lindstedt G, Lindstedt S. Studies on the biosynthesis of carnitine. J Biol Chem 1965; 240:316–321.
37. Rebouche CJ. Comparative aspects of carnitine biosynthesis in microorganisms and mammals with attention to carnitine biosynthesis in man. In: Frenkel RA, McGarry JD, eds. Carnitine Biosynthesis, Metabolism, and Functions. New York: Academic, 1980:57–72.
38. Borum PR, Broquist HP. Lysine deficiency and carnitine in male and female rats. J Nutr 1977; 107:1209–1215.
39. Rebouche CJ, Broquist HP. Carnitine biosynthesis in *Neurospora crassa*: enzymatic conversion of lysine to ε-N-trimethyllysine. J Bacteriol 1976; 126:1207–1214.
40. Paik WK, Kim S. Protein methylation: chemical, enzymological, and biological significance. Adv Enzymol Relat Areas Mol Biol 1975; 42:227–286.
41. Rebouche CJ, Paulson DJ. Carnitine metabolism and function in humans. Ann Rev Nutr 1986; 6:41–66.
42. Labadie J, Dunn WA, Aronson NN Jr. Hepatic synthesis of carnitine from protein-bound trimethyl-lysine. Lysosomal digestion of methyl-lysine-labelled asialo-fetuin. Biochem J 1976; 160:85–95.
43. Hulse JD, Ellis SR, Henderson LM. Carnitine biosynthesis. β-Hydroxylation of trimethyllysine by an α-ketoglutarate-dependent mitochondrial dioxygenase. J Biol Chem 1978; 253:1654–1659.
44. Rebouche CJ, Engel AG. Tissue distribution of carnitine biosynthesis enzymes in man. Biochim Biophys Acta 1980; 630:22–29.
45. Hulse JD, Henderson LM. Carnitine biosynthesis. Purification of 4-N-trimethylaminobutyraldehyde dehydrogenase from beef liver. J Biol Chem 1980; 225:1146–1151.
46. Bohmer T. Conversion of butyrobetaine to carnitine in the rat in vivo. Biochim Biophys Acta 1974; 343:551–557.
47. Cederblad G, Holm J, Lindstedt G, Lindstedt S, Nordin J, Schersten T. γ-Butyrobetaine hydroxylase activity in human and bovine liver and skeletal muscle tissue. FEBS Lett 1979; 98:57–60.
48. Cox RA, Hoppel CL. Carnitine and trimethylaminobutyrate synthesis in rat tissue. Biochem J 1974; 142:699–701.
49. Englard S. Hydroxylation of γ-butyrobetaine to carnitine in human and monkey tissues. FEBS Lett 1979; 102:297–300.
50. Brooks DE, McIntosh JEA. Turnover of carnitine in rat tissues. Biochem J 1975; 148:439–445.
51. Cederblad G, Lindstedt S, Lundholm K. Concentration of carnitine in human muscle tissue. Clin Chim Acta 1974; 53:311–321.
52. Brooks DE. Carnitine in the male reproductive tract and its relation to the metabolism of the epididymis and spermatozoa. In: Frenkel RA, McGarry JD, eds. Carnitine Biosynthesis, Metabolism, and Functions. New York: Academic, 1980:219–235.

53. Rebouche CJ. Carnitine function and requirements during the life cycle. FASEB J 1992; 6:3379–3386.
54. Kahn L, Bamji MS. Tissue carnitine deficiency due to dietary lysine deficiency: triglyceride accumulation and concomitant impairment in fatty acid oxidation. J Nutr 1979; 109:24–31.
55. Tanphaichitr V, Broquist HP. Lysine deficiency in the rat: concomitant impairment in carnitine biosynthesis. J Nutr 1973; 130:80–87.
56. Nelson PJ, Pruit RE, Henderson LL, Jeness R, Henderson LM. Effect of ascorbic acid deficiency in the in vivo synthesis of carnitine. Biochim Biophys Acta 1981; 672:123–127.
57. Rebouche CJ, Lehmann LJ, Olson AL. ϵ-N-Trimethyllysine availability regulates the rate of carnitine biosynthesis in the growing rat. J Nutr 1986; 116:751–759.
58. Rebouche CJ, Bosch EP, Chenard CA, Schabold KJ, Nelson SE. Utilization of dietary precursors for carnitine biosynthesis in human adults. J Nutr 1989; 119: 1907–1913.
59. Sandor A, Hoppel CL. Butyrobetaine availability in liver is a regulatory factor for carnitine biosynthesis in rat. Flux through butyrobetaine hydroxylase in fasting state. Eur J Biochem 1989; 185:671–675.
60. Heinonen OJ. Carnitine: effect on palmitate oxidation, exercise capacity, and nitrogen balance. An experimental study with special reference to carnitine depletion and supplementation. PhD dissertation, University of Turku, Turku, 1992.
61. Rebouche CJ, Chenard CA. Metabolic fate of dietary carnitine in human adults: identification und quantification of urinary and fecal metabolites. J Nutr 1991; 121: 539–546.
62. Rebouche CJ, Mack DL, Edmonson PF. L-Carnitine dissimilation in the gastrointestinal tract of the rat. Biochemistry 1984; 23:6422–6426.
63. Seim H, Schulze J, Strack E. Catabolic pathways for high-dosed L(−)- or D(+)-carnitine in germ-free rats? Biol Chem Hoppe-Seylers 1985; 366:1017–1021.
64. Strack E, Seim H. The formation in vivo of γ-butyrobetaine from exogenous L(−)-carnitine in the mouse and the rat. Hoppe-Seyler's Z Physdiol Chem 1979; 360: 207–215.
65. Seim H, Strack E. Reduction of crotonobetaine and D-carnitine to γ-butyrobetaine, and the metabolism of L-carnitine in the mouse and rat. Hoppe-Seyler's Z Physiol Chem 1980; 361:1059–1067.
66. Rebouche CJ, Engel AG. Kinetic compartmental analysis of carnitine metabolism in the human carnitine deficiency syndromes. Evidence for alterations in tissue carnitine transport. J Clin Invest 1984; 73:857–867.
67. Seim H. The role of catabolic reactions and nutrition for the etiopathogenesis of carnitine deficiency syndromes. In: H Seim, H Löster, eds. Carnitine—Pathobiochemical Basis and Clinical Applications. Bochum: Ponte, 1996:123–140.
68. Gross CJ, Henderson LM. Absorption of D- and L-carnitine by the intestine and kidney tubule in the rat. Biochim Biophys Acta 1984; 772:209–219.
69. Gudjonsson H, Li BUK, Shug Al, Olsen WA. In vivo studies of intestinal carnitine absorption in rats. Gastroenterology 1985; 88:1880–1887.
70. Gudjonsson H, Li BUK, Shug AL, Olsen WA. Studies of carnitine metabolism in relation to intestinal absorption. Am J Physiol 1985; 248:G 313–G 319.

71. Shaw RD, Li BUK, Hamilton JW, Shug AL, Olsen WA. Carnitine transport in rat small intestine. Am J Physiol 1983; 245:G 378–G 381.
72. Hamilton JW, Li BUK, Shug AL, Olsen WA. Carnitine transport in human intestinal biopsy specimens. Demonstration of an active transport system. Gastroenterology 1986; 91:10–16.
73. Hamilton JW, Li BUK, Shug AL, Olsen WA. Studies of L-carnitine absorption in man. Gastroenterology 1983; 84:1180–1185.
74. BUK Li, Lloyd ML, Gudjonsson H, Shug AL, Olsen WA. The effect of enteral carnitine administration in humans. Am J Clin Nutr 1992; 55:838–845.
75. McLoud E, Ma TY, Grant KE, Mathis RK, Said HM. Uptake of L-carnitine by a human intestinal epithelial cell line, Caco-2. Gastroenterology 1996; 111:1534–1540.
76. Borum PR, Fisher KD. Health effects of dietary carnitine. Report of the Life Sciences Research Office, Federation of American Societies for Experimental Biology, Maryland, 1983.
77. Li BUK, Bummer PM, Hamilton JW, Gudjonsson H, Zografi G, Olsen WA. Uptake of L-carnitine by rat jejunal brush border microvillous membrane vesicles. Evidence of passive diffusion. Digest Dis Sci 1990; 35:333–339.
78. Gross CJ, Savaiano DA. Effect of development and nutritional state on the uptake, metabolism and release of free and acetyl-L-carnitine by the rodent small intestine. Biochim Biophys Acta 1993; 1170:265–274.
79. Gross CJ, Henderson LM, Savaiano DA. Uptake of L-carnitine, D-carnitine and acetyl-L-carnitine by isolated guinea-pig enterocytes. Biochim Biophys Acta 1986; 886:425–433.
80. Engel AG, Rebouche CJ. Carnitine metabolism and inborn errors. J Inherit Metab Dis 1984; 7(suppl 1):38–43.
81. Carter L, Abney TO, Lapp DF. Biosynthesis and metabolism of carnitine. J Child Neurol 1995; 10(suppl):2S3–2S7.
82. Bremer J. The role of carnitine in intracellular metabolism. J Clin Chem Clin Biochem 1990; 28:297–301.
83. Rebouche CJ, Engel AG. Carnitine metabolism and deficiency syndromes. Mayo Clin Proc 1983; 58:533–540.
84. Christiansen RZ, Bremer J. Active transport of butyrobetaine and carnitine into isolated liver cells. Biochim Biophys Acta 1976; 448:562–577.
85. Kispal GY, Melegh B, Alkonyi I, Sandor A. Enhanced uptake of carnitine by perfused rat liver following starvation. Biochim Biophys Acta 1987; 896:96–102.
86. Rebouche CJ, Seim H. Carnitine metabolism and its regulation in microorganisms and mammals. Annu Rev Nutr 1998; 18:39–61.
87. Hokland BM. Uptake, metabolism and release of carnitine and acylcarnitine in the perfused liver. Biochim Biophys Acta 1998; 961:234–241.
88. Sandor A, Kispal GY, Melegh B, Alkonyi I. Ester composition of carnitine in the perfusate of liver and in the plasma of donor rats. Eur J Biochem 1987; 170:443–445.
89. Sandor A, Kispal GY, Melegh B, Alkonyi I. Release of carnitine from the perfused rat liver. Biochim Biophys Acta 1985; 835:83–91.

90. Bohmer T, Eiklid K, Jonsen J. Carnitine uptake into human heart cells in culture. Biochim Biophys Acta 1977; 465:627–633.
91. Vary TC, Neely JR. Characterization of carnitine transport in isolated perfused adult rat hearts. Am J Physiol 1982; 242:H585–H592.
92. Martinuzzi A, Vergani L, Rosa M, Angelino C. L-Carnitine uptake in differentiating human cultured muscle. Biochim Biophys Acta 1991; 1095:217–222.
93. Rebouche CJ. Carnitine movement across muscle cell membranes. Studies in isolated rat muscle. Biochim Biophys Acta 1977; 471:145–155.
94. Stieger B, O'Neill D, Krähenbühl S. Characterization of L-carnitine transport by rat kidney brush-border-membrane vesicles. Biochem J 1995; 309:643–647.
95. Rebouche CJ, Mack DL. Sodium gradient-stimulated transport of L-carnitine into renal brush border membrane vesicles: kinetics, specifity, regulation by dietary carnitine. Arch Biochem Biophys 1984; 235:393–402.
96. Cederblad G, Lindstedt S. Metabolism of labeled carnitine in the rat. Arch Biochem Biophys 1976; 175:173–180.
97. Seim H, Strack E. Acetylcarnitine in the blood and urine of the mouse after injection of L-carnitine and several D-acyl-L-carnitines. Hoppe-Seyler's Z Physiol Chem 1977; 358:675–683.
98. Wolff L, Müller D, Strack E. Toxicität von L(−)-Carnitin und einigen O-Azylcarnitinen. Acta Biol Med Germ 1971; 26:1237–1241.
99. Löster H, Seim H, Strack E. Self-decomposition of DL[methyl-^{14}C] carnitine to labelled β-methylcholine and acetonyltrimethylammonium. J Lab Cmpd Radiopharm 1983; 20:1035–1045.
100. Haeckel R, Kaiser E, Oellerich M, Siliprandi N. Carnitine: metabolism, function and clinical application. J Clin Chem Clin Biochem 1990; 28:291–295.
101. Kleber H-P. Bacterial carnitine metabolism. FEMS Microbiol Lett 1997; 147: 1–9.
102. Kleber H-P, Seim H, Aurich H, Strack E. Verwertung von Trimethylammoniumverbindungen durch *Acinetobacter calcoaceticus*. Arch Microbiol 1977; 112:201–206.
103. Seim H, Löster H, Claus R, Kleber H-P, Strack E. Splitting of the C-N-bound in carnitine by an enzyme (trimethylamine forming) from membranes of *Acinetobacter calcoaceticus*. FEMS Microbiol Lett 1982; 15:165–167.
104. Ditullio D, Anderson D, Chen CS, Shih CJ. L-Carnitine via enzyme-catalyzed oxidative kinetic resolution. Bioorg Med Chem 1994; 6:415–420.
105. Seim H, Ezold R, Kleber H-P, Strack E. Stoffwechsel des L-Carnitins bei Enterobakterien. Z Allg Mikrobiol 1980; 20:591–594.
106. Seim H, Löster H, Claus R, Kleber H-P, Strack E. Formation of γ-butyrobetaine and trimethylamine from quaternary ammonium compounds structure-related to L-carnitine and choline by *Proteus vulgaris*. FEMS Microbiol Lett 1982; 13:201–205.
107. Seim H, Löster H, Claus R, Kleber H-P, Strack E. Stimulation of the anerobic growth of *Salmonella typhimurium* by reduction of L-carnitine, derivatives and structure-related trimethylammonium compounds. Arch Microbiol 1982; 132:91–95.
108. Hamilton JJ, Hahn P. Carnitine and carnitine esters in rat bile and human duodenal fluid. Can J Physiol Pharmacol 1987; 65:1816–1820.

109. Munteanu M, Seim H. Radiochemical enzymatic method for determination of L(−)-carnitine fractions in body fluids including bile. Eur J Clin Chem Biochem 1995; 33:A79.
110. Heinonen OJ. Carnitine and physical exercise. Sports Med 1996; 22:109–132.
111. Engel AG, Rebouche CJ, Wilson DM, Glasgow AM, Romshe CA, Cruse RP. Primary systemic carnitine deficiency. II. Renal handling of carnitine. Neurology 1981; 31:819–825.
112. Rebouche CJ, Lombard KA, Chenard CA. Renal adaptation to dietary carnitine in humans. Am J Clin Nutr 1993; 58:660–665.
113. Hockland BM, Bremer J. Metabolism and excretion of carnitine and acylcarnitines in the perfused rat kidney. Biochim Biophys Acta 1986; 886:223–230.
114. Rebouche CJ. Role of carnitine biosynthesis and renal conservation of carnitine in genetic and acquired disorders of carnitine metabolism. In: H Seim, Löster, eds. Carnitine—Pathobiochemical Basis and Clinical Applications. Bochum: Ponte, 1996:111–121.
115. Stadler DD, Chenard CA, Rebouche CJ. Effect of dietary macronutrient content on carnitine excretion and efficiency of carnitine reabsorption. Am J Clin Nutr 1993; 58:868–872.
116. Bremer J. The role of carnitine in cell metabolism. In: DeSimone C, Famularo G, eds. Carnitine Today. New York: Springer, 1997:1–37.
117. McGarry JD, Woeltje KF, Kuwajima M, Foster DW. Regulation of ketogenesis and the renaissance of carnitine palmitoyltransferase. Diabetes/Metabolism Rev 1989; 5:271–284.
118. Saggerson D, Ghadiminejad I, Awan M. Regulation of mitochondrial carnitine palmitoyl transferases from liver and extrahepatic tissues. Advan Enzyme Regul 1992; 32:285–306.
119. Brady PS, Ramsay RR, Brady LJ. Regulation of the long-chain carnitine acyltransferases. FASEB J 1993; 7:1039–1044.
120. Sugden MC, Holness MJ. Interactive regulation of the pyruvate dehydrogenase complex and the carnitine palmitoyltransferase system. FASEB J 1994; 8:54–61.
121. Eaton S, Bartlett K, Pourfarzam M. Mammalian mitochondrial β-oxidation. Biochem J 1996; 320:345–357.
122. Ramsay RR. The role of the carnitine system in peroxisomal fatty acid oxidation. Am J Med Sci 1999; 318:28–35.
123. Breningstall GN. Carnitine deficiency syndromes. Pediatr Neurol 1990; 6(2):75–81.
124. Famularo G, Matricardi F, Nucera E, Santini G, DeSimone C. Carnitine deficiency: Primary and secondary syndromes. In: DeSimone C, Famularo G, eds. Carnitine Today. New York: Springer, 1997:119–161.
125. Karpati G, Carpenter S, Engel AG, Watters G, Allen J, Rothman S, Klassen G, Mamer OA. The syndrome of systemic carnitine deficiency. Clinical morphologic, biochemical, and pathophysiologic features. Neurology 1975; 25:16–24.
126. Kerner J, Hoppel C. Genetic disorders of carnitine metabolism and their nutritional management. Annu Rev Nutr 1998; 18:179–206.
127. Seim H. Carnitine. In: Thomas L, ed. Clinical Laboratory Diagnostics. Use and Assessment of Clinical Laboratory Results. Frankfurt: TH-Books, 1998:202–207.

128. Mesmer OT, Lo LCY. Hexose transport properties of myoblasts isolated from a patient with suspected muscle carnitine deficiency. Biochem Cell Biol 1990; 68: 1372–1379.
129. Campos Y, Huertas R, Lorenzo G, Bautista J, Gutierrez E, Aparicio M, Alesso L, Arenas J. Plasma carnitine insufficiency and effectiveness of L-carnitine therapy in patients with mitochondrial myopathy. Muscle Nerve 1993; 16:150–153.
130. Sewell A, Böhles HJ. Acylcarnitines in intermediary metabolism. Eur J Pediatr 1995; 154:871–877.
131. Tanphaichitr V, Leelahagul P. Carnitine metabolism and human carnitine deficiency. Nutrition 1993; 9:246–254.
132. Pons R, De Vivo DC. Primary and secondary carnitine deficiency syndromes. J Child Neurol 1995; 10:S 8–S 24.
133. Verderio E, Cavadini P, Montermini L, Wang H, Lamantea E, Finocchiaro G, DiDonato S, Gellera C, Taroni F. Carnitine palmitoyltransferase II deficiency: structure of the gene and characterization of two novel disease-causing mutations. Hum Mol Genet 1995; 4:19–29.
134. Yang BZ, Ding JH, Dewese T, Roe D, He G, Wilkinson J, Day DW, Demaugre F, Rabier D, Brivet M, Roe C. Identification of four novel mutations in patients with carnitine palmitoyltransferase II (CPT II) deficiency. Mol Genet Metab 1998; 64:229–236.
135. Wataya K, Akanuma J, Cavadini P, Aoki Y, Kure S, Invernizzi F, Yoshida I, Kira J, Taroni F, Matsubara Y, Narisawa K. Two CPT2 mutations in three Japanese patients with carnitine palmitoyltransferase II deficiency: functional analysis and association with polymorphic haplotypes and two clinical phenotypes. Hum Mutat 1998; 11:377–386.
136. Taggart RT, Smail D, Apolito C, Vladutiu GD. Novel mutations associated with carnitine palmitoyltransferase II deficiency. Hum Mutat 1999; 13:210–220.
137. Taroni F, Verderio E, Dworzak F, Willems PF, Cavadini P, DiDonato S. Identification of a common mutation in the carnitine palmitoyltransferase II gene in familial recurrent myoglobinuria patients. Nat Genet 1993; 4:314–320.
138. Hug G, Bove KE, Soukup S. Lethal neonatal multiorgan deficiency of carnitine palmitoyltransferase II. N Engl J Med 1991; 325:1862–1864.
139. Murthy MSR, Pande SV. Molecular biology of carnitine palmitoyltransferases and role of carnitine in gene transcription. In: DeSimone C, Famularo G, eds. Carnitine Today. New York: Springer, 1997:39–70.
140. Britton CH, Schultz RA, Zhang B, Esser V, Foster DW, McGarry JD. Human liver mitochondrial carnitine palmitoyltransferase I: characterization of its cDNA and chromosomal localization and partial analysis of the gene. Proc Natl Acad Sci USA 1995; 92:1984–1988.
141. Yamazaki N, Shinohara Y, Shima A, Yamanaka Y, Terada H. Isolation and characterization of cDNA and genomic clones encoding human muscle type carnitine palmitoyltransferase I. Biochim Biophys Acta 1996; 1307:157–161.
142. Britton CH, Mackey DW, Esser V, Foster DW, Burns DK. Fine chromosome mapping of the genes for human liver and muscle carnitine palmitoyltransferase I (CPT1A and CPT1B). Genomics 1997; 40:209–211.
143. van der Leij FR, Takens J, van der Veen AY, Terpstra P, Kuipers JR. Localization

and intron usage analysis of the human CPT1B gene for muscle type carnitine palmitoyltransferase I. Biochim Biophys Acta 1997; 1352:123–128.
144. Brown NF, Hill JK, Esser V, Kirkland JL, Corkey BE, Foster DW, McGarry JD. Mouse white adipocytes and 3T3-L1 cells display an anomalous pattern of carnitine palmitoyltransferase (CPT) I isoform expression during differentiation. Inter-tissue and inter-species expression of CPT I and CPT II enzymes. Biochem J 1997; 327: 225–231.
145. Cook GA, Park EA. Expression and regulation of carnitine palmitoyltransferase-Ialpha and -Ibeta genes. Am J Med Sci 1999; 318:43–48.
146. Xia Y, Buja LM, McMillin JB. Change in expression of heart carnitine palmitoyltransferase I isoforms with electrical stimulation of cultured rat neonatal cardiac myocytes. J Biol Chem 1996; 271:12082–12087.
147. Yu GS, Lu YC, Gulick T. Rat carnitine palmitoyltransferase Ibeta mRNA splicing isoforms. Biochim Biophys Acta 1998; 1393:166–172.
148. McGarry JD, Brown NF. The mitochondrial carnitine palmitoyltransferase system. From concept to molecular analysis. Eur J Biochem 1997; 244:1–14.
149. Berman AJ, Donckerwolcke RA, Duran M, Smeitink JA, Mousson B, Vianey-Saban C, Poll-The BT. Rate-dependent distal renal tubular acidosis and carnitine palmitoyltransferase I deficiency. Pediatr Res 1994; 36:582–588.
150. Schaefer J, Jackson S, Taroni F, Swift P, Turnbull DM. Characterisation of carnitine palmitoyltransferase deficiency: implications for diagnosis and therapy. J Neurol Neurosurg Psychiatry 1997; 62:169–176.
151. Demaugre F, Bonnefont JP, Mitchell G, Nguyen-Hoang N, Pelet A, Rimoldi M, S Di Donato, Saudubray JM. Hepatic and muscular presentations of carnitine palmitoyl transferase deficiency: two distinct entities. Pediatr Res 1988; 24:308–311.
152. Brivet M, Boutron A, Slama A, Costa C, Thuillier L, Demaugre F, Rabier D, Saudubray JM, Bonnefont JP. Defects in activation and transport of fatty acids. J Inherit Metab Dis 1999; 22:428–441.
153. Hostetler KY, Hoppel CL, Romine JS, Sipe JC, Gross SR, Higginbottom PA. Partial deficiency of muscle carnitine palmitoyltransferase with normal ketone production. N Engl J Med 1978; 298:553–557.
154. Pande SV. Carnitine-acylcarnitine translocase deficiency. Am J Med Sci 1999; 18: 22–27.
155. Indiveri C, Iacobazzi V, Giangregorio N, Palmieri F. The mitochondrial carnitine carrier protein: cDNA cloning, primary structure and comparison with other mitochondrial transport proteins. Biochem J 1997; 321:713–719.
156. DiDonato S, Rimoldi M, Moise A, Bertagnoglio B, Uziel G. Fatal ataxic encephalopathy and carnitine acetyltransferase deficiency: a functional defect of pyruvate oxidation? Neurology 1979; 29:1578–1583.
157. AC Bach. Carnitine in human nutrition. Z Ernährungswiss 1982; 21:257–265.
158. Leibovitz BE. L-Carnitine. Basel: Edition Lonza, 1993:7–12.
159. Marzo A, Rescigno A, Arrigoni Martelli E. Some pharmacokinetic considerations about homeostatic equilibrium of endogenous substances. Eur J Drug Metab Pharmacokinet 1993; 18:215–219.
160. Matsuda K, Yuasa H, Watanabe J. Fractional absorption of L-carnitine after oral

administration in rats: evaluation of absorption site and dose dependency. Biol Pharm Bull 1998; 21:752–755.
161. Matsuda K, Yuasa H, Watanabe J. Physiological mechanism-based analysis of dose-dependent gastrointestinal absorption of L-carnitine in rats. Biopharm Drug Dispos 1998; 19:465–472.
162. Harper P, Elwin CE, Cederblad G. Pharmacokinetics of bolus intravenous and oral doses of L-carnitine in healthy subjects. Eur J Clin Pharmacol 1988; 35:69–75.
163. Segre G, Bianchi E, Corsi M, D'Iddio S, Ghirardi O, Maccari F. Plasma and urine pharmacokinetics of free and of short-chain carnitine after administration of carnitine in man. Arznei-Forsch/Drug Res 1988; 38(II):1830–1834.
164. Rizza V, Lorefice R, Rizza N, Calabrese V. Pharmacokinetics of L-carnitine in human subjects. In: R Ferrari, S DiMauro, G Sherwood, eds. L-Carnitine and Its Role in Medicine: From Function to Therapy. London: Academic, 1992:63–77.
165. Uematsu T, Itaya T, Nishimoto M, Tagiguchi Y, Mizuno A, Nakashima M, Yoshinobu K, Hasebe T. Pharmacokinetics and safety of L-carnitine infused i.v. in healthy subjects. Eur J Clin Pharmacol 1988; 34:213–216.
166. Sahajwalla CG, Helton ED, Purich ED, Hoppel CL, Cabana BE. Multiple-dose pharmacokinetics and bioequivalence of L-carnitine 330-mg tablet versus 1-g chewable tablet versus enteral solution healthy adult male volunteers. J Pharm Sci 1995; 84:627–633.
167. Jager W, Koch HP. Pharmacokinetics and organ distribution of liposome-encapsulated L-carnitine in rats. Arzneimittelforschung 1993; 43:974–977.
168. Brass EP. Pharmacokinetic considerations for the therapeutic use of carnitine in hemodialysis patients. Clin Ther 1995; 17:176–185.
169. Shenai JP, Borum PR. Tissue carnitine reserves of newborn infants. Pediatr Res 1984; 18:679–682.
170. Penn D, Ludwigs B, Schmidt-Sommerfeld E, Pascu F. Effect of nutrition on tissue carnitine concentrations in infants of different gestational ages. Biol Neonate 1985; 47:130–135.
171. Scholte HR, Stinis JT, Jennekens FG. Low carnitine levels in serum of pregnant women. N Engl J Med 1978; 299:1079–1080.
172. Bargen-Lockner C, Hahn P, Wittmann B. Plasma carnitine in pregnancy. Am J Obstet Gynecol 1981; 140:412–414.
173. Cederblad G, Fahraeus L, Lindgren K. Plasma carnitine and renal-carnitine clearance during pregnancy. Am J Clin Nutr 1986; 44:379–383.
174. Schoderbeck M, Auer B, Legenstein E, Genger H, Sevelda P, Salzer H, Marz R, Lohninger A. Pregnancy-related changes of carnitine and acylcarnitine concentrations of plasma and erythrocytes. J Perinat Med 1995; 23:477–485.
175. Lohninger A, Laschan C, Auer B, Linhart L, Salzer H. Animal experiment and clinical studies of the significance of carnitine for energy metabolism in pregnant patients and the fetus during the pre- and perinatal period. Wien Klin Wochenschr 1996; 108:33–39.
176. Schmidt-Sommerfeld E, Werner D, Penn D. Carnitine plasma concentrations in 353 metabolically healthy children. Eur J Pediatr 1988; 147:356–360.
177. Warshaw JB, Curry E. Comparison of serum carnitine and ketone body concentrations in breast- and in formula-fed newborn infants. J Pediatr 1980; 97:122–125.

178. Sandor A, Pecsuvac K, Kerner J, Alkonyi I. On carnitine content of the human breast milk. Pediatr Res 1982; 16:89–91.
179. Rubaltelli FF, Orzali A, Rinaldo P, Donzelli F, Carnielli V. Carnitine and the premature. Biol Neonate 1987; 52:65–77.
180. Borum PR. Carnitine in neonatal nutrition. J Child Neurol 1995; 10:S25–31.
181. Schmidt-Sommerfeld E, Penn D. Carnitine deficiency in infants and children: metabolic effects of carnitine supplementation. In: Seim H, Löster H, eds. Carnitine—Pathobiochemical Basics and Clinical Applications. Bochum: Ponte, 1996:141–155.
182. Arenas J, Rubio JC, Martin MA, Campos Y. Biological roles of L-carnitine in perinatal metabolism. Early Hum Dev 1998; 53:S43–50.
183. Helms RA, Mauer EC, Hay WW Jr, Christensen ML, Storm MC. Effect of intravenous L-carnitine on growth parameters and fat metabolism during parenteral nutrition in neonates. J Parenter Enteral Nutr 1990; 14:448–453.
184. Bonner CM, DeBrie KL, Hug G, Landrigan E, Taylor BJ. Effects of parenteral L-carnitine supplementation on fat metabolism and nutrition in premature neonates. J Pediatr 1995; 126:287–292.
185. Delanghe J, Slypere JP, De Buyzere M, Robbrecht J, Wieme R, Vermeulen A. Normal reference values for creatine, and carnitine are lower in vegetarians. Clin Chem 1989; 35:1802–1803.
186. Lombard KA, Olson AL, Nelson SE, Rebouche CJ. Carnitine status of lactoovovegetarians and strict vegetarian adults and children. Am J Clin Nutr 1989; 50:301–306.
187. Richter V, Purschwitz K, Bohusch A, Seim H, Weisbrich C, Reuter W, Sorger D, Rassoul F. Lipoproteins and other clinical-chemistry parameters under the conditions of lacto-ovo-vegetarian nutrition. Nutr Res 1999; 19:545–554.
188. Slonim EA, Borum PR, Tanaka K, Stanley CA, Kasselberg AG, Greene HL, Burr IM. Dietary-dependent carnitine deficiency as a cause of nonketotic hypoglycemia in an infant. J Pediatr 1981; 99:551–556.
189. Kanaka C, Schütz B, Zuppinger KA. Risks of alternative nutrition in infancy: a case report of severe iodine and carnitine deficiency. Eur J Pediatr 1992; 151:786–788.
190. Novak M, Wieser PB, Buch M, Hahn P. Acetylcarnitine and free carnitine in body fluids before and after birth. Pediatr Res 1979; 13:10–15.
191. Penn D, Schmidt-Sommerfeld E, Wolf E. Carnitine deficiency in premature infants receiving total parenteral nutrition. Early Hum Dev 1980; 4:23–28.
192. Hahn P, Allardyce DB, Frohlich J. Plasma carnitine levels during total parenteral nutrition of adult surgical patients. Am J Clin Nutr 1982; 36:569–572.
193. Schäfer J, Reichmann H. Subnormal carnitine levels and their correction in artificially fed patients from neurological intensive care unit: a pilot study. J Neurol 1990; 237:213–215.
194. Bowyer BA, Fleming CR, Ilstrup D, Nelson J, Reek S, Burnes J. Plasma carnitine levels in patients receiving home parenteral nutrition. Am J Clin Nutr 1986; 43: 85–91.
195. Berner YN, Larchian WA, Lowry SF, Nicroa RR, Brennan MF, Shike M. Low

plasma carnitine in patients on prolonged total parenteral nutrition: association with low plasma lysine. J Parenter Enteral Nutr 1990; 14:255–258.
196. Richter T, Müller DM, Rotzsch C, Seim H. Carnitine deficiency in children with long term tube feeding via percutaneous endoscopicaly controlled gastrostomy (PEG). Monatsschr Kinderheilkd 1996; 144:716–721.
197. Richter T, Seim H, Rotzsch C, Müller DM. Carnitine deficiency and fatty acid oxidation in patients with long term formula feeding. In: Seim H, Löster H, eds. Carnitine—Pathobiochemical Basics and Clinical Applications. Bochum: Ponte, 1996:264.
198. Demmelmair H, Sauerwald T, Koletzko B, Richter T. New insights into lipid and fatty acid metabolism via stable isotopes. Eur J Pediatr 1997; 156:S70–74.
199. Kelly GS. L-Carnitine: therapeutic applications of a conditionally-essential amino acid. Altern Med Rev 1998; 3:345–160.
200. Delattre J. Etude de la lactacidemie et de l'electrocardigramme, lors du traitement de la fatigue sportive par Aminox. Med Sport 1971; 45:132–133.
201. Leclercq J, Andrivet R, Chignon J-C. Traitement des etats de fatigue du sportif. Gaz Med France 1969; 31:6460–6461.
202. Brouns F, van der Vusse GJ. Utilization of lipids druing exerise in human subjects: metabolic and dietary constraints. Br J Nutr 1998; 79:117–128.
203. Cerretelli P, Marconi C. L-Carnitine supplementation in humans. The effects on physical performance. Int J Sports Med 1990; 11:1–14.
204. Clarkson PM. Nutrition for improved sports performance. Current issues on ergogenic aids. Sports Med 1996; 21:393–401.
205. Hawley JA, Brouns F, Jeuckendrup A. Strategies to enhance fat utilisation during exercise. Sports Med 1998; 25:241–257.
206. Kanter MM, Williams MH. Antioxidants, carnitine and choline as putative ergogenic aids. Int J Sport Nutr 1995; 5S:S120–S131.
207. Wagenmakers AJM. L-Carnitine supplementation and performance. In: Brouns F, ed. Advances in Nutrition and Top Sport. Vol. 32. Basel: Karger, 1991:110–127.
208. Neumann G. Effect of L-carnitine on athletic performance. In: Seim H, Löster H, eds. Carnitine—Pathobiochemical Basics and Clinical Applications. Bochum: Ponte, 1996:61–72.
209. Rokitzki L, Andree N, Sagredos N, Reuβ F, Büchner M, Keul J. Acute changes in vitamin B_6 status in endurance athletes before and after a marathon. Int J Sports Nutr 1994; 4:154–165.
210. Föhrenbach R, März M, Lohrer H, Siekmeier R, Evangeliou A, Böhles H. Der Einfluβ von L-Carnitin auf den Lipidstoffwechsel von Hochleistungssportlern. Dtsch Z Sportmed 1993; 44:349–356.
211. Arenas J, Ricoy JR, Encinas AR, Pola P, SD'Iddio, Zeviani M, Didonato S, Corsi M. Carnitine in muscle, serum and urine of non-professional athletes: effects of physical exercise, training and L-carnitine administration. Muscle Nerve 1991; 14: 598–604.
212. Carlin JI, Reddan WG, Sanjak M, Hodach R. Carnitine metabolism during prolonged exercise und recovery in humans. J Appl Physiol 1986; 61:1275–1278.
213. Marconi C, Sassi G, Carpinelli A, Cerretelli P. Effects of L-carnitine loading on

the aerobic and anaerobic performance of endurance athletes. Eur J Appl Physiol 1985; 54:131–135.
214. Soop K, Bjorkman O, Cederblad G, Hagenfeldt H, Wahren J. Influence of carnitine supplementation on muscle substrate and carnitine metabolism during exercise. Eur J Appl Physiol 1988; 64:2394–2399.
215. Brass EP, Hiatt WR. Carnitine metabolism during exercise. Life Sci 1994; 54: 1383–1393.
216. Harris RC, Forster CV, Hültman E. Acetylcarnitine formation during intense muscular contraction in humans. J Appl Physiol 1987; 63:440–442.
217. Hiatt ER, Regensteiner JG, Wolfel EE, Ruff L, Brass EP. Carnitine and acylcarnitine metabolism during exercise in humans. J Clin Invest 1989; 84:1167–1173.
218. Ramsay RR, Arduini A. The carnitine acyltransferases and their role in modulating acyl-CoA pools. Arch Biochem Biophys 1993; 302:307–314.
219. Barnett C, Costill DL, Vukovich MD, Cole KJ, Goodpaster BH, Trappe SW, Fink WJ. Effect of L-carnitine supplementation on muscle and blood carnitine content and lactate accumulation during high-intensity sprint cycling. Int J Sport Nutr 1994; 4:280–288.
220. Salatin B, Astrand PO. Free fatty acids and exercise. Am J Clin Nut 57:752S–757S, discussion 1993; 757S–758S.
221. Gunzman M, Sabborido A, Castro J, Molano F, Megias A. Treatment with anabolic steroids increase the activity of the mitochondrial outer carnitine palmitoyltransferase in rat liver and fast twitch muscle. Biochem Pharmacol 1991; 41:833–835.
222. Fritz IB, Wong K, Burdzy K. Clustering of erythrocytes by fibrinogen is inhibited by carnitine: Evidence that sulfhydryl groups on red blood cell membranes are involved in carnitine actions. J Cell Physiol 1991; 149:269–276.
223. Arduini A, Mancinelli G, Ramsay RR. Palmitoyl-L-carnitine, a metabolic intermediate of a the fatty acid incorporation pathway in erythrocyte membrane phospholipids. Biochem Biophys Res Commun 1990; 173:212–217.
224. Arduini A, Gorbunow N, Arrigoni-Martelli E, Dottori S, Molajoni F, Russo F, Federici G. Effects of L-carnitine and its acetate and propionate esters on the molecular dynamics of human erythrocyte membrane. Biochim Biophys Acta 1993; 1146: 229–235.
225. Reichmann H, Lindeneiner R. Carnitine analysis in normal human red blood cells, plasma, and muscle tissue. Eur Neurol 1994; 34:40–43.
226. Billigmann P-W, Künzel U, Bertsch S. Wie wirkt sich L-Carnitin auf die physische Maximalbelastung aus? Therapiewoche 1990; 40:1866–1872.
227. Borum PR. Plasma carnitine compartment and red blood cell carnitine compartment of healthy adults. Am J Clin Nutr 1987; 46:437–441.
228. Maebashi M, Kawamura N, Sato M, Yoshinaga K, Suzuki M. Urinary excretion of carnitine in man. J Lab Clin Med 1976; 87:760–766.
229. Costell M, O'Connor JE, Grisolia S. Age-dependent decrease of carnitine content in muscle of mice and humans. Biochim Biophys Res Commun 1989; 161:1135–1143.
230. Ziegler R. Faszination L-Carnitin: entmystifiziert und praxisgerecht positioniert. Therapiewoche 1994; 44:2–3.

231. Bowman BAB. Acetyl-carnitine and Alzheimer's disease. Nutrition Rev 1992; 50: 142–143.
232. Calvani M, Carta A, Caruso G, Benedetti N, Iannuccelli M. Action of acetyl-L-carnitine in neurodegeneration and Alzheimer's disease. In: Franceschi C, Crepaldi G, Critofalo VJ, Vijg J, eds. Aging and Cellular Defense Mechanisms. Vol. 663. New York: The New York Academy of Science, 1992:483–486.
233. Spagnoli A, Lucca U, Menasce G, Bandera L, Cizza G, Forloni G, Tettamanti M, Frattura L, Tiraboschi P, Comelli M, Senin U, Longo A, Petrini A, Brambill G, Belloni A, Negri C, Cavazzuti F, Salsi A, Calogero P, Parma E, Stramba-Badiale M, Vitali S, Andreoni G, Inzoli MR, Santus G, Caregnato R, Peruzza M, Favaretto M, Bozeglav C, Alberoni M, Leo DD, Serraiotto L, Baiocchi A, Scoccia S, Culotta P, Ieracitano D. Long-term acetyl-L-carnitine treatment in Alzheimer's disease. Neurology 1991; 41:1726–1732.
234. Janiri L, Falcone M, Persico A, Tempesta E. Activity of L-carnitine and L-acetylcarnitine on cholinoceptive neocortical neurons of the rat in vivo. J Neural Transm Gen Sect 1991; 86:135–146.
235. Castorina M, Ferraris L. Acetyl-L-carnitine affects aged brain receptorial system in rodents. Life Sci 1994; 54:1205–1214.
236. Castorina M, Ambrosini AM, Pacifici L, Ramacci MT, Angelucci L. Age-dependent loss of NMDA receptors in hippocampus, striatum and frontal cortex of the rat: prevention by acetyl-L-carnitine. Neurochem Res 1994; 19:795–798.
237. Costa A, Martignoni E, Bono G, Sinforiani E, Petraglia F, Genazzani A, Nappi G. Pituitary-adrenal function and cognitive performance in demented patients on acetyl-L-carnitine treatment. Med Sci Res 1993; 21:589–591.
238. Davis S, Markowska AL, Wenk GL, Barnes CA. Acetyl-L-carnitine: behavioral, electrophysiological, and neurochemical effects. Neurobiol Aging 1993; 14:107–115.
239. Salvioli G, Neri M. L-Acetylcarnitine treatment of mental decline in the elderly. Drugs Exp Clin Res 1994; 20:169–176.
240. Taglialatela G, Navarra D, Cruciani R, Ramacci MT, Alema GS, Angelucci L. Acetyl-L-carnitine treatment increases nerve growth factor levels and choline acetyltransferase activity in the central nervous system of aged rats. Exp Gerontol 1994; 29:55–66.
241. Ames BN. Micronutrients prevent cancer and delay ageing. Toxicol Lett 1998; 102–103:5–18.
242. Hagen TM, Wehr CM, Ames BN. Mitochondrial decay in ageing: reversal through supplementation of acetyl-L-carnitine and N-tert-butyl-2-phenylnitrone. Ann NY Acad Sci 1999; 854:214–223.
243. Scholte HR, de Jonge PC. Metabolism, function and transport of carnitine in health and disease. In: Gitzelmann R, Baerlocher K, Steinmann B, eds. Carnitin in der Medizin. Stuttgart: Schattauer, 1987:21–60.
244. Lindstedt G, Lindstedt S. Cofactor requirement of γ-butyrobetaine hydroxylase from rat liver. J Biol Chem 1970; 245:4178–4186.
245. Holme E, Lindstedt S, Nordin J. Uncoupling in the γ-butyrobetaine hydroxylase reaction by D- and L-carnitine. Biochim Biophys Res Commun 1982; 107:518–524.

246. Rebouche CJ. Effect of dietary carnitine isomers and γ-butyrobetaine on L-carnitine biosynthesis and metabolism in the rat. J Nutr 1983; 113:1906–1913.
247. Sandor A. Butyrobetaine is equal to L-carnitine in elevating L-carnitine levels in rats. Biochim Biophys Acta 1991; 1083:135–138.
248. Olson AL, Rebouche CJ. γ-Butyrobetaine hydroxylase activity is not rate limiting for carnitine biosynthesis in the human infant. J Nutr 1987; 117:1024–1031.
249. Berardi S, Stieger B, Wachter S, Oneill B, Krähenbühl S. Characterisation of a sodium-dependent transport system for butyrobetaine into rat liver plasma membrane vesicles. Hepatology 1998; 28:521–525.

13
Conjugated Linoleic Acid

Werner G. Siems
Herzog-Julius Hospital, Harzburg, Germany

Tilman Grune
Humboldt University of Berlin, Berlin, Germany

Oliver Hasselwander and Klaus Krämer
BASF Aktiengesellschaft, Ludwigshafen, Germany

I. CHEMICAL STRUCTURE OF CONJUGATED LINOLEIC ACID

Conjugated linoleic acid (CLA) isomers are natural fatty acids that occur preferentially in foods derived from ruminants. They are a mixture of positional and geometric isomers of linoleic acid (C18:2), one of the ω-6-polyunsaturated fatty acids (PUFA).

Linoleic acid represents a PUFA with a chain length of 18 carbon atoms and two double bonds at the positions 9 and 12, both of which have *cis* configuration. Linoleic acid is present in plant oils including corn, sweet corn, linseed, and cotton seed oils. Linoleic acid is an essential fatty acid for mammals.

CLA isomers are formed by "translocation" of one double bond from linoleic acid into the *trans* position. The reaction responsible for this isomerization is of great importance, as the new position of the double bond is associated with new structural and functional properties.

Both double bonds within the CLA molecule are located at the positions 9 and 11 or at the positions 10 and 12 along the carbon chain, thus always forming a conjugated diene. Each double bond can be in *cis* or *trans* configuration. Therefore, theoretically, eight geometric isomers of the 9,11- and the 10,12-octadeca-

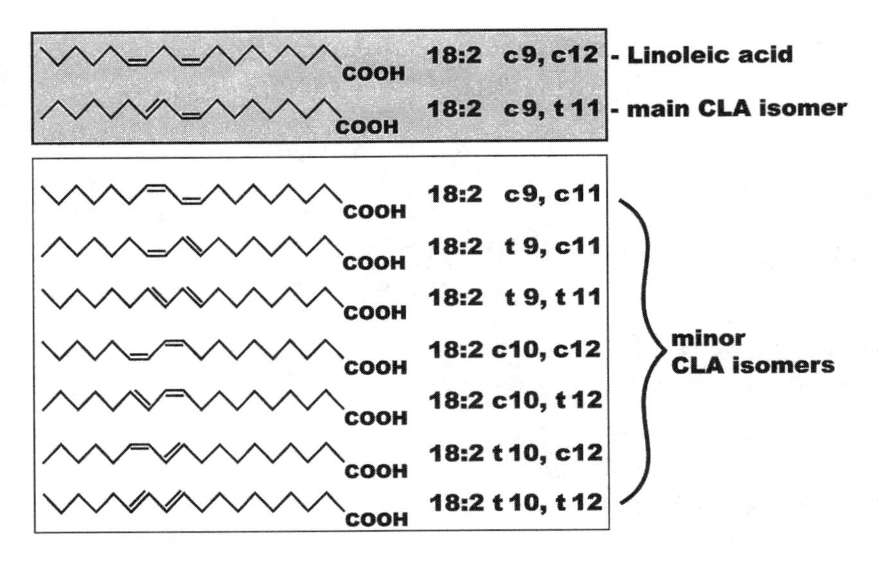

Figure 1 Chemical structure of linoleic acid (*cis*-9,*cis*-12-octadecadienoic acid) and of eight CLA isomers. Linoleic acid and the main CLA isomer in animal tissues (*cis*-9,*trans*-11-octadecadienoic acid) are highlighted.

dienoic acids could be formed. All eight isomers are shown in Figure 1. For the 9,11-octadecadienoic acid these are the following isomers: c9,c11; c9,t11; t9,c11; t9,t11. For the 10,12-octadecadienoic acid these are c10,c12; c10,t12; t10,c12; t10,t12. One can distinguish the main CLA isomer, the 18:2 c9,t11 (referred to as 18:2 c9,t11 or simply as c9,t11-isomer) from so-called minor CLA isomers such as 18:2 t9,c11, 18:2 t9,t11, and 18:2 c9,c11. Other minor CLA isomers are 18:2 t10,c12, 18:2 t10,t12, 18:2 c10,t12, and 18:2 c10,c12. The term CLA relates to mixtures of these eight isomers of linoleic acid. In many studies, however, the term CLA only refers to the group of 18:2 9,11 derivatives.

To study the physical and biological properties of individual geometric CLA isomers, Lie Ken Jie et al. analyzed nuclear magnetic resonance (NMR) properties of CLA isomers, particularly the four 9,11 derivatives (1).

II. HISTORY OF CLA RESEARCH

Table 1 represents milestones of CLA research. It starts with the discovery of fatty acids with conjugated double bonds by Kass and Burr in 1939. Riel reported that the amount of conjugated dienoic fatty acids in milk fat varies from 0.24 to

Table 1 History of CLA Research

Year	Milestone	Ref.
1939	Fatty acids with conjugated double bonds	—
1963	Conjugated dienoic fatty acids in milk fat: 0.24–2.81%	2
1970	CLA generated by rumen bacterium *Butyrivibrio fibrisolvens*	3
1973	CLA produced during oil processing, i.e., in margarine manufacture	4
1979	A ground beef factor inhibits mutagenesis. Is it anticarcinogenic?	5
1985	An organic solvent extract from ground beef inhibits tumor growth	6
1987	CLA identified and recognized as an anticarcinogen	7
1991	CLA inhibits mammary cancers in rats	8
1993	CLA preserves growth in immune-induced growth depression	9
1994	CLA improves nutrient utilization and enhances body mass	10
1996	CLA reduces body fat	11
1996	Tonalin as commercially available form of CLA (PharmaNutrients)	—
1997	Start of clinical trials with CLA	12

2.81% (2). CLA appears to be a common, although usually minor, naturally occurring product of microbial lipid metabolism. It was found that a number of bacterial species that reside in the rumen (the first compartment in the stomach of ruminants) generate CLA from linoleic acid. This implies that these bacteria possess enzymes with linoleate isomerase activity, a phenomenon first described for the strict anaerobe bacterium *Butyrivibrio fibrisolvens* by Kepler et al. (3). Additionally, various CLA isomers may be formed during oil processing, for example, during margarine production (4).

Pariza et al. (5) studied the formation of mutagens in ground (minced) beef during grilling using the Ames test, a bacterial mutagenesis assay system. In addition to mutagens, they found that ground beef also contained a factor that could inhibit mutagenesis. Unlike the mutagens, which were generated during cooking, that inhibitor was present both in raw and grilled beef. In 1979 Pariza et al. published the results and postulated that ''it may also be found that the mutagenic inhibitory activity inhibits carcinogenesis'' (5). This hypothesis was subsequently verified by the same research group. In 1985 Pariza and Hargraves demonstrated that an organic solvent extract from ground beef inhibits tumor growth (6). In 1987 CLA was identified (7). In 1991 it was shown that CLA inhibits the growth of mammary cancers in rats (8). In the following years, new aspects of the biological activity of CLA were discovered: CLA preserves growth in immune-induced growth depression initiated by endotoxin injection (9). CLA also improves nutrient utilization and enhances body mass by improving feed efficiency (10). Additionally, it was found in 1996 that CLA may reduce body fat accumulation (11). In the same year, Tonalin, a commercially available form of CLA, was launched as a supplement ingredient by PharmaNutrients. In 1997, the first clinical trials were started in order to evaluate effects of CLA in humans (12).

III. NATURAL AND ARTIFICIAL FORMATION OF CLA

CLA are generated via natural pathways in the stomach of ruminants such as cattle, sheep, and goats and are intermediates of bacterial biohydration of unsaturated fatty acids. Hence, CLA are normal isomerization products of linoleic acid metabolism of rumen bacteria. The first step of the biohydration is the isomerization of linoleic acid (18:2 c9,c12), preferentially to 18:2 c9,t11. This reaction is catalyzed by the anaerobic bacterium *Butyrivibrio fibrisolvens*, a bacterium present in the first compartment of the stomach of ruminants, which possesses high linoleic acid isomerase activity. Figure 2 demonstrates the isomerase reaction converting linoleic acid to the c9,t11 CLA isomer. The isomerase reaction was intensively studied (3,13,14). The c9,t11 isomer of CLA makes up at least three quarters of CLA in beef and has also been suggested to represent the biologically

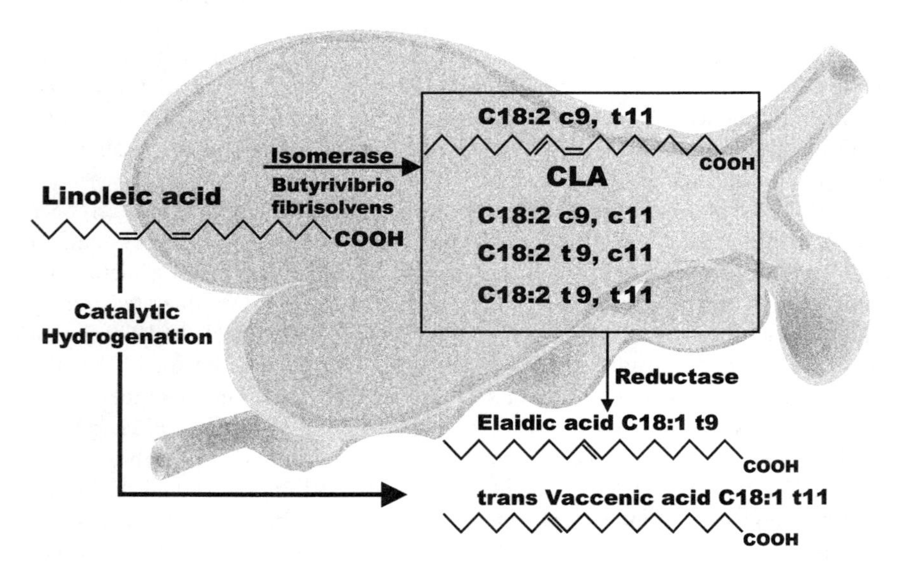

Figure 2 Formation of CLA 18:2 c9,t11 by the isomerase reaction of rumen bacteria (*Butyrivibrio fibrisolvens*) and subsequent hydration leading to the formation of *trans* vaccenic acid (18:1 t11), elaidic acid (18:1 t9), and stearic acid (18:0). These reactions had in principle already been discovered by Kepler et al. (13).

active CLA compound in the prevention of carcinogenesis. The selective accumulation of the c9,t11 isomer is in agreement with the finding of Hughes et al. (15), who demonstrated that rumen bacteria transform linoleic acid preferentially to the c9,t11 configuration. After the isomerization, hydrogenation to *trans*-vaccenic acid (18:1 t11) and elaidic acid (18:1 t9) and finally to stearic acid (18:0) occurs (13) (Fig. 2). This conversion results in the formation of fat containing between 2 and 9% *trans* fatty acids (TFA) (16,17), as measured in fat of cheese, milk, and beef. Ruminants living in symbiosis with rumen bacteria are not the only source for the biosynthesis of CLA. It was demonstrated that pork and poultry also contain CLA (18), albeit in smaller quantities than meat from ruminants.

TFA are also formed during the industrial hydrogenation of plant oils. Catalytic hydrogenation by means of nickel catalysts increases the oxidative and heat stability of the oils. This is of special importance for PUFA such as linolenic acid (18:3 n-3). Under extreme conditions of industrial hydrogenation, completely hardened oil without any TFA content is formed.

CLA can also be generated by the autoxidation of linoleic acid in presence of hydrogen donors. Such autoxidation processes can contribute to the accelerated formation of CLA during processing of meat.

Cooking, grilling, and further meat-processing procedures applying high temperatures contribute to the increase of CLA concentration of meat. It was reported that the CLA content of beef was increased fivefold by grilling (19). The mechanisms of the conversion of linoleic acid to CLA during cooking, grilling, and further food processing are not completely understood. Many factors can modulate the conversion: oxidizing environment, pH value, increased temperature, and others (19).

Dormandy and Wickens reported that CLA in humans or animals come not only from food but also from endogenously carbon-centered oxidation of linoleic acid, which is initiated by free radicals (20). Ip et al. produced CLA for their experiments on the prevention of breast cancer in Sprague-Dawley rats by the reaction of linoleic acid with NaOH in a nitrogen atmosphere (8).

IV. ANALYTICAL METHODS FOR CLA MEASUREMENT

Gas chromatography (GC) separation is mainly used for the analysis of fatty acids and fatty acid derivatives after their extraction [see the classical Folch method (21)]. Derivatization resulting in the formation of fatty acid methyl esters (FAMEs) is generally achieved by transesterification (22). The analysis of TFA and CLA was previously reviewed excellently and in detail by Fritsche and Steinhart (23). This article will therefore only present an overview of the basic principles of CLA analysis. Figure 3 shows different methods for CLA analysis.

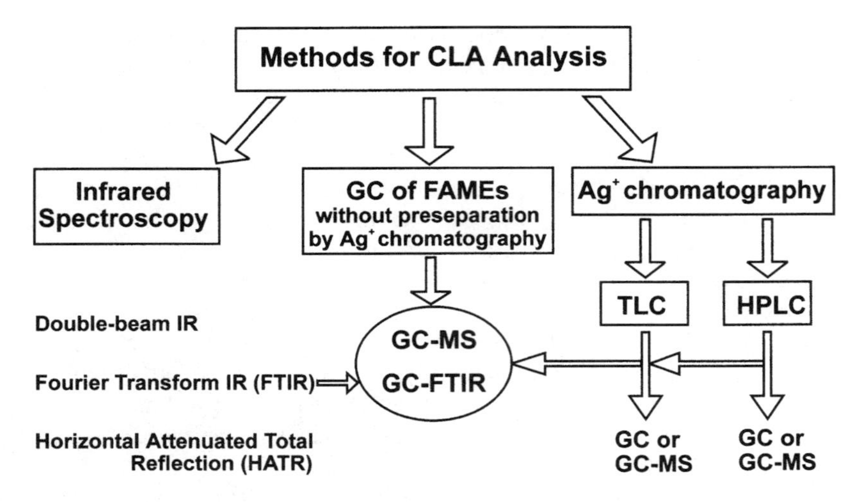

Figure 3 Methods for CLA analysis.

The total TFA content of foods or tissues can be measured by means of infrared (IR) spectroscopy. Generally IR measurements are carried out with FAMEs. The absorption of isolated double bonds is measured at 966 cm^{-1} and derives from the C-H out-of-plane deformation band for *trans* R_1-HC=CH-R_2 groups accompanied by the CH_3 in-plane rocking band at 1121 cm^{-1} for saturated FAMEs (17,23). The IR spectrophotometers used are double-beam IR or Fourier transform IR (FTIR) equipment. An IR spectrum is received by scanning from 1050 to 900 cm^{-1} (23). Details of methodology relate to the interference between the absorption of isolated *trans* double bond and conjugated *trans* double bonds, the subsequent elimination of this interference and inclusion of correction factors aiming at the compensation for the lower absorption of FAMEs in comparison with the nonesterified compounds, or to the single-beam horizontal attenuated total reflection (HATR) method (23).

GC is used for the separation of different FAMEs, which are detected by flame ionization detection (FID). The GC separation without preseparation by Ag^+ chromatography (direct GC method) is based on the assumption that the *cis* and *trans* isomers can be separated completely by means of high polar capillary columns, e.g., coated with cyanoalkylsiloxane stationary phases. Duchateau et al. developed an optimized GC separation of *cis* and *trans* isomers suitable for hydrogenated and for refined processed oils (24). Methodological details on the GC of CLA are given in Refs. 8, 10, 25–28.

The complete separation of *trans* and *cis* isomers without any thin-layer chromatography (TLC) or high-performance liquid chromatography (HPLC) preseparation is often impossible. In such cases argentation chromatography may be helpful. Argentation chromatography can separate fatty acids according to the configuration and the number of double bonds and also according to the position of the double bonds (29). Ag^+ chromatography has most often been used in conjunction with TLC, with silver nitrate being incorporated into a silica gel layer. Using Ag^+ TLC, FAMEs can be separated by the number of their *cis* and *trans* double bonds but not by the location of *cis* and *trans* double bonds. Details of FAME separation by argentation TLC are described in Refs. 25, 29, 30.

The advantages of Ag^+ HPLC methods are the ability to control chromatographic parameters such as flow rate and separation temperature, as well as the reusability of the column, short separation times, and high recoveries (>95%) in comparison with about 60% for Ag^+ TLC, etc. (23,31). Further information on CLA analysis by Ag^+ HPLC separation is given in Refs. 32–35.

Another method for the analysis of TFA or CLA is the coupling of the IR spectroscopic determination or FTIR with capillary GC, then referred to as GC-FTIR. Possible interference or *cis-trans* overlapping effects do not disturb this approach (36). GC-FTIR also allows the analysis of double-bond configuration. The double-bond configuration can be confirmed by nuclear magnetic resonance (NMR) spectroscopy if sufficient amounts of compounds are available. The GC-FTIR method possesses a high sensitivity, hence, only a few ng of sample are necessary for quantitative determinations (37). A further reduction of the minimum identifiable quantity is achieved by the use of matrix isolation or direct deposition techniques (23,38,39).

Mass selective detectors are useful for the determination of CLA. The use of a mass spectrometer in connection with GC is common. Double-bond positions can be determined if the unsaturated fatty acids are converted into suitable derivatives. Different derivatives have been used, such as pyrrolidine, picolinyl, and 4,4-dimethyloxazoline (DMOX) derivatives. By means of this derivatization and the combined application of GC-FTIR and GC-MS, complete characterization of the structure is possible (also for fatty acids/fatty acid derivatives at very low concentration). This is important for the structural analysis of the so-called minor CLAs in biological samples or in food.

For all analytical approaches given above, the availability of different standard compounds is essential (26).

V. CLA SOURCES IN HUMAN NUTRITION

A. General Overview on CLA Content in Foods

CLA was found for the first time in grilled beef and characterized in 1987 (7). In the same year Ha et al. (7) isolated an anticarcinogenic substance from extracts of grilled ground beef and established that it consisted of a series of conjugated dienoic isomers of linoleic acid. The mixture was referred to as CLA. In 1989 CLA was found in cheese, and later in other dairy products such as yogurt. CLA is widespread in biological materials, including plant and animal tissues, that are usually consumed by humans. CLA is present particularly in food products from ruminant animals, e.g., in cheese, butter, beef, and beef products. High total CLA concentrations are found in ground beef with 4.3 mg/g of fat corresponding to 0.4%, veal with 2.7 mg/g of fat, lamb with 5.6 mg/g of fat, milk with 3.4–8.0 mg/g of fat (see Sec. V.B), cheddar cheese with 3.6 mg/g of fat, mozzarella cheese with 4.9 mg/g of fat, and yogurt with 4.8 mg/g of fat. Figure 4 shows data on the total CLA content given as mg CLA/g of fat and additionally the c9,t11 content of CLA for a variety of foods produced in the United States, such as meat, fish, dairy products, edible oils, and fats (40). Table 2 presents data on the fat content and the CLA content as mg/g fat and as mg/100 g of food for foods produced in Germany (39).

The CLA content of various types of cheese differs greatly. Values between 3 and 9 mg/g of fat have been reported (40,41). In milk and cheese, practically

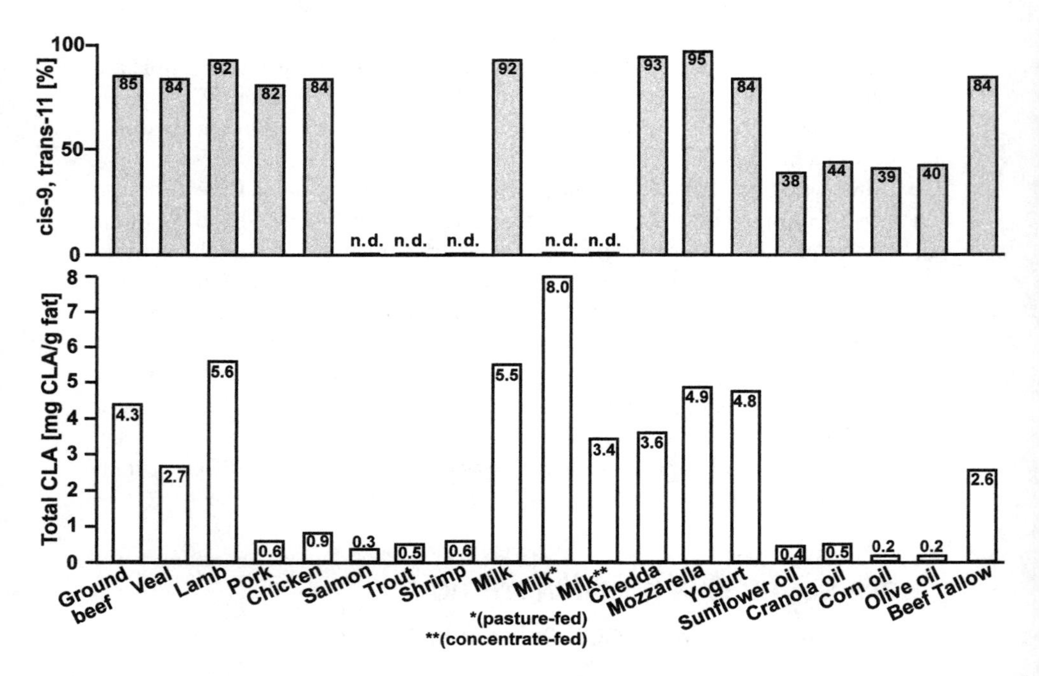

Figure 4 Total CLA content in mg CLA/g fat and the c9,t11 content of CLA in food produced in the United States: meat, fish, dairy products, edible oils, and fat. n.d. = Not determined. (Data from Ref. 40.)

Table 2 Mean Fat and CLA Content of Food Produced in Germany

	Fat content (g/100 g food)	CLA content (mg/g fat)	CLA content (mg/100 g food)
Butter	80.0	4.7	376
Condensed milk	10.0	7.0	70
Milk, homogenized	3.5	5.5	19
Yogurt, natural	3.5	5.1	17
Cottage cheese	4.3	4.5	19
Mozzarella cheese	11.5	4.7	54
Gouda cheese	30.0	6.3	189
Beef tallow	96.5	2.6	251
Roast beef	8.9	2.9	26
Ground meat	14.0	4.3	60
Veal, chop	3.1	5.6	17
Lamb, chop	32.0	2.7	86
Pork, chop	13.0	0.6	8

Source: Data from Ref. 47.

all CLA is present as triacylglycerol esters (40,41). In all types of food the C18:2 *cis*9,*trans*11 isomer accounts for at least 84% of the total CLA (40).

CLA is also detectable in meat of nonruminants, but at much lower concentrations. CLA levels between 3 and 6 mg CLA/g of fat were measured in meat of ruminants, but CLA contents of less than 1 mg/g of fat were measured in pork and poultry (40).

During the cooking process the CLA content of meat increases. An approximate fivefold CLA increase in beef was measured during grilling (19). The mechanisms of the conversion of linoleic acid to CLA during cooking, grilling, and further processing are under discussion. Besides the oxidative environment, temperature and other factors such as protein quality seem to play a role (19). An increase in CLA content during processing and storage of dairy products was also described (42). The total CLA content of butter increased significantly during storage, but there was no change of the ratio between c9,t11 and total CLA during storage of both salted and nonsalted butter (42).

In edible oils such as refined or unrefined sunflower, olive, corn, rapeseed, soybean, avocado, and peanut oil, only minute amounts of TFA and CLA occur (Fig. 4) (16,23,40). The CLA content in these oils is always lower than 1 mg/g of fat, i.e., lower than 0.01%.

Seafood, namely fish, also contains only very low amounts of CLA (Fig. 4). The highest values in seafood were measured in shrimp with 0.6 mg/g of fat.

B. CLA Content in Milk and Dairy Products

CLA concentrations in milk and dairy products as important components of human nutrition are in the range of 3–10 mg/g of fat (43). The conjugated c9,t11 C18:2 isomer was detected as early as 1977 by Parodi in milk fat (44). The dependence of milk CLA content on the specific feeding conditions was described in detail by Jiang et al. (45). Precht and Molkentin previously analyzed a representative number of different milk fats based on different feed composition and different lactation conditions (25,26). Furthermore, these authors analyzed the amount of *trans* C18:2 isomers with at least one *trans* double bond in more than 120 kinds of German margarine, baking, cooking, and diet fats, all of which were produced in the northern part of Germany in August 1994 (26). For milk fat mean contents of t9,t12, c9,t13 (+t8,c12), t8,c13, c9,t12, t9,c12, and t11,c15 were measured to be 0.09, 0.11, 0.11, 0.10, 0.07, and 0.33%, respectively. The content of all *trans* C18:2 isomers (except c9,t11) was 0.99%. In 238 milk fat samples a mean value of 0.81% CLA c9,t11 isomer corresponding to 8.1 mg/g of fat was determined. The maximal content of the CLA isomer c9,t11 in milk fat in that study was 1.95% corresponding to 19.5 mg/g of fat. In contrast to these values, in margarine and baking and cooking fats of plant origin only traces of c9,t11 were found. In margarine, for the isomers t9,t12, c9,t13 (+t8,c12), c9,t12, and t9,c12 contents of 0.03, 0.04, 0.29, and 0.23%, respectively, as well as a mean content of all *trans* C18:2 isomers of 0.61% were measured. Furthermore, the frequency distribution of all *trans* C18:2 isomers was determined and correlated to the *trans* C18:1 position isomers *trans*6 to *trans*16 were derived by these authors (26). The very low CLA content of plant oils was also reported by Chin et al. (40) with values in the range of 0.1–0.7 mg/g fat. In this paper only small differences between refined and unrefined products were found (40). The fat of butter contained 6.1 mg of CLA/g of fat with the c9,t11 isomer accounting for about 90% (40). Jiang et al. measured a c9,t11 isomer content of 2.5–17.7 mg/g of fat in Swedish milk fat (45). Already in 1963, Riel reported a wide variation of the CLA content in milk produced in Canada (2). The lowest CLA value in his study was 2.4 mg/g of milk fat; the highest was 21.8 mg/g of milk fat (2). In agreement with the CLA content of 0.81% corresponding to 8.1 mg/g of milk fat in milk produced in Germany ($n = 238$) (26), Henninger and Ulberth measured a mean CLA content of 0.85% equivalent to 8.5 mg/g of milk fat in milk produced in Austria ($n = 31$) (46).

C. Is There a Deficiency in Dietary CLA Intake?

Although CLA isomers exist in many types of animal food, there might be an insufficient mean intake by humans. Steinhart et al. (17) reported that the TFA contents of most kinds of margarine decreased—sometimes drastically—within the previous 5 years. That should be the case for margarine produced both in Germany and in other European countries (Danish, French, and Belgian products confirm this trend) (17). Within the same time interval the consumption of beef and beef products also declined. One reason for this may be the topical warning related to bovine spongiform encephalopathy (BSE). Therefore, the intake of one of our most important CLA sources declined. The authors estimated a decline of TFA intake in Germany of about 40% between 1992 and 1998 (17). This decline of TFA intake is much greater in 2000 and 2001 due to the rising BSE problems in Europe.

TFA intake by a male population was estimated to be 2.3 g/day (16). Compared with the estimated daily TFA intake, the actual intake of CLA in male Germans is approximately one fifth and calculated to be 0.43 g per day (39). In the same paper a CLA intake of 0.35 g per day was stated for German women (39). Jahreis presented a CLA intake value of 0.31 g per day (47), but for an Australian population values between 0.5 and 1.5 g per person and day were reported (48).

Fritsche and Steinhart published a complete list of estimated daily TFA and CLA intake values in different countries (23). Daily TFA intakes in that list ranged from 1.5 to 12.8 g, and correspond to an estimated CLA intake between 0.3 g and 2.6 g.

The CLA (TFA) intake in the United States is probably higher in comparison to the intake in Europe, possibly due to the higher total fat intake there. But the total TFA and CLA intake in the United States declined within the last two decades. The per capita availability of TFA from margarine and spreads has decreased slightly since 1984. This was caused by the continuing popularity of tub margarine, which has lower TFA content than stick margarine (39,49). On the other hand, the per capita TFA consumption from meat and dairy products in the United States remained relatively constant during the 1980s and was estimated to be 1.34 g per person per day in 1989 (49). Tendencies for a reduced contribution of TFA from fast food are related to the switch from the use of solid partially hydrogenated vegetable oils to liquid oils with lower amounts of TFA and CLA.

The most important contributions to the daily CLA intake for the male German population in the year 1991 were calculated to come from butter (92 mg), milk and milk products (72 mg), meat and meat products (41 mg), bread, cakes, and pastries (21 mg), and oils and baking/cooking fats (17 mg) (Fig. 5). Together with traces from other foods, this amounts to only about 250 mg CLA, which is even less than the 430 mg CLA intake per day given above. Some important reasons for the low or even declining CLA intake in human nutrition are summarized in Figure 6.

It should be mentioned that CLA almost exclusively occurs in animal food. Margarine and oils derived from plants, which are rich in essential unsaturated fatty acids, contain only traces of CLA. The preference of plant fats in comparison

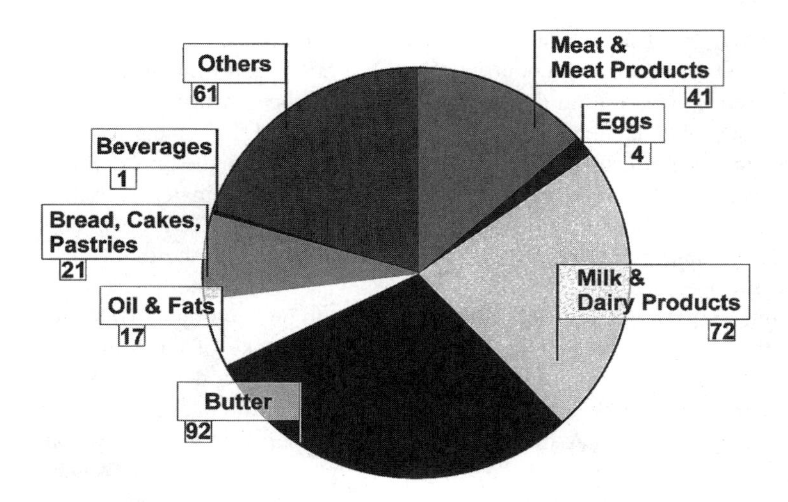

Figure 5 Foods contributing to the daily CLA intake in the male German population in the year 1991. The total CLA intake was estimated to be 309 mg/day. (Calculated from data given in National Food Intake Survey.)

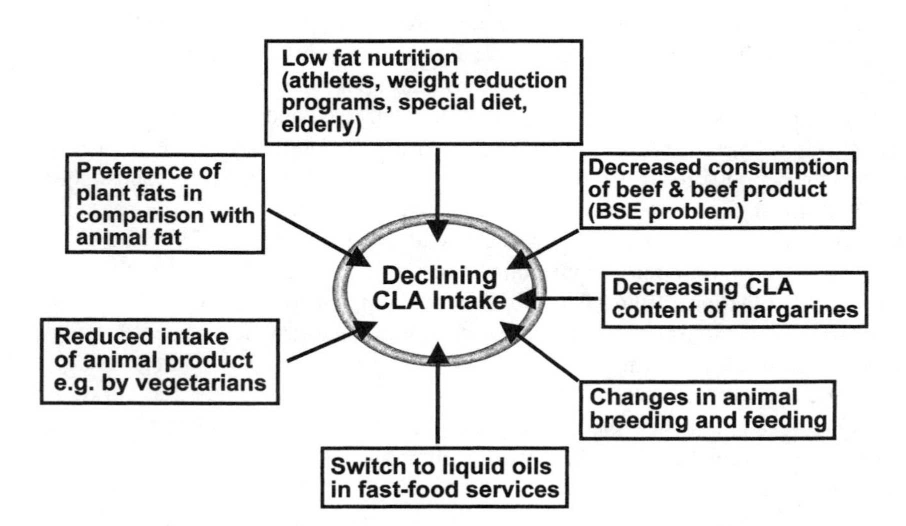

Figure 6 Important reasons for low or declining CLA intake in human nutrition.

with animal fats on one side is useful, e.g., for the intake of PUFA, but on the other side contributes to an additional decline in CLA intake.

An especially low CLA intake is estimated for people on a very low-fat diet such as athletes, obese people during weight-reduction periods, people on special diets, and the elderly. The CLA intake of these persons seems to be even lower than the already insufficient intake of the average population. Ip et al. tried to estimate the CLA intake by humans required to exert anticarcinogenic effects (18). A rat with a body weight of 300 g fed with an efficient 0.1% containing CLA diet (this level has been proven to reduce the incidence of rat mammary tumors) needs about 15 mg of CLA per day. The direct extrapolation to a man with a body weight of 70 kg results in a required CLA intake of 3.5 g of CLA per day, which is markedly higher than the already high CLA intake in the U.S. population (approximately 1 g per person per day—overestimation of this value was discussed) and much higher than the CLA intake in Germany (about 0.5 g per person per day).

The dosage for the CLA intake desirable or necessary according to the estimation of Ip et al. is not so high that its realization would lead to technical (supplementation of food with CLA) or clinical (unimpaired digestion, no incompatibilities, etc.) difficulties. Therefore, according to Ip et al. CLA could become a prototype of a new generation of designer food (18). This would be beneficial to humans who favor protection against cancer achieved by modified food composition instead of a drastic change of eating habits. Ip et al. wrote: ''The challenge of future research will be to define the potential benefit of CLA in our diet, to characterize its anticancer activity, to elucidate its mechanism of action at the subcellular level, and to design new strategies for enriching foods with CLA if this approach is deemed appropriate'' (18).

VI. CLA LEVELS IN HUMAN TISSUES AND BODY FLUIDS

Analysis of TFA in human adipose tissues resulted in concentrations of 2.6% of total fatty acids (GC) or of 3.1% of total fatty acids (IR) (50). The CLA content measured in human adipose tissue (GC) was $0.47 \pm 0.11\%$ (sum of 18:2 c9,t11 and 18:2 t9,t11). Fritsche et al. detected traces of the so-called minor CLA isomers in human adipose tissue: 18:2 t9,t11, 18:2 c9,c11, and 18:2 t9,c11 (37). The authors measured methyl esters and the 4,4-dimethyloxazolin (DMOX) derivatives of isomers by GC-DD-FTIR (gas chromatography–direct deposition–Fourier transform infrared spectroscopy) and GC-EIMS (gas chromatography–electron ionization mass spectrometry).

C18:1 TFA levels were measured in different human tissues and organs. Values higher than those in human plasma were found in the aorta, heart, and liver (51). A value in the range of TFA plasma values was measured in kidneys, and very low TFA levels were determined in the brain (52).

The data on TFA contents (total TFA, 18:1 *trans*, 18:2 *trans*) measured in human milk from different countries indicate a wide variation caused by different eating habits. The monounsaturated isomers, mainly 18:1 isomers, contribute to about 70–80% of the total TFA content in human milk (23,39). The TFA content of human milk reflects the TFA content of the diet of the previous day (53).

CLAs were identified and measured in different body fluids of the human organism: in blood serum/plasma, in gall bladder fluid, and in intestinal fluid (54–57). The ratio between the 18:2 c9,t11 isomer and the 18:2 c9,c12 compound, i.e., between the main CLA isomer and linoleic acid as the common 18:2 fatty acid, was proposed as a diagnostic parameter for clinical chemical investigations (20).

VII. BIOLOGICAL EFFECTS OF CLA

A. Summary of Biological Effects of CLA

CLAs exert a multitude of biological effects. Some of the established and effects under discussion are summarized in Figure 7.

Probably the most important biological—and pathophysiological—effects may be the beneficial influence of CLA on the development of atherosclerosis (antiatherogenicity) and cancer (anticarcinogenicity). Furthermore, increased

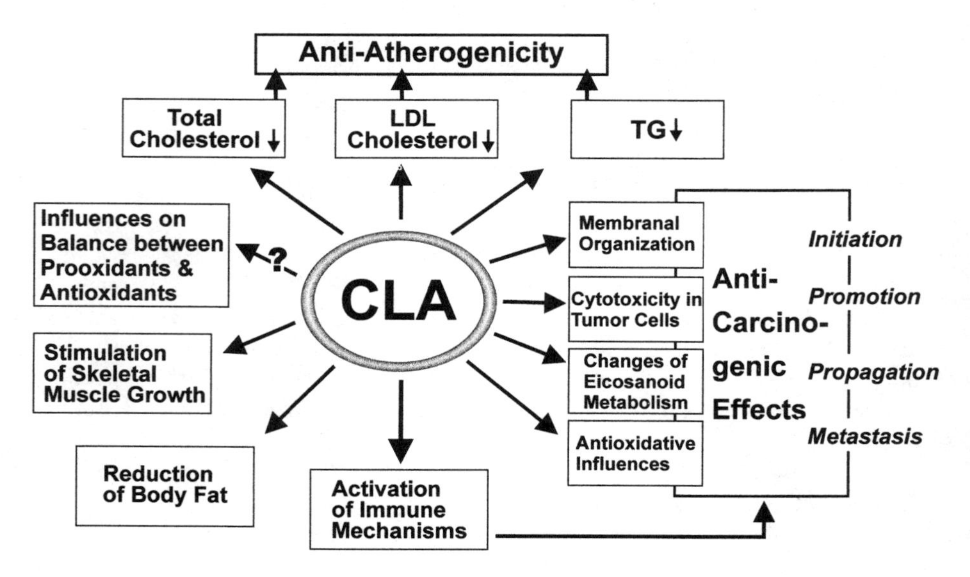

Figure 7 Known and discussed biological effects of CLA.

CLA intake leads to a reduction of body fat and to a stimulation of skeletal muscle growth. There is also evidence for immune-stimulating effects such as activation of the immune system. These immune-stimulating effects may also contribute to the anticarcinogenic properties of CLA. Additionally, antioxidative protective effects have been discussed. The last point needs further clarification, because it seems unclear whether direct antioxidative effects of CLA are possible. Therefore, in Figure 7 this point has been referred to as ''influence on the balance between antioxidants and prooxidants.'' An excellent overview on the multitude of biological effects of CLA was given by Belury (58).

B. Antiatherogenic Effects and Other Influences on Lipid Metabolism

Investigations of TFA/CLA effects on lipid metabolism, namely the cholesterol concentration in blood plasma and correlations between TFA/CLA intake, TFA/CLA level in the adipose tissue, and frequency and seriousness of myocardial infarctions, have increased since 1993. Willett et al. reported an increased risk for coronary heart disease after increased TFA intake (59). Subsequent clinical investigations showed increases of total serum cholesterol and low-density lipoprotein (LDL) cholesterol and a decrease of high-density lipoprotein (HDL) cholesterol following a high TFA intake. Additionally an effect on the lipoprotein A content was discussed in these studies (60). The findings on TFA effects on plasma lipids, however, do not reflect the effects of CLA on lipid metabolism, as has been shown by the following studies.

Data on the beneficial influence of CLA on the LDL/HDL ratio in rabbits disagree with results reported by Willett et al. (59). Lee et al. fed 12 rabbits a semi-synthetic diet containing 14% fat and 0.1% cholesterol for 22 weeks. The diet of 6 rabbits was supplemented with 0.5 g of CLA per animal per day (61). After 12 weeks, total cholesterol, LDL cholesterol, triglyceride levels, and LDL/HDL ratio were markedly lower in the CLA-fed animals (61). These changes were also seen at the end of the experiment, i.e., after 22 weeks. There were no differences in hepatic cholesterol levels in CLA-fed and control animals, but the examination of the aortas of the CLA-fed rabbits showed less atherosclerosis in comparison with the aortas of control animals (histological investigation; lipid deposition; connective tissue evaluation). The cholesterol concentration of aortas was 13.2 mg/g in animals fed with CLA-supplemented diet compared to 18.8 mg/g in animals with the nonsupplemented diet (61). The plaque : artery wall volume ratio was markedly lower in CLA-fed animals in comparison with the control animals. The authors suggest antioxidative effects of CLA as reason for the prevention/reduction of atherosclerosis in CLA-fed rabbits. In agreement with the beneficial antiatherosclerotic CLA effects in rabbits were analogous experiments in hamsters. In these hypercholesterolemic animals, CLA supplementation led to a drastic reduction of plasma lipoprotein levels and to the prevention of atherosclerosis (62).

Chaloner et al. (63) investigated the effect of oral supplementation with micronutrient antioxidants on the TFA content of lipoproteins in healthy humans. The persons were supplemented with 200 μg of selenium, 1800 IU of β-carotene, 180 mg of ascorbic acid, and 90 IU of α-tocopherol for 20 days. The subjects showed increased β-carotene contents of LDL and HDL, decreased phospholipid oleic acid, and elevated c9,t11 octadecadienoic acid in HDL phospholipids. The authors related these results to the induction and inhibition of atherosclerosis (63).

Unexpected results were found in clinical investigations including the analysis of adipose tissue samples of 671 patients who suffered myocardial infarction compared with a control group of 717 healthy persons. The TFA content of adipose tissues was without significant difference in both groups (60).

Although there is evidence that TFA increase cardiovascular risk (64,65), it seems that CLA has unique antiatherogenic properties. The reason for these discrepancies and the exact antiatherogenic mechanism of CLA remains to be elucidated.

C. Anticarcinogenic Effects

The most beneficial and impressive effects of CLA in the prevention of cancer were demonstrated in both in vitro and in vivo studies, particularly the prevention of chemically induced tumorigenesis. Therefore, among the many natural substances with anticarcinogenic activities, CLA seems to be the only one of animal origin. CLA is an example of a fat component present in meat, milk, and dairy products with anticancer properties (18,66). Numerous studies were carried out to investigate the nature of the anticarcinogenic effects of CLA.

CLA acts not only at the initiation stage (mutation), but also during promotion (cell proliferation, leading to the development of tumors) and progression (increase of the tumor size including the spreading to other organs), possibly also inhibiting metastasis formation. According to Pariza, CLA may inhibit carcinogenesis at each of its major stages (67,68).

The anticarcinogenic effect of CLA has been validated in various animal species. It was also described for human tumor cells (in cultivation).

The mechanism of the anticarcinogenic effect of CLA has not been clarified as yet. Under discussion are antioxidative properties, cytotoxic effects in tumor cells following CLA incorporation into the phospholipids of their membranes, modulatory influences on eicosanoid metabolic pathways, and the activation of immunological defense mechanisms. For the discussion of the different mechanisms, see the review of Belury (69).

We would like to focus on the high number of articles that discuss a causal relationship between increased fat consumption and a high intake of (ω-6) PUFA, especially of linoleic acid, and the stimulation of tumorigenesis, e.g., of breast cancer (70–74). In 1985, Ip et al. carried out experiments in which the influence of increasing linoleic acid concentration of food on dimethylbenz(α)anthracene (DMBA)–induced breast cancer was investigated in an animal model (75). The authors found that the frequency of tumor development increased with increasing intake of linoleic acid, starting with a linoleic acid content in the diet of 0.5% to 4% (75). These results were confirmed by experiments with dietary linoleic acid between 0.8 and 8% carried out by Fischer et al. (76). Ip (77) tried to elucidate the relationship between high calorie and high fat supply, including different lipid components and their respective carcinogenic effects. He discriminated between the impact of fat and calories as independent risk factors during breast cancer development by interpolation of data obtained under defined experimental conditions (fat supply, supply of calories). Ip reported that the restriction of calorie supply, even under conditions of high fat intake, is more important in the prevention of breast cancer development than a restriction of fat supply (77). Therefore, in his opinion, total energy consumption is considered to be the risk-determining component (18,66,77,78). Ip proposed dual effects of fat in breast cancer carcinogenesis: (1) fats can represent the source for a surplus of calories; (2) single fatty acids can exert specific effects including the proven carcinogenic effect of linoleic acid (18,66).

In contrast to the carcinogenic effect of linoleic acid, the preventive function of fish oils or a diet rich in (ω-3) PUFA, e.g., eicosapentaenoic acid C20:5, docosahexaenoic acid C22:6, is emphasized in studies on breast cancer (79–81). In order to achieve significant anticarcinogenic effects by eicosapentaenoic acid and docosahexaenoic acid in human nutrition, a fish oil content in the diet of higher than 10% would be necessary (18,66).

The significant anticarcinogenic activity of CLA isomers derived from linoleic acid was demonstrated for epidermal and stomach cancer in studies with rats and mice and also for breast cancer in studies with rats. In these experiments, both the frequency of tumor development and the growth of tumors were suppressed (58). An effective concentration of CLA between 0.1 and 1% in the diet was reported to prevent rat breast cancer (66). This amount is similar to CLA concentrations in human food (66). The anticarcinogenic effect of CLA was demonstrated in different animal model systems (7,8,18,66,68,78,82–85). Thus, CLA inhibits benzo(α)pyrene-induced mouse stomach cancer by 46–67%, in comparison to control animals fed adequate amounts of olive oil or linoleic acid instead of CLA (82). CLA supplementation was carried out 4 and 2 days before the treatment with benzo(α)pyrene in the first week of the experiments; the sequence of CLA and benzo(α)pyrene application was then continued for a further 4 weeks.

Pariza and Hargraves reported that the number of papillomas in mice induced by 7,12-dimethylbenz(α)anthracene was reduced by supplying a partially purified mixture of CLA from beef (6). Shultz et al. (84) showed that CLA is cytotoxic against MCF-7 cells (human breast cancer cells). The cells were treated with CLA for 12 hours in comparison to cells treated with linoleic acid. Ip et al. demonstrated a positive effect of CLA in the methylnitrosourea (MNU) model of breast cancer in rats (78). Other authors demonstrated that CLA acts against chemically induced colon carcinoma in rats (84).

To test the anti-initiation activity of CLA, Ha et al. (7) used synthetically prepared CLA in the two-stage mouse epidermal carcinogenesis system. Mice were treated with 7,12-dimethylbenz(α)anthracene (DMBA/10 mg) to induce cancer and after that with 12-O-tetradecanoylphorbol-13-acetate to promote tumor growth. Mice that were treated topically with CLA 5 minutes prior to DMBA gavage developed, in agreement with Ref. 6, about half as many papillomas and exhibited a lower tumor incidence compared with the control mice (7). In this model, CLA was supplied in different doses for longer periods of time, simulating the intake of CLA in humans. The studies demonstrate that CLA exerts anticarcinogenic effects both following acute supplementation of high amounts of CLA and during repetitive CLA supplementation for longer periods of time.

CLA can also inhibit the growth and the metastasis of human mammary carcinoma cells (87). Furthermore, CLA is also able to inhibit colon tumorigenesis. In a study of Shultz et al. (84), effects of physiological CLA concentrations (18–71 μM) and of β-carotene against human cancer cells were tested: MCF-7 cells (mammary carcinoma cells) grown in the presence of CLA incorporated smaller amounts of [^{3}H]leucine (45%), [^{3}H]uridine (63%), and [^{3}H]thymidine (46%) in comparison with control cultures. M21-HPB (malignant melanoma) and HT-29 (colorectal carcinoma) cells cultivated in the presence of CLA incorporated smaller amounts of [^{3}H]leucine (25–30%) in comparison with the control cultures. The proliferation of tumor cells in the presence of CLA was in some cases drastically reduced in comparison with control cells in culture (18–100%). The viability/cell mortality of M21-HPB (malignant melanoma) and of MCF-7 (breast cancer cells) cells depended on time and CLA concentration. β-Carotene only inhibited the proliferation and the incorporation rate of MCF-7 cells (breast cancer cells). Figure 8 summarizes the data of Shultz et al. (84) on the inhibitory effects of CLA in vitro on the growth of three human tumor cell types: M21-HPB, HT-29, and MCF-7. These results suggest that CLA and β-carotene may also be cytotoxic to human tumor cells types in vivo.

Preventive effects of CLA in animal models of breast cancer were reported by different research groups. Ip et al. used the DMBA-induced breast cancer model in Sprague-Dawley rats (8). CLA supplementation of the diet (0.5, 1.0, or 1.5% of total food weight) was carried out 2 weeks before exposure to DMBA and continued until the end of the experiments (6 months after exposure to

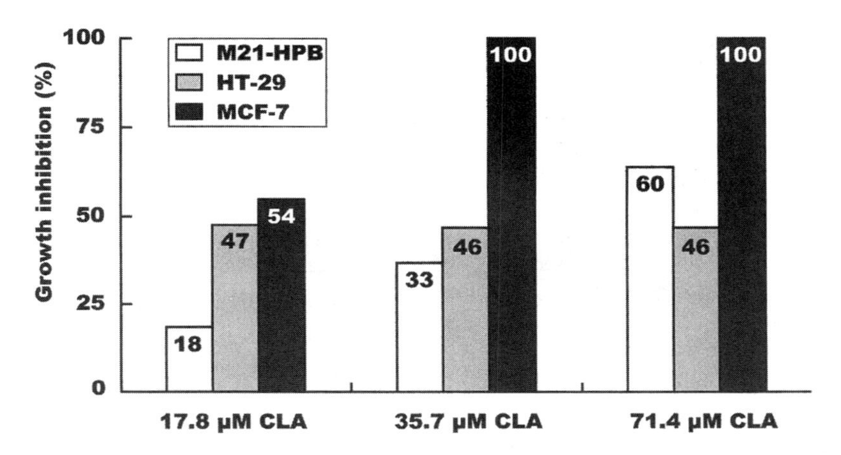

Figure 8 The effects of CLA on growth of human tumor cell types M21-HPB, HAT-29, and MCF-7 in vitro. Percentage of growth inhibition following 8 (M21-HPB), 9 (HAT-29), and 12 (MCF-7) days in CLA-supplemented culture media. (Data from Ref. 85.)

DMBA). All rats were exposed to a high dosage of DMBA (10 mg). This well-defined and reproducible model has the disadvantage that one cannot discriminate the extent to which CLA affects tumor initiation and/or tumor promotion. The decision to add CLA before, during, and after the DMBA exposition maximized the possibility to observe any protective CLA effect (8). The experiments demonstrated that the total number of breast carcinomas in the 0.5, 1.0, and 1.5% CLA groups was reduced by 32, 56, and 60%, respectively, in comparison to the non–CLA-treated control group. Hence, CLA intake was associated with a drastic decrease of tumor incidence. Furthermore, the cumulative tumor weight was markedly lower in the CLA-treated groups. The authors interpreted the results as a CLA dose-dependent protection at CLA contents up to 1%. At higher CLA intakes the authors could not observe a further improvement of protection. Chronic CLA supplementation did not induce any damaging side effects (8). Figure 9A demonstrates the reduction of tumor rate of palpable mammary adenocarcinomas after DMBA administration in rats by a CLA-containing diet (CLA content differed from 0.5 to 1.5%).

This study also looked at the effect of reduced DMBA dosage for tumor induction (5 mg). Thus, the time for tumor development increased. In this part of the experiments, lower CLA dosages were used: 0.05, 0.1, 0.25, and 0.5%, starting 2 weeks before exposure to DMBA for a period of 9 months (66). A marked dose-dependent CLA effect was also found in these experiments: the number of palpable tumors was reduced by 22, 36, 50, and 58%. The data from

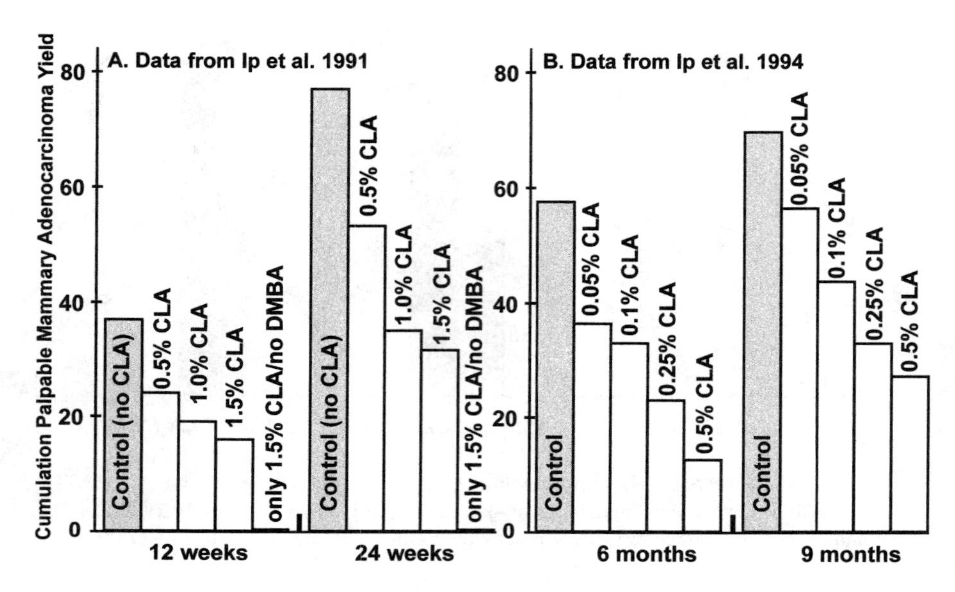

Figure 9 Reduction in palpable mammary adenocarcinomas by a CLA containing diet as a function of time following DMBA administration. (A) High DMBA dosage of 10 mg, CLA 0.5–1.5%. (B) Lower DMBA dosage of 5 mg, CLA 0.05–0.5% starting at 2 weeks before DMBA administration and continuing for 36 weeks until the end of the experiment. (Fig. 9A from Ref. 8; Fig. 9B from Ref. 66.)

these experiments are shown in Figure 9B. CLA supplementation (1% CLA) also showed significant anticarcinogenic effects in the cancer model using methylnitrosourea for tumor induction (66).

Important findings in the relation to the anticarcinogenic effects of CLA are based on the comparison of the amount of fatty acid/fatty acid derivatives in food necessary to obtain such effects. In order to obtain significant anticarcinogenic effects by eicosapentaenoic acid and docosahexaenoic acid, the fish oil content of the diet has to be higher than 10% (66), whereas a CLA content of 0.1% is sufficient to achieve a significant reduction in the number of mammary tumors in the DMBA animal model. This implies highly specific anticarcinogenic effects of CLA. Thus, CLA is much more efficient in the modulation of tumorigenesis and tumor growth than any other fatty acid. In some of the studies discussed above, it has been suggested that the anticarcinogenic potential of CLA was attributable to its antioxidative (8,82,83). It has also been hypothesized that the anticancer properties of CLA may be due to the formation of autoxidation products. The possible cyclization of CLA to furane fatty acids, which are known to exhibit various inhibitory effects, was postulated.

D. Incorporation into Mammary Tissue

It is known that all CLA isomers occur preferentially in triglycerides, with the exception of the c9,t11 isomer, which is mainly found in membrane phospholipids. To study the distribution of CLA isomers in detail, Ip et al. (66) investigated CLA incorporation into the mammary gland of experimental animals. The phospholipid fraction represents only about 1% of the total amount of extractable fat, which complicates the analysis. However, it is of special interest what amount of CLA is incorporated into the membrane phospholipids of mammary epithelial cells. For that purpose, epithelial cells were harvested by means of collagenase and dispase, followed by the commonly used centrifugation and washing procedures. CLA incorporation experiments were carried out with these freshly prepared epithelial cells. The phospholipids were extracted and the fatty acids were analyzed by HPLC and GC. In cells of rats fed a normal diet not supplemented with CLA, there were no detectable amounts of CLA in phospholipids. In cells of rats fed a diet supplemented with 1% CLA, the incorporation of c9,t11 was about 1.5–2.0 μg/mg of phospholipid. Other CLA isomers were not detected.

The authors aimed to address the question of whether the CLA content of phospholipids in target organ or cells is a marker for the resistance of the tissue against carcinogenesis (66). However, this question cannot be answered as yet.

The question as to whether CLA also influences the proliferative activity of the mammary gland in rats not treated with tumor inducers has already been answered. In 1994, Ip et al. found that dietary CLA supplementation resulted in a reduction of proliferative activity of the lobuloalveolar compartment of 25% (18,66).

E. Influences on Body Fat Content and Skeletal Muscle Growth

Another generally accepted effect of enhanced CLA intake is related to regulative aspects of energy and protein metabolism (88). The reduction of body fat content and the stimulation of skeletal muscle growth has been demonstrated. Such results were obtained in animal experiments (e.g., in mice or chickens). In catabolic situations CLA prevents skeletal muscle loss. Pariza et al. previously showed in humans that CLA prevents muscle decomposition even under extreme catabolic conditions such as during disease or during intoxication, which would otherwise lead to muscle hypotrophy (''anticatabolic effect'') (11). The stimulation of skeletal muscle growth is accompanied by increased protein synthesis in muscle tissue and by increased nitrogen retention. Mice were fed a control diet or a CLA-supplemented diet (0.5% CLA) for 32 days. During the whole experiment there was no difference in body weight between control and CLA-fed animals. After 32 days, marked differences in fat and water content of the animals were measured (89–91). In contrast to the fat content of control animals, which was 10.1%, the fat content in CLA-treated animals was only 4.3%. Thus, the fat content of the mice was reduced by 57% (Fig. 10). The water content increased to 71% after CLA supplementation in comparison to 66% in control animals. Water content may correlate with increased skeletal muscle mass (if one takes into account a water content of skeletal muscle of about 75% in comparison with a water content of adipose tissue in the range of 30–35%). Furthermore, in animals fed the CLA-supplemented diet, the protein content increased slightly (18.6% vs. 17.8%). This may also correlate with increased muscle weight.

In the same paper, in animals fed the CLA-fortified diet, increased activity of carnitine-palmitoyl-transferase was measured in muscle and adipose tissues after one week of CLA treatment. Carnitine-palmitoyl-transferase is the rate-limiting enzyme of the β-oxidation of fatty acids (Fig. 11). In contrast to the increased enzyme activity in adipose tissue and muscle following CLA supplementation, there were no differences in enzyme activity in the liver in either fasted or fed animals.

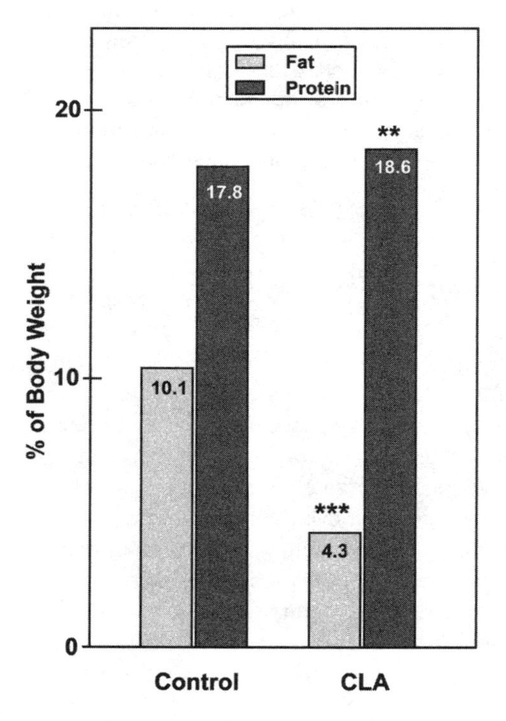

Figure 10 CLA-induced changes in body composition of mice. (Data from Ref. 89.)

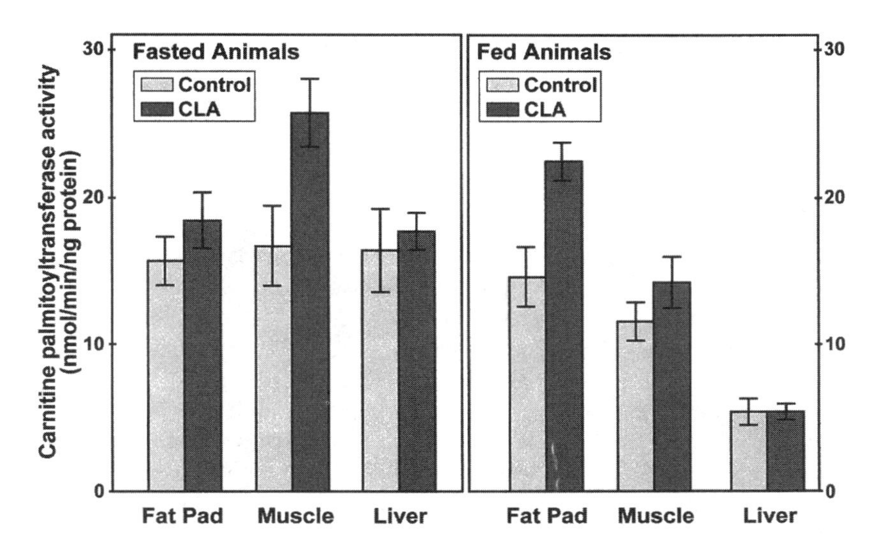

Figure 11 Carnitine-palmitoyl-transferase activity in adipose tissue, skeletal muscle, and liver of animals fed a CLA-supplemented diet in comparison to a not-supplemented control diet; fasted and fed animals were investigated. (Data from Ref. 89.)

The reduction of body fat content by CLA without affecting energy intake has previously been confirmed in mice (91,92).

Another study on CLA supplementation of mice showed an increased lipid concentration of the liver. The lipid concentration of the liver (without CLA supplementation)—approximately 75 mg/g wet weight—increased to about 100 mg/g at 0.5% CLA supplementation, to about 115 mg/g at 1.0% CLA supplementation, and to about 135 mg/g liver at 1.5% CLA supplementation after 6 weeks (69).

In 3T3-L1 adipocyte cultivation, an inhibition of lipoprotein lipase (LPL) activity by CLA was observed. CLA treatment was tested in comparison to a control treatment without CLA and to linoleic acid treatment at the same concentration (100 μM). LPL activity was decreased by 70% to 30% of the control. In the presence of linoleic acid there was no decrease in enzyme activity (89,90).

The ability of CLA to prevent growth suppression induced by endotoxin was investigated by Miller et al. (93). Mice fed a basal diet or a diet containing 0.5% of fish oil lost twice the amount of weight following an endotoxin injection in comparison to mice fed a CLA-supplemented diet. Thus, CLA supplementation prevented the drastic body weight loss induced by the endotoxin injection. Furthermore, blastogenesis of splenocytes was activated in the presence of CLA.

A study with the CLA preparation Tonalin, which was carried out as placebo-controlled double-blind study with 20 healthy volunteers with normal body weight, also led to a reduction of whole body fat. During the experimental period of 3 months, a significant body fat reduction of 20% was measured. This effect was not observed in the placebo group (12).

F. Influence on the Balance Between Antioxidants and Prooxidants

Antioxidative effects of CLA have been reported by Ha et al. in vitro (82), and by Ip et al. in vivo (8). Ip et al. (66) speculated that the close environment (microenvironment) at all sites where CLA is incorporated, e.g., in the adipocytes of the mammary gland, can be protected against oxidation. We, however, feel that these findings do not prove direct antioxidant action of CLA. Hence, up to now no direct antioxidative effects of CLA have been measured. Lee et al. found no differences in plasma TBARS in rabbits fed a CLA-supplemented or control diet (1.67 ± 0.11 nmol/mL in control animals; 1.64 ± 0.12 nmol/mL in CLA-fed animals) (61). Ip et al. (8) found no differences in TBARS in the liver of rats with and without CLA supplementation, but markedly decreased TBARS in the mammary gland of rats fed CLA. These findings do not demonstrate a direct antioxidative action of CLA, but argue for influences of CLA on the balance between antioxidants and prooxidants.

Van den Berg et al. (94) found that the formation of conjugated dienes increased during oxidative loading of membranes, which are composed predominantly of 1-palmitoyl-2-linoleolyl phosphatidylcholine, if CLA replaced linoleic acid (94). The authors mentioned that the oxidative sensitivity of CLA is higher than that of linoleic acid. The inhibition of palmitoyl-linoleolyl-phosphatidylcholine oxidation at higher CLA concentrations is probably due to a competitive rather than an antioxidative effect (94). CLA (1–50 μM) did not show direct antioxidative effects under the conditions tested. CLA was not an efficient free radical scavenger in comparison with vitamin E and BHT.

Nothing is known about the peroxidation of TFA and CLA or the formation of secondary lipid peroxidation products, which might have prooxidative effects comparable to other lipid peroxidation products such as malondialdehyde (MDA) or 4-hydroxy-2,3-trans-nonenal (HNE). These secondary peroxidation products could exert antiproliferative effects (95).

In conclusion, there are no fundamental data on antioxidative or prooxidative influences of CLA as yet.

G. Activation of Immunological Functions

CLA seems to contribute to the activation of immunological functions as shown by experimental data in mice, rats, and chickens (9,96). Chew et al. (97) studied the effects of CLA in combination with β-carotene on immunological functions, which may also be of importance in the prevention of cancer. Porcine blood lymphocytes and murine peritoneal macrophages were incubated in the presence of CLA or/and β-carotene. CLA alone stimulated mitogen-induced lymphocyte proliferation, lymphocyte cytotoxic activity, and macrophage bactericidal activity. The combination of CLA and β-carotene markedly enhanced lymphocyte cytotoxicity and spontaneous lymphocyte proliferation.

VIII. EPIDEMIOLOGICAL STUDIES: CLA INTAKE AND MORBIDITY RISK

As discussed in Sec. VII.B, there is some evidence that an increased TFA intake may increase cardiovascular risk (59,64,65).

Although a high consumption of meat and especially of animal fat has often been associated with a number of diseases, some epidemiological studies associate a high consumption of meat and fat with decreased morbidity risk for gastric (98,99) and for esophageal cancer (100,101). Furthermore, a prospective epidemiological study in Japan demonstrated a three- to fourfold reduced mortality risk of colon carcinoma in patients consuming meat and green/yellow vegetables daily in higher amounts in comparison to patients who consumed preferably only meat or only vegetables (102). However, there are no epidemiological studies in relation to CLA consumption and increased or decreased morbidity rate for various diseases.

IX. CONCLUSIONS

CLA exerts beneficial biological effects such as anticarcinogenicity and antiatherogenicity. Furthermore, it can reduce body fat content and stimulate skeletal muscle growth. Within the last decade the daily intake of TFA and CLA decreased. This is only partially due to the decreasing TFA content in most kinds of margarine. There are other reasons for the declining human CLA intake, including decreased consumption of beef, which is partly related to the BSE problem. Supplementation of CLA may be an effective way of improving cancer protection.

CLA supplementation of human food implies a lack of toxic side effects. From animal experiments (see the experiments on rat mammary carcinoma development described in Ref. 8), it can be concluded that the continuous application of 0.5, 1.0, and 1.5% CLA did not result in any damaging side effects. The authors carried out a separate experiment to investigate possible side effects. For that purpose rats were fed with 1.5% CLA for 36 weeks. The growth of animals, feed intake, and organ weights did not deviate from control animals. After the experimental time of 36 weeks, 15 different tissues/organs of the animals fed a CLA-supplemented diet were investigated in the department of pathology. No histomorphological abnormalities were found. The authors concluded that CLA does not exert negative side effects and that CLA could be consumed safely in relatively high amounts and for long periods of time (8,66).

Nevertheless, more information on effects of CLA in humans is required. In particular, the safety of CLA needs to be guaranteed before it is used for food fortification (i.e., as a nutraceutical).

REFERENCES

1. Lie Ken Jie MSF, Pasha MK, Alam MS. Synthesis and nuclear magnetic resonance-properties of all geometrical isomers of conjugated linoleic acids. Lipids 1997; 32: 1041–1044.
2. Riel RR. Physico-chemical characteristics of Canadian milk fat. J Dairy Sci 1963; 46:102–106.
3. Kepler CR, Tucker WP, Tove SB. Biohydrogenation of unsaturated fatty acids. IV. Substrate specificity and inhibition of linoleate delta-12-cis, delta-11-trans-isomerase from *Butyrivibrio fibrisolvens*. J Biol Chem 1970; 245:3612–3620.
4. Carpenter DL, Slover HAT. Lipid composition of selected margarines. J Am Oil Chem Soc 1973; 50:372–376.
5. Pariza M, Ashoora S, Chuab F, Lundb D. Effects of temperature and time on mutagen formation in pan-fried hamburger. Cancer Lett 1979; 7:63–69.
6. Pariza MW, Hargraves WA. A beef-derived mutagenesis modulator inhibits initiation of mouse epidermal tumors by 7,12-dimethylbenz[α]anthracene. Carcinogenesis 1985; 6:591–593.
7. Ha YL, Grimm NK, Pariza MW. Anticarcinogens from fried ground beef: heat-altered derivatives of linoleic acid. Carcinogenesis 1987; 8:1881–1887.
8. Ip C, Chin SF, Scimeca JA, Pariza MW. Mammary cancer prevention by conjugated dienoic derivatives of linoleic acid. Cancer Res 1991; 51:6118–6124.
9. Cook ME, Miller CC, Park Y, Pariza M. Immune modulation by altered nutrient metabolism: Nutritional control of immune-induced growth depression. Poultry Sci 1993; 72:1301–1305.
10. Chin SF, Storkson JM, Albright KJ, Cook ME, Pariza MW. Conjugated linoleic acid is a growth factor for rats as shown by enhanced weight gain and improved feed efficiency. J Nutrition 1994; 124:2344–2349.
11. Pariza M, Park Y, Cook M, Albright K, Liu W. Conjugated linoleic acid (CLA) reduces body fat. FASEB J 1996; 10:A560.
12. Thom E. A pilot study with the aim of studying the efficacy and tolerability of Tonalin CLA on the body composition in humans. Thesis, Medstat Research Ltd., Lillestrom, Norway, 1997.
13. Kepler CR, Hirons KP, McNeil JJ, Tove SB. Intermediates and products of the biohydrogenation of linoleic acid by *Butyrivibrio fibrisolvens*. J Biol Chem 1966; 241:1350–1354.

14. Kepler CR, Tove SB. Biohydrogenation of unsaturated fatty acids. J Biol Chem 1967; 242:5686–5692.
15. Hughes PE, Hunter WJ, Tove SB. Biohydrogenation of unsaturated fatty acids: purification and properties of cis-9, trans-11 octadecadienoate reductase. J Biol Chem 1982; 257:3643–3649.
16. Fritsche J, Steinhart H. Contents of trans fatty acids (TFA) in German food and estimation of daily intake. Fett/Lipid 1997; 99:314–318.
17. Steinhart H, Fritsche J, Mossoba MM, Yurawecz MP, Roach JAG, Sehat N, Ku Y. Determination of trans-fatty acids and conjugated linoleic acid isomers (CLA) and their amounts in foods. GIT Labor-Fachzeitschrift 1998; 4/98:359–361.
18. Ip C, Scimeca JA, Thompson HJ. Conjugated linoleic acid. A powerful anticarcinogen from animal fat sources. Cancer 1994; 74:1050–1054.
19. Ha YL, Grimm NK, Pariza MW. Newly recognized anticarcinogenic fatty acids: identification and quantification in natural and processed cheeses. J Agr Food Chem 1989; 37:75–81.
20. Dormandy TL, Wickens DG. The experimental and clinical pathology of diene conjugation. Chem Phys Lipids 1987; 45:353–364.
21. Folch J, Lees M, Sloane Stanley GH. A simple method for the isolation and purification of total lipids from animal tissues. J Biol Chem 1957; 226:497–509.
22. Park PH, Goins RE. In situ preparation of fatty acid methyl esters for analysis of fatty acid composition in foods. J Food Sci 1994; 59:1262–1266.
23. Fritsche J, Steinhart H. Analysis, occurrence, and physiological properties of trans fatty acids (TFA) with particular emphasis on conjugated linoleic acid isomers (CLA)—a review. Fett/Lipid 1998; 100:190–210.
24. Duchateau GSMJE, van Oosten HJ, Vasconcellos MA. Analysis of cis- and trans-fatty acid isomers in hydrogenated and refined vegetable oils by capillary gas-liquid chromatography. J Am Oil Chem Soc 1996; 73:275–282.
25. Precht C, Molkentin J. Vergleich der Fettsäuren und der Isomerenverteilung der trans-C18:1-Fettsäuren von Milchfett, Margarine, Back-, Brat- und Diätfetten. Kieler Milchwirtsch Forschungsber 1997; 49:17–34.
26. Precht D, Molkentin J. Trans-geometrical and positional isomers of linoleic acid including conjugated linoleic acid (CLA) in German milk and vegetable fats. Fett/Lipid 1997; 99:319–326.
27. Ulberth F, Henninger M. Quantitation of trans fatty acids in mild fat using spectroscopic and chromatographic methods. J Dairy Res 1994; 61:517–527.
28. Chin SF, Storkson JM, Liu W, Albright KJ, Pariza MW. Conjugated linoleic acid (9,11- and 10,12-oxtadecadienoic acid) is produced in conventional but not germ-free rats fed linoleic acid. J Nutr 1994; 124:694–701.
29. Dobson G, Christie WW, Nikolova-Damyanova B. Silver ion chromatography of lipids and fatty acids. J Chromatogr B 1995; 671:197–222.
30. Molkentin J, Precht D. Isomeric distribution and rapid determination of trans-oxtadecenoic acids in German brands of partially hydrogenated edible fats. Nahrung-Food 1996; 40:297–304.
31. Aveldano MI, van Rollins M, Horrocks LA. Separation and quantitation of free fatty acids and fatty methyl esters by reversed phase high pressure liquid chromatography. J Lipid Res 1983; 24:83–93.

32. Nikolova-Damyanova B, Herslof BG, Christie WW. Silver ion high-performance liquid chromatography of isomeric fatty acids. J Chromatogr 1992; 609:133–140.
33. Christie WW, Breckenridge GHM. Separation of cis and trans isomers of unsaturated fatty acids by HPLC in the silver ion mode. J Chromatogr 1989; 489:261–269.
34. Adlof RO. Separation of cis and trans unsaturated fatty acid methyl esters by silver ion high-performance liquid chromatography. J Chromatogr 1994; 659:95–99.
35. Sehat N, Yurawecz MP, Roach JAG, Mossoba MM, Kramer JKG, Ku Y. Silver-ion high-performance liquid chromatographic separation and identification of conjugated linoleic acid isomers. Lipids 1998; 33:217–221.
36. Ratnayake WMN, Beare-Rogers JL. Problems of analyzing C18 cis and trans-fatty acids of margarine on the SP-2340 capillary column. J Chromatogr Sci 1990; 28: 633–639.
37. Fritsche J, Mossoba MM, Yurawecz MP, Roach JAG, Sehat N, Ku Y, Steinhart H. Conjugated linoleic acid isomers in human adipose tissue. Z Lebensm Unters Forsch 1997; 205:415–419.
38. Bourne S, Haefner AM, Norton KL, Griffiths PR. Performance characteristics of a real-time direct deposition gas chromatography/Fourier transform infrared spectrometry. Anal Chem 1990; 62:2448–2452.
39. Fritsche J, Steinhart H. Amounts of conjugated linoleic acid (CLA) in German foods and evaluation of daily intake. Z Lebensm Unters Forsch A 1998; 206:77–82.
40. Chin SF, Liu W, Storkson JM, Ha YL, Pariza MW. Dietary sources of conjugated dienoic isomers of linoleic acid, a newly recognized class of anticarcinogens. J Food Compos Anal 1992; 5:185–197.
41. Shanta NC, Decker EA, Ustunol Z. Conjugated linoleic acid concentration in processed cheese. J Am Oil Chem Soc 1992; 69:425–428.
42. Shanta NC, Ram LN, O'Leary J, Hicks CL, Decker EA. Conjugated linoleic acid concentrations in dairy products as affected by processing and storage. J Food Sci 1995; 60:695–697.
43. Jahreis G, Fritsche J, Steinhart H. Monthly variations of milk composition with special regard to fatty acids depending on season and farm management systems conventional versus ecological. Fett Wiss Technol Fat Sci Technol 1996; 98:356–359.
44. Parodi PW. Conjugated octadecadienoic acids of milk fat. J Dairy Sci 1977; 60: 1550–1553.
45. Jiang J, Bjoerck I, Fondén R, Emanuelson M. Occurrence of conjugated cis-9-trans-11-octadecadienoic acid in bovine milk: effects of feed and dietary regimen. J Diary Sci 1996; 79:438–445.
46. Henninger M, Ulberth F. Trans fatty acid content of bovine milk fat. Milchwissenschaft 1994; 49:555–558.
47. Jahreis G. Krebshemmende Fettsäuren in Milch und Rindfleisch. Ernährungs-Umschau 1997; 44:168–172.
48. Parodi PW. Conjugated linoleic acid: an anticarcinogenic fatty acid present in mild fat. Austr J Dairy Technol 1994; 49:93–97.

49. Hunter JE, Applewhite TH. Reassessment of trans fatty acid availability in the US diet. Am J Clin Nutr 1991; 54:363–369.
50. Fritsche J, Steinhart H, Mossoba MM, Yurawecz MP, Sehat N, Ku Y. Rapid determination of trans-fatty acids in human adipose tissue. Comparison of attenuated total reflection infrared spectroscopy and gas chromatography. J Chromatogr B 1998; 705:177–182.
51. Adlof RO, Emken EA. Distribution of hexadecanoic, octadecadienoic trans unsaturated fatty acids in the adipose tissue lipids. Lipids 1986; 21:543–547.
52. Siguel EN, Lerman RH. Trans fatty acid patterns in patients with angiographically documented coronary artery disease. Am J Cardiol 1993; 71:916–920.
53. Craig-Schmidt M, Weete JD, Faircloth SA, Wickwire MA, Livant EJ. The effect of hydrogenated fat in the diet of nursing mothers on lipid composition and prostaglandin content of human milk. Am J Clin Nutr 1984; 39:778–786.
54. Cawood P, Wickens DG, Iversen SA, Braganza JM, Dormandy TL. The nature of diene conjugation in human serum, bile and duodenal juice. FEBS Lett 1983; 162: 239–243.
55. Fink R, Clemens MR, Marjot DH, Patsalos P, Cawood P, Norden AG, Iversen SA, Dormandy TL. Increased free-radical activity in alcoholics. Lancet 1985; 2(8450): 291–294.
56. Iversen SA, Cawood P, Madigan MJ, Lawson AM, Dormandy TL. A diene-conjugated isomer of linoleic acid, 18:2(9,11), in human plasma phospholipids. Life Chem Rep 1985; 3:45–48.
57. Szebeni J, Eskelson C, Sampliner R, Hartmann B, Griffin J, Dormandy T, Watson RR. Plasma fatty acid pattern including diene-conjugated linoleic acid in ethanol users and patients with ethanol related liver disease. Metab Clin Exp Res 1986; 10:647–650.
58. Belury MA. Conjugated dienoic linoleate: a polyunsaturated fatty acid with unique chemoprotective properties. Nutr Rev 1995; 53:83–89.
59. Willett WC, Stampfer MJ, Manson MJ, Colditz GA, Speizer FE, Rosner BA, Sampson LA, Hennekens CH. Intake of trans fatty acids and risk of coronary heart disease among women. Lancet 1993; 341:581–585.
60. Aro A, Kardinaal AFM, Kark JD, Riemersma RA, Delgado-Rodriguez M, Gamez-Aracena J, Huttunen JK, Kohlmeier L, Martin-Moreno BC, Mazaev VP, Ringstad J, Thamin M, Van't Veer P, Kok FJ. Adipose tissue isomeric trans-fatty acids and risk of myocardial infarction in nine countries: the EURAMIC study. Lancet 1995; 345:273–277.
61. Lee KN, Kritchevsky D, Pariza MW. Conjugated linoleic acid and atherosclerosis in rabbits. Atherosclerosis 1994; 108:19–25.
62. Nicolosi RJ, Rogers EJ, Kritchevsky D, Scimeca JA, Huth PJ. Dietary conjugated linoleic acid reduces plasma lipoproteins and early aortic atherosclerosis in hypercholesterolemic hamsters. Artery 1997; 22:266–277.
63. Chaloner C, Mackness MI, Durrington PN, Branganza JM. Effect of oral supplementation with micronutrient antioxidants on trans fatty acid content of lipoproteins in healthy humans. Biochem Soc Trans 1996; 24:191S.
64. Lichtenstein AH, Ausman LM, Jalbert SM, Schaefer EJ. Effects of different forms of dietary hydrogenated fats on serum lipoprotein cholesterol levels. N Engl J Med 1999; 340:1933–1940.

65. Ascherio A, Katan MB, Zock PL, Stampfer MJ, Willett WC. Trans fatty acids and coronary heart disease. N Engl J Med 1999; 340:1994–1998.
66. Ip C, Singh M, Thompson HJ, Scimeca JA. Conjugated linoleic acid suppresses mammary carcinogenesis and proliferative activity of the mammary gland in the rat. Cancer Res 1994; 54:1212–1215.
67. Pariza MW. Conjugated linoleic acid, a newly recognized nutrient. Chem Indust 1997; 464–466.
68. Pariza MW. CLA, a new cancer inhibitor in dairy products. Bull Int Dairy Fed 1991; 257:29–30.
69. Belury MA, Kempa-Steczko A. Conjugated linoleic acid modulated hepatic lipid composition in mice. Lipids 1997; 32:199–204.
70. Freedman LS, Clifford C, Messina M. Analysis of dietary fat, calories, body weight, and development of mammary tumors in rats and mice: a review. Cancer Res 1990; 50:5710–5719.
71. Welsch CW. Relationship between dietary fat and experimental mammary tumorigenesis: a review and critique. Cancer Res 1992; 52:2040S–2048S.
72. Carroll KK, Braden LM. Dietary fat and mammary carcinogenesis. Nutr Cancer 1985; 6:254–259.
73. Karmali RA, Marsh J, Fuchs C. Effect of ω-3 fatty acids on growth of a rat mammary tumor. J Natl Cancer Inst 1984; 73:457–461.
74. Cohen LA, Chen-Backlund J-Y, Sepkovic DW, Sugie S. Effect of varying proportions of dietary menhaden and corn oil on experimental rat mammary tumor promotion. Lipids 1993; 28:449–456.
75. Ip C, Carter CA, Ip MM. Requirement of essential fatty acid for mammary tumorigenesis in the rat. Cancer Res 1985; 45:1997–2001.
76. Fischer SM, Conti CJ, Locniskar M, Belury MA, Maldve RE, Lee ML. The effect of dietary fat on the rapid development of mammary tumors induced by 7,12-dimethylbenz(a)anthracene in SENCAR mice. Cancer Res 1992; 52:662–666.
77. Ip C. Quantitative assessment of fat and calorie as risk factors in mammary carcinogenesis in an experimental model. Prog Clin Biol Res 1990; 346:107–117.
78. Ip C, Scimeca JA, Thompson H. Effect of timing and duration of dietary conjugated linoleic acid on mammary cancer prevention. Nutr Cancer 1995; 24:241–247.
79. Caygill CPJ, Charlett A, Hill MJ. Fat, fish, fish oil and cancer. Br J Cancer 1996; 74:159–164.
80. Kaizer F, Boyd NF, Kriukow V, Trichler D. Fish consumption and breast cancer risk: an ecological study. Nutr Cancer 1989; 12:61–68.
81. Dolecek TA, Granditis G. Dietary polyunsaturated fatty acids and mortality in the multiple risk factor intervention trial (MRFIT). World Rev Nutr Diet 1991; 66: 205–216.
82. Ha YL, Storkson J, Pariza MW. Inhibition of benzo(α)pyrene-induced mouse forestomach neoplasia by conjugated dienoic derivatives of linoleic acid. Cancer Res 1990; 50:1097–1101.
83. Pariza MW, Ha YL, Benjamin H, Sword JT, Gruter A, Chin SF, Starkson J, Faith N, Albright K. Formation and action of anticarcinogenic fatty acids. In: Friedman

M, ed. Nutritional and Toxicological Consequences of Food Processing. New York: Plenum Press; 1991:269–272.

84. Shultz TD, Chew BP, Seaman WR. Differential stimulatory and inhibitory responses of human MCF-7 breast cancer cells to linoleic acid and conjugated linoleic acid in culture. Anticancer Res 1992; 12:2143–2146.
85. Shultz TD, Chew BP, Seaman WR, Luedecke LO. Inhibitory effect of conjugated dienoic derivatives of linoleic acid and β-carotene on the in vitro growth of human cancer cells. Cancer Lett 1992; 63:125–133.
86. Liew C, Schut HAJ, Chin SF, Pariza MW, Dashwood RH. Protection of conjugated linoleic acids against 2-amino-3-methylimidazo[4,5-f]quinoline-induced colon carcinogenesis in the F344 rat: a study of inhibitory mechanisms. Carcinogenesis 1995; 16:3037–3043.
87. Visonneau S, Cesano A, Tepper SA, Scimeca JA, Santoli D, Kritchevsky D. Conjugated linoleic acid suppresses the growth of human breast adenocarcinoma cells in SCID mice. Anticancer Res 1997; 17:969–974.
88. Haumann BF. Conjugated linoleic acid offers research promise. INFORM 1996; 7:152–159.
89. Park Y, Albright KJ, Liu W, Storkson JM, Cook ME, Pariza MW. Effect of conjugated linoleic acid on body composition in mice. Lipids 1997; 32:853–858.
90. Park Y. Regulation of energy metabolism and the catabolic effects of immune stimulation by conjugated linoleic acid (antioxidants). Diss Abstr Int B 1996; 57(2): 788.
91. Park Y, Storkson JM, Albright KJ, Liu KJ, Pariza MW. Evidence that the trans-10,cis-12 isomer of conjugated linoleic acid induces body composition changes in mice. Lipids 1999; 34:235–241.
92. Delany JP, Blohm F, Truett AA, Scimeca JA, West DB. Conjugated linoleic acid rapidly reduces body fat content in mice without affecting energy intake. Comp Physiol 1999; 45:R1172–R1179.
93. Miller CC, Park Y, Pariza MW, Cook ME. Feeding conjugated linoleic acid to animals partially overcomes catabolic responses due to endotoxin injection. Biochem Biophys Res Comm 1994; 198:1107–1112.
94. van den Berg JJM, Cook NE, Tribble DL. Reinvestigation of the antioxidant properties of conjugated linoleic acid. Lipids 1995; 30:599–615.
95. Esterbauer H, Schaur RJ, Zollner H. Chemistry and biochemistry of 4-hydroxynonenal, malondialdehyde and related aldehydes. Free Radic Biol Med 1991; 4: 81–128.
96. Hayek MG, Han SN, Wu DY, Watkins BA, Meydani M, Dorsey JL, Smith DE, Meydani SN. Dietary conjugated linoleic acid influences the immune response of young and old C57BL/6NCr1BR mice. J Nutr 1999; 129:32–38.
97. Chew BP, Wong TS, Shultz TD, Magnuson NS. Effects of conjugated dienoic derivatives of linoleic acid and β-carotene in modulating lymphocyte and macrophage function. Anticancer Res 1997; 17:987–994.
98. Geboers J, Joossens JV, Kesleloot H. Epidemiology of stomach cancer. In: Joossens JV, Hill MJ, Geboers J, eds. Diet and Human Carcinogenesis. New York: Elsevier, 1995:81–115.
99. Hill MJ. Dietary fat and human cancer. Anticancer Res 1987; 7:281–292.

100. Ziegler RG, Morris LE, Blott WJ, Pottern LM, Hoover R, Fraumeni JF Jr. Esophageal cancer among black men in Washington, DC. J Natl Cancer Inst 1981; 67: 1199–1206.
101. Tuyns A, Ribotti E, Doornbos G, Pequignot. Diet and esophageal cancer in Calvados (France). Nutr Cancer 1987; 9:81–92.
102. Hirayama T. Diet and cancer: feasibility and importance of prospective cohort study. In: Joossens JV, Hill MJ, Geboers J, eds. Diet and Human Carcinogenesis. New York: Elsevier, 1985:191–198.

14
Contributions of Different Types of Evidence

Charles Hennekens
University of Florida School of Medicine, Miami, Florida

Each research discipline makes a critical contribution to the totality of evidence that permits the evaluation of risks and benefits of agents such as antioxidants (1). Advances in medical knowledge proceed on several fronts, optimally simultaneously. First, basic researchers provide unique and crucial information about mechanisms that explains why a particular agent averts premature death or disability. Second, clinicians provide enormous benefits to patients through advances in diagnosis and treatment and, in addition, formulate hypotheses from their own clinical experiences—i.e., case reports and case series. Clinical investigators test the relevance of basic research to healthy individuals and approved patients. Finally, epidemiologists and biostatisticians formulate hypotheses from descriptive studies and test hypotheses in observational studies, either case-control or cohort, or, where necessary, in randomized trials to answer the unique and crucial question of whether a particular agent can prevent premature death or disability.

In evaluating the effects of an agent, basic research has the unique advantage of precision, afforded by its ability to achieve virtually complete control of exposures, environment, and even genetics. On the other hand, results may differ so greatly from those that apply to free-living humans as to render them of questionable direct relevance. The inability to predict the applicability of findings from a particular species of animals to humans was underscored by John Cairns, who wrote: ''Who could have guessed that *Homo sapiens* would share with the humble guinea pig the unenviable distinction of being incapable of synthesizing ascorbic acid, or share with armadillos a susceptibility to the bacterium that causes leprosy, or that intestinal cancer usually occurs in the large intestine of humans and the small intestine of sheep?'' (2).

Another major concern about the extrapolation of the findings of animal studies to humans relates to differences in dosages and routes of administration. For example, animal experiments clearly indicated that Canadian rats fed daily the equivalent of 15 gallons of saccharin-containing beverages developed bladder cancer. However, observational studies of humans that followed showed no increase in bladder cancer for adults consuming usual amounts of saccharin-containing diet foods and beverages (3).

While the findings from animals are limited in their ability to provide a reliable quantitative estimate of human risk, their precision provides crucial information to set priorities for epidemiological research. Unfortunately, however, while epidemiology has the unique advantage of direct relevance to free-living humans, it also has the unique and troubling disadvantage of far greater imprecision. Unlike basic research, epidemiology is crude and inexact, since even careful observations on free-living humans can never take place under the rigidly controlled conditions possible in a laboratory. The results of a single observational study provide reliable evidence of whether there is a valid statistical association, but support for a judgment of causality derives from consideration of a number of studies using different methods at various times in a variety of geographic or cultural settings and among different populations and that yield consistent evidence.

Epidemiological studies can be either descriptive (case reports, case series, correlational studies, and cross-sectional surveys) or analytical (observational studies, either case-control or cohort, and randomized trials). Descriptive studies are primarily useful for the formulation of hypotheses, while analytical studies are useful for hypothesis testing. Observational studies are often criticized because of their potential for bias, case-control studies because of the selection of individuals participating in the study and their recall of prior events, and cohort studies because of losses to follow-up. Nonetheless, even at worst, observational studies, if well designed and conducted, will contribute importantly relevant information to a totality of evidence, which provides a firm rationale for testing in randomized trials. At best, such observational studies can provide reliable evidence to test hypotheses. Indeed, many, if not most, exposure-disease relationships have been well established from observational evidence, sometimes well ahead of an understanding of biological mechanisms.

For example, in 1950 Doll and Hill in the United Kingdom (4) and Wynder and Graham in the United States (5) conducted case-control studies clearly establishing a valid association between smoking and lung cancer. Doll and Hill went on to examine this question further in a prospective cohort study of British doctors (6) and after a decade of follow-up reported results consistent with the earlier case-control studies. Since the biggest impact of these findings was, in fact, on the behavior of the British doctors themselves, after a second decade follow-up

(7), Doll and Peto were able to evaluate the effect of smoking cessation on decreasing risks of lung cancer as well as to quantitate the greater importance of duration than dose. On the basis of the totality of evidence, which included their case-control study, Doll and Hill in 1950 judged smoking to be a cause of lung cancer but at that time postulated arsenic as a possible etiologic factor (4). In 1964 the U.S. Surgeon General also judged smoking a definite cause of this disease (8), still years before there was any clear understanding of the actual mechanism of alterations in DNA by initiators or promoters of cancer.

Thus, while basic research and theoretical speculation are crucial to identifying mechanisms that may explain causal or preventive factors, direct answers to the question of whether factors play a causal or preventive role must come from straightforward observation of what actually happens in human populations.

There are a number of situations in which observational studies are particularly advantageous (9). The first relates to the evaluation of interventions that require long duration. Another particular strength of observational studies lies in evaluating associations where the relative risk (RR) is moderate to large in size—greater than 1.5. In observational studies, information can be collected on any potential confounding variables known to the investigator and then used in the data analysis to adjust for unknown confounding variables.

When a large effect is seen, such as with smoking and lung cancer, the amount of uncontrolled confounding may affect the magnitude of the RR estimate, making it as high as 25 or as low as 10. However, it is unlikely that it would change the conclusion that there is a strong relationship between smoking and lung cancer. Even in the case of smoking and coronary heart disease (CHD), uncontrolled confounding may mean that the observed effect is as small as an RR of 1.6 or as large as an RR of 2.0, instead of the RR of 1.8 most consistently seen in observational studies. That range of uncertainty, however, will not materially affect the conclusion that current cigarette smoking clearly increases the risk of CHD. On the other hand, when the most plausible effect size is 20–30%, as is the case with many promising interventions, a small amount of uncontrolled confounding could mean the difference between an RR of 0.8, which indicates a 20% decreased risk, 1.0, which indicates no effect, or even 1.2, which suggests a 20% increased risk. For this reason, reliable inferences about interventions likely to confer only small to moderate benefits can emerge only from large-scale randomized trials.

By allocating subjects to the exposure of interest at random, clinical trials eliminate the confounding that may be introduced in observational studies by self-selection. The unique strength of randomized trials is that, if the sample is large enough, on average the two study groups will be comparable with respect not only to those confounding variables known to the investigators, but also to any unknown factors that might be related to risk of the disease. Thus, randomized trials achieve a degree of control of confounding that is simply not possible with any observational design strategy and thus allow for the testing of small effects that are beyond the ability of observational studies to detect reliably.

In summary, basic research and epidemiological studies provide crucial and complementary information. In epidemiology, some investigators who conduct observational studies maintain that there is little need for trials, which they claim are overused and overemphasized. Similarly, clinical trialists occasionally state that the only way to answer reliably any research question is to perform a randomized trial. In fact, each discipline, and every research strategy within a discipline, contributes importantly relevant and complementary information to a totality of evidence upon which rational clinical decision making and public policy can be reliably based. In this context, observational evidence has provided and will continue to make unique and important contributions to this totality of evidence upon which to support a judgment of proof beyond a reasonable doubt in the evaluation of interventions.

REFERENCES

1. Hennekens CH, Buring JE. Epidemiology in Medicine. Boston: Little, Brown, 1987.
2. Cairns J. The treatment of diseases and the war against cancer. Sci Am 1985; 253: 51.
3. Morrison AS, Buring JE. Artificial sweeteners and cancer of the lower urinary tract. N Engl J Med 1980; 302:537.
4. Doll R, Jill AB. Smoking and carcinoma of the lung. Br Med J 1950; 2:739.
5. Wynder EL, Graham EA. Tobacco smoking as a possible etiologic factor in bronchiogenic carcinoma. A study of 684 proved cases. JAMA 1950; 143:329.
6. Doll R, Hill AB. Mortality in relation to smoking: ten years' observations of British doctors. Br Med J 1964; 1:1399–1410, 1460–1467.
7. Doll R, Peto R. Mortality in relation to smoking: 20 years' observations on male British doctors. Br Med J 1976; 2:1525–1536.
8. U.S. Department of Health, Education and Welfare. Smoking and Health. Report of the Advisory Committee to the Surgeon General of the Public Health Service. PHS Publication No. 1103. Washington, DC: Government Printing Office, 1964.
9. Hennekens CH, Buring JE. Observational evidence. In: Warren KS, Mosteller F, eds. Doing More Good Than Harm: The Evaluation of Health Care Interventions. Ann NY Acad Sci 1993:1824.

15
The Brave New World of Foods That Make Health-Related Claims

Stephen H. McNamara
Hyman, Phelps & McNamara, P.C., Washington, D.C.

I. THRESHOLD PROBLEM: NEED TO AVOID "DRUG" STATUS

In pertinent part, section 201(g)(1) of the Federal Food, Drug, and Cosmetic Act (FDC Act), 21 U.S.C. § 321(g)(1), states:

> The term "drug" means . . .
> (B) articles intended for use in the diagnosis, cure, mitigation, treatment, or prevention of disease . . . ; and
> (C) articles (other than food) intended to affect the structure or any function of the body. . . .

Pursuant to this definition, in general, no claim should be made in labeling for a food that represents that the food is intended to "cure," "mitigate," "treat," or "prevent" any "disease." Under section 201(g)(1)(B), such a claim can cause a food to become subject to regulation as a "drug." "Drug" status would trigger numerous requirements applicable to "drugs" (including the possibility of a requirement for U.S. Food and Drug Administration [FDA] approval of a "new drug application" [NDA] prior to marketing) (21 U.S.C. §§ 321(g)(1)(B), 321(p), 355). In most cases, "drug" status for a food would constitute illegality for the product, since, as a putative food, the product almost certainly would not be in compliance with all applicable "drug" requirements.

Nevertheless, notwithstanding the "drug" definition and the need to avoid triggering "drug" status, the law authorizes several different types of explicit health-related claims to appear in food labeling. In Sec. II, I review the various provisions of the law that are most likely to be useful to manufacturers or distributors who want to consider the available possibilities for inclusion of explicit claims about health-related benefits in labeling for their food products.

Some of the types of claims described below may on first impression appear to risk triggering ''drug'' status because they implicitly suggest that a food will have a mitigating or preventative effect with respect to a disease. Nevertheless, all of the types of claims described below are exempt from ''drug'' status provided that all of the applicable requirements for each type of claim are met. Failure to comply with all of the applicable requirements for any particular type of health-related claim described below may cause FDA to assert that the subject food is, either, a ''misbranded'' (mislabeled and therefore illegal) food or a product that is an illegal ''drug'' for failure to comply with all applicable ''drug'' requirements.

II. HEALTH-RELATED CLAIMS THAT MAY BE USED IN FOOD LABELING

A. Claims That "Characterize the Relationship" of a Food "to a Disease or Health-Related Condition" ("Health Claims")

1. The Basic Rules Concerning Use of "Health Claims" (Requirements for FDA Approval)

As an exemption from ''drug'' status, pursuant to amendments to the FDC Act established by the Nutrition Labeling and Education Act (NLEA) of 1990, FDA regulations allow a food's labeling to bear a claim that ''characterizes the relationship of any substance to a disease or health-related condition'' if the claim is first approved by an FDA regulation (21 C.F.R. § 101.14). Such claims are called ''health claims.''

''Health claims'' that FDA has approved generally have been claims to the effect that inclusion of a substance in the diet on a regular basis ''may help to reduce the risk'' of a named disease. As two examples, (1) FDA has approved the use of a ''health claim'' concerning calcium and osteoporosis, to the effect that adequate calcium intake may help certain women reduce their risk of osteoporosis (21 C.F.R. § 101.72), and (2) FDA has approved the use of a ''health claim'' concerning folate and neural tube defects, to the effect that adequate dietary intake of folate may reduce a woman's risk of having a child with a brain or spinal cord birth defect (21 C.F.R. § 101.79).

However, except for a limited authorization provided by the FDA Modernization Act (FDAMA) for the use of certain claims based on an ''authoritative statement'' by a ''scientific body,'' reviewed below, it generally is not permitted to use a ''health claim'' in labeling for a food unless FDA has first approved the use of the claim in a ''health claim'' regulation (21 C.F.R. § 101.14(e)).

One moderating aspect of this preclearance requirement is that not all claims about health are ''health claims'': in general, it is claims that ''characterize the relationship'' of a substance to ''disease,'' ''damage,'' or ''dysfunction'' of the human body that come within the definition of a ''health claim'' (21 C.F.R. § 101.14(a)(1), (6)). A claim that links a nutrient solely to the normal, healthy structure or function of the human body, e.g., ''protein helps build strong and healthy muscles,'' is not a ''health claim'' under these regulations and, therefore, does not require FDA preclearance in order to be used. (See Sec. II.E for further discussion about the use of such ''structure/function'' claims.)

One may petition FDA to issue a regulation to approve a ''health claim,'' but FDA will issue such a regulation

> only when it determines, based on the totality of publicly available scientific evidence (including evidence from well-designed studies conducted in a manner which is consistent with generally recognized scientific procedures and principles), that there is significant scientific agreement, among experts qualified by scientific training and experience to evaluate such claims, that the claim is supported by such evidence (21 C.F.R. § 101.14(c)).

In other words, there is a very high standard of scientific proof that will be required before FDA can be expected to issue such a regulation.*

Note that an approved ''health claim'' may be used in labeling for any food that meets the qualifications set forth in the approving regulation; the approval is not limited to the petitioner who requested the regulation.

---

* On January 15, 1999, in *Durk Pearson and Sandy Shaw, American Preventive Medical Association and Citizens for Health* v. *Donna Shalala, Secretary, United States Department of Health and Human Services* et al., No. 98-5043 (consolidated with No. 98-5084), the United States Court of Appeals for the District of Columbia Circuit, in a unanimous three-judge opinion, ruled that FDA had acted improperly in denying four particular ''health claims,'' including the claims ''consumption of antioxidant vitamins may reduce the risk of certain kinds of cancers'' and ''consumption of omega-3 fatty acids may reduce the risk of coronary heart disease.'' The Court did not authorize the use of the claims but instead sent the matter back to FDA for further consideration in light of particular rulings by the Court. In addition to ruling that FDA may not deny approval of a ''health claim'' simply by stating that the agency does not believe that there is ''significant scientific agreement'' to support the claim without a sufficiently detailed explanation to enable meaningful judicial review, the Court also ruled that FDA must consider the possibility of approving ''health claims'' that incorporate qualified representations or ''disclaimers.'' For example, with respect to FDA's denial of approval for the proposed health claim ''consumption of antioxidant vitamins may reduce the risk of certain kinds of cancers,'' the Court stated that FDA should consider whether the claim should be approved ''by adding a prominent disclaimer to the label along the following lines'': ''The evidence is inconclusive because existing studies have been performed with foods containing antioxidant vitamins, and the effect of those foods on reducing the risk of cancer may result from other components in those foods.''

2. Exceptional Use of a "Health Claim" Pursuant to FDAMA (Use of a Health Claim Based on an "Authoritative Statement")

The FDAMA was signed into law by President Clinton on November 21, 1997. Section 303 of the FDAMA amends section 403(r)(3) of the FDC Act to add new subparagraphs (C) and (D), authorizing food labeling to include certain ''health claims'' *without* approval by an FDA regulation. Such a ''health claim'' must be the subject of a ''published . . . authoritative statement, which is currently in effect,'' issued by

> a scientific body of the United States Government with official responsibility for public health protection or research directly relating to human nutrition (such as the National Institutes of Health or the Centers for Disease Control and Prevention) or the National Academy of Sciences or any of its subdivisions. . . . (§ 403(r)(3)(C)(i) of the FDC Act; 21 U.S.C. § 343(r)(3)(C)(i)).

At least 120 days ''before the first introduction into interstate commerce of the food with a label containing the claim,'' the following information must be submitted to FDA: (1) ''a notice of the claim, which shall include the exact words used in the claim and shall include a concise description of the basis . . . for determining'' that the requirements for use of the claim have been satisfied, (2) a copy of the ''authoritative statement'' upon which the claim is premised, and (3) a ''balanced representation of the scientific literature'' relating to the claim (§ 403(r)(3)(C)(ii) of the FDC Act; 21 U.S.C. § 343(r)(3)(C)(ii)).

The claim must be stated ''in a manner so that the claim is an accurate representation of the authoritative statement'' and ''so that the claim enables the public to comprehend the information provided in the claim and to understand the relative significance of such information in the context of a total daily diet'' (§ 403(r)(3)(C)(iv) of the FDC Act; 21 U.S.C. § 343(r)(3)(C)(iv)).

Such a ''health claim'' remains subject to the requirement of section 403(r)(3)(A)(ii) of the FDC Act, 21 U.S.C. § 343(r)(3)(A)(ii), i.e., the claim may be made only if the food

> does not contain, as determined by [FDA] by regulation, any nutrient in an amount which increases to persons in the general population the risk of a disease or health-related condition which is diet related, taking into account the significance of the food in the total daily diet. . . . (§ 403(r)(3)(C)(iii) of the FDC Act; 21 U.S.C. § 343(r)(3)(C)(iii); § 403(r)(3)(A)(ii), of the FDC Act; 21 U.S.C. § 343(r)(3)(A)(ii)).

FDA has already established these ''disqualifying nutrient levels'' in 21 C.F.R. § 101.14(a)(5).*

In addition, the ''health claim'' may not be ''false or misleading in any particular'' (which includes a prohibition on being misleading by failure to reveal facts that are ''material in the light of'' the claim) (§§ 201(n), 403(a)(1), (r)(3)(C)(iii) of the FDC Act; 21 U.S.C. §§ 321(n), 343(a)(1), (r)(3)(C)(iii)).

FDA will continue to be the final arbiter about whether such a ''health claim'' may be made because the claim may be made only until, either (1) FDA issues a regulation prohibiting or modifying the claim or finding that the requirements to make the claim have not been met or (2) a district court of the United States finds in an enforcement proceeding that the requirements to make the claim have not been met (§ 403(r)(3)(D)(i–ii) of the FDC Act; 21 U.S.C. § 343(r)(3)(D)(i–ii)).

Moreover, note that FDA may publish a proposed regulation to prohibit or modify such a ''health claim'' pursuant to the provisions of new § 403(r)(7) of the FDC Act, 21 U.S.C. § 343(r)(7), established by § 301 of the FDAMA, which authorizes FDA to make a proposed ''health claim'' regulation effective immediately upon the date of publication of the proposal (§ 403(r)(7) of the FDC Act; 21 U.S.C. § 343(r)(7)). In other words, FDA could terminate the right to use a ''health claim'' simply by publishing a proposal for public comment in the Federal Register, without needing first to complete the rule making and to issue a final rule.†

---

* For example, for most foods these levels are

> 13.0 grams (g) of fat, 4.0 g of saturated fat, 60 milligrams (mg) of cholesterol, or 480 mg of sodium, per reference amount customarily consumed, per label serving size, and, only for foods with reference amounts customarily consumed of 30 g or less or 2 tablespoons or less, per 50 g (21 C.F.R. § 101.14(a)(5)).

† In the Federal Register of June 11, 1998 (63 Fed. Reg. 32102), FDA announced the availability of guidelines entitled ''Guidance for Industry: Notification of a Health Claim or Nutrient Content Claim Based on an Authoritative Statement of a Scientific Body.'' The referenced document expresses generally conservative interpretations of the FDAMA provisions that allow a ''health claim'' or ''nutrient content claim'' to be used without an approving FDA regulation based on an ''authoritative statement'' by a ''scientific body.'' Among other provisions, the FDA guidance expresses the view that an ''authoritative statement'' should ''reflect a consensus within the identified scientific body if published by a subdivision of one of the Federal scientific bodies'' and should ''be based on a deliberative review by the scientific body of the scientific evidence.'' FDA states, ''Not all pronouncements by the designated scientific bodies would meet these criteria.''

In addition, in the Federal Register of June 22, 1998 (63 Fed. Reg. 34084-34117), FDA published nine ''interim final rules'' to prohibit use of a series of ''health claims'' about which notifications had been submitted to the agency pursuant to FDAMA. Comments were invited, and in the Federal Register of September 10, 1998 (63 Fed. Reg. 48428), FDA published a notice ''reopening to October 8, 1998, the comment period for the nine interim final rules.'' In general,

B. Claims That "Characterize the Level" of a Nutrient (e.g., Claims That a Food Is a "Good Source" of, or "High" in, a Particular Nutrient) ("Nutrient Content Claims")

1. The Basic Rules Concerning Use of "Nutrient Content Claims" (Requirements for FDA Approval)

A claim in food labeling that ''expressly or implicitly characterizes the level of a nutrient,'' e.g., ''high in vitamin C'' or ''low in sodium,'' is known as a ''nutrient content claim'' (21 C.F.R. § 101.13(b)). Such a claim generally may not be used in food labeling unless the claim is made in accordance with authorizing FDA regulations. (However, see the new developments resulting from the FDAMA concerning the use of ''nutrient content claims'' based on an ''authoritative statement'' by a ''scientific body,'' reviewed below.)

FDA has authorized certain ''nutrient content claims'' for substances for which the agency has established ''daily reference values'' (DRVs) or ''reference daily intakes'' (RDIs) (21 C.F.R. § 101.54 et seq.). For example, generally, a food's labeling may claim that the food is ''high in,'' ''rich in,'' or an ''excellent source of'' a vitamin or mineral for which FDA has established an RDI if the food provides 20% or more of the RDI per reference amount customarily consumed (21 C.F.R. § 101.54(b)). FDA has published regulations authorizing (and establishing detailed requirements for) ''good source,'' ''more,'' and ''light'' (or ''lite'') ''nutrient content claims'' for ''nutrient content claims'' about calorie content, for ''nutrient content claims'' about sodium content, and for ''nutrient content claims'' about fat, fatty acid, and cholesterol content (21 C.F.R. §§ 101.54–101.62).

However, if one were to want to make a claim about a food's being a good source of an additional nutrient for which no DRV or RDI and no FDA ''nutrient content claim'' regulation already exists, one might not be able to make the claim at all in labeling (even if the claim would be truthful and not misleading) unless and until FDA could be persuaded to issue an approving ''nutrient content claim'' regulation to authorize use of the claim. For example, FDA has stated that ''. . . a claim such as 'contains lycopene' would be an unauthorized nutrient

---

the FDA actions in these interim final rules reflect a conservative interpretation of the FDAMA's authorization for the use of ''health claims'' based upon ''authoritative statements.'' For example, FDA concluded that the statement ''Garlic is well-known for its medicinal benefits: Lowering blood cholesterol, fighting off infections and boosting the immune system,'' which was contained in a United States Department of Agriculture (USDA) press release, was not an ''authoritative statement'' for the purposes of FDAMA (63 Fed. Reg. at 34111). FDA stated that USDA had advised FDA that the statement was ''not an authoritative statement of USDA because it was not based upon a deliberative review of the scientific evidence. . . .''

content claim because lycopene does not have an RDI'' (62 Fed. Reg. 49868, 49873).

Nevertheless, one should note that FDA also has said that a labeling statement can be made to the effect that a food provides a stated amount of lycopene per serving, although any claim that suggests that the amount is substantial would not be permitted. For example, the agency has said that a label statement such as

> '''x' mg of lycopene per serving'' is permitted under [21 C.F.R. § 101.13 (i)(3)], which allows for the use of amount or percentage statements that do not implicitly characterize the level of the nutrient in a food (e.g., claims that do not imply whether the amount is high or low based on an established RDI or DRV value), so long as the statement is not misleading in any way (62 Fed. Reg. at 49873).

One may petition FDA to issue a regulation that defines and permits a particular ''nutrient content claim'' (21 C.F.R. § 101.69). The petition must show, for example, ''why use of the food component characterized by the [proposed] claim is of importance in human nutrition by virtue of its presence or absence at the levels that such claim would describe'' (21 C.F.R. § 101.69(m)(1)(B)).

Furthermore, note that, once issued, a ''nutrient content claim'' regulation approves the use of a claim by any company whose product contains the referenced nutrient at the required level, i.e., such a regulation is not an exclusive license that applies only to the person who has petitioned for the issuance of the regulation.

2. Exceptional Use of a "Nutrient Content Claim" Pursuant to FDAMA (Use of a "Nutrient Content Claim" Based on an "Authoritative Statement")

As in the case of ''health claims'' (see Sec. A.2), the FDAMA also amends the FDC Act to authorize the use in labeling of certain ''nutrient content claims'' that are the subject of a ''published . . . authoritative statement'' by ''a scientific body'' of the U.S. Government or the National Academy of Sciences (§ 403 (r)(2)(G) and (H) of the FDC Act; 21 U.S.C. § 343(r)(2)(G) and (H)).

Such a ''nutrient content claim'' must use a term (e.g., ''high'' in, ''good source'' of) that is already defined by FDA in its regulations and must conform to certain other technical requirements that are set forth at section 403(r)(2)(A) and (B) of the FDC Act, 21 U.S.C. § 343(r)(2)(A) and (B). (See also § 403 (r)(2)(G)(iii) of the FDC Act; 21 U.S.C. § 343(r)(2)(G)(iii).)

As is also the case with "health claims," the FDAMA authorizes FDA to exercise its discretion to allow use of a new "nutrient content claim" at the time that FDA publishes a proposal to permit use of the claim for public comment.

C. Claims to Provide Dietary Management of a Disease Under a Doctor's Supervision ("Medical Foods")

If a food is "specially formulated" for the feeding of a "patient" who has "special medically determined nutrient requirements," "the dietary management of which cannot be achieved by the modification of the normal diet alone," and the food is labeled to be used under the supervision of a "physician" (or under "medical" supervision), the food's labeling may bear information about its usefulness for the "dietary management" of a disease or medical condition "for which distinctive nutritional requirements, based on recognized scientific principles, are established by medical evaluation." Such foods are known as "medical foods" (21 U.S.C. § 360ee(b)(3); 21 C.F.R. § 101.9(j)(8)).

If a food qualifies as a "medical food," it is exempt from the requirements that otherwise generally apply for approval of "health claims" and "nutrient content claims" used in labeling (21 C.F.R. §§ 101.13(q)(4)(ii) and 101.14(f)(2)).

A company that is responsible for a "medical food" must possess data that are sufficient to show that no claim made on the label or in other labeling is either "false" or "misleading in any particular" (21 U.S.C. § 343(a)(1)). However, there is no requirement to obtain FDA approval or even to notify FDA that one is manufacturing or marketing a "medical food."

Note that a "medical food" is not authorized to bear a claim to cure, mitigate, treat, or prevent a disease; as discussed in Sec. I, such a claim would create "drug" status for the product. Instead, a "medical food" is permitted to make a claim to address a patient's special dietary needs that exist because of a disease; this type of claim is distinguished from a claim to treat the disease. The distinction should be kept in mind in developing any labeling claims for a "medical food."

As an example (assuming, of course, that one has data that show that the claim is truthful and not misleading), a claim of the following type would be appropriate for a "medical food": "For use under medical supervision [enter brand name of product] can be helpful in the dietary management of [enter name of a disease or medical condition] by [explain the special dietary usefulness of the product for a patient with the disease or medical condition]."

At first impression, the "medical food" provision may appear to be outside the scope of interest for a company that wants to sell conventional-type foods. However, it should be recognized that the number of consumers who are "patients'' and for whom particular types of ''medical foods'' might be of interest is substantial and growing.

''Medical food'' status can also be an initial ''bridge'' mechanism for introducing a product that is subsequently promoted to a wider segment of the population. Ensure® appears to have gained its foothold in the marketplace in this manner.*

D. Claims That a Dietary Supplement Has a Beneficial Effect ("Statements of Nutritional Support")

1. Basic Rules Concerning Use of "Statements of Nutritional Support" in Labeling for Dietary Supplement Products

Dietary supplements are food products that (1) are intended to be ingested in the form of a tablet, capsule, powder, softgel, gelcap, or liquid droplet (or, if not intended for ingestion in such a form, that are not ''represented'' to be useful either as a ''conventional food'' or as ''a sole item of a meal or the diet'') and (2) provide a ''vitamin,'' ''mineral,'' ''herb or other botanical,'' ''amino acid,'' or other ''dietary substance'' (including a concentrate, metabolite, constituent, extract, or combination of any of the above) (21 U.S.C. § 321(ff)(1)).† There are

---

* In the Federal Register of November 29, 1996 (61 Fed. Reg. 60661–60671), FDA published an ''advance notice of proposed rulemaking'' ''to initiate a reevaluation of . . . the regulation of . . . medical foods.'' This ''advance notice'' has not yet led to publication of any proposed new regulations by FDA.

† It is not always clear whether a particular product is properly subject to regulation as a ''dietary supplement.'' For example, on February 16, 1999 in *Pharmanex, Inc.* versus *Donna Shalala*, Case No. 2: 97 CV 0262 K, the U.S. District Court for the District of Utah ruled that FDA had improperly decided that the product Cholestin was a drug and not a dietary supplement. The Court stated that Cholestin is a ''capsule consisting solely of milled red yeast rice, a traditional food that has been eaten and valued for its health benefits in China and elsewhere for centuries and in the United States for decades,'' and that Cholestin is ''intended for use, along with diet and exercise, in helping maintain a healthy cholesterol level.'' FDA had held that Cholestin was a drug, and not a dietary supplement, on the grounds (1) that the milled red yeast rice in Cholestin contains the substance mevinolin, which is ''chemically indistinguishable from lovastatin, a pure, crystallized, and synthetic substance which is the active ingredient in the prescription drug Mevacor, . . . [which is] . . . indicated for treatment of hypercholesterolemia (elevated blood serum cholesterol and triglyceride levels) . . .'' and (2) that in marketing the dietary supplement, Pharmanex was really marketing lovastatin because (FDA alleged) ''Pharmanex manufactures and markets Cholestin in a manner that emphasizes'' the mevinolin/lovastatin constituent. The Court concluded that FDA was in error because Cholestin was materially different from the ''article'' Mevacor/lovastatin that FDA had ''approved as a new drug,'' and accordingly, that Cholestin is a proper dietary supplement and not a drug. FDA has appealed this decision to the U.S. Court of Appeals for the Tenth Circuit. In other recent developments concerning the proper interpretation of the meaning of ''dietary supplement,'' FDA has advised two manufacturers of margarine-type products that their products should not be

particular rules about certain health-related claims that may be made in labeling for dietary supplement products.

(Note that dietary supplements may be of interest even for food manufacturers or distributors who are engaged primarily in selling conventional-type foods. For example, insofar as FDA concedes that a particular claim does not create ''drug'' status when made for a dietary supplement, a good argument often can be made that the same type of claim may also be made for a conventional food without triggering ''drug'' status. Furthermore, a product that is in the physical form of a conventional-type food [a product that ''simulates'' a conventional food] may be able to be sold as a ''dietary supplement'' if it is not ''represented'' for use as a ''conventional food.'')

As described in Sec. II.A, it generally is not permitted to make a ''health claim'' in labeling for a food (including a dietary supplement) unless the claim meets the FDA approval or FDAMA requirements for ''health claims.'' However, for dietary supplement products only, there is an exception to the usual requirements for use of ''health claims'' that permits four types of ''statements of nutritional support'' to be made in labeling without complying with the usual requirements for ''health claims.'' These exceptional ''statements of nutritional support'' are as follows (21 U.S.C. § 343(r)(6)):

A statement that ''claims a benefit related to a classical nutrient deficiency disease and discloses the prevalence of such disease in the United States''

A statement that ''describes the role of a nutrient or dietary ingredient intended to affect the structure or function in humans''

A statement that ''characterizes the documented mechanism by which a nutrient or dietary ingredient acts to maintain such structure or function''

A statement that ''describes general well-being from consumption of a nutrient or dietary ingredient''

Any of the above four types of ''statements of nutritional support'' may be made in labeling for a dietary supplement, without the approval of a ''health claim'' regulation, if (21 U.S.C. § 343(r)(6)):

The manufacturer ''has substantiation that such statement is truthful and not misleading''

The labeling contains, prominently displayed, the following additional text, ''This statement has not been evaluated by the Food and Drug Administration. This product is not intended to diagnose, treat, cure, or prevent any disease''

---

marketed as ''dietary supplements'' because the products were to be represented to be used like ''conventional'' margarine-type spread products.

The manufacturer notifies the FDA ''no later than 30 days after the first marketing of the dietary supplement with such statement that such a statement is being made''

After this legislation (part of the Dietary Supplement Health and Education Act [DSHEA]) was passed in 1994, it appeared at first that there might be reluctance within the industry to use the ''statement of nutritional support'' exemption from ''health claim'' clearance requirements because of the mandated ''disclaimer'' labeling. However, it appears that more than 3000 ''statements of nutritional support'' have now been filed with FDA by companies that have told the agency that they are using the statements in labeling.

It is important to note that not all claims that describe ''the role of a nutrient or dietary ingredient intended to affect the structure or function'' need to comply with the requirements for ''statements of nutritional support'' when used in labeling for a dietary supplement. The provisions of DSHEA concerning ''statements of nutritional support'' were intended to provide an alternative mechanism for allowing the use in labeling for dietary supplements of certain claims that otherwise would have been required to comply with ''health claim'' requirements. Accordingly, *if* a labeling claim about the effect of a nutrient on the structure or function of the human body does *not* come within FDA's definition of a ''health claim'' in 21 C.F.R. § 101.14 (see Sec. II.A.1. of this paper, above), the claim can be used in labeling for a dietary supplement *without* needing to comply with the requirements for ''statements of nutritional support.'' For example, a claim such as ''calcium helps build strong bones'' is a claim about the effect of a nutrient on the structure or function of the human body, but can be made in labeling for a dietary supplement of calcium without compliance with requirements for ''health claims''/''statements of nutritional support''—because such a claim is not a ''health claim'' under the FDA definition since it is not a claim that ''characterizes the relationship'' of a substance to ''disease,'' ''damage,'' or ''dysfunction'' of the human body. 21 C.F.R. § 101.14(a)(1)–(6). For a detailed discussion of the use of ''structure/function'' claims in dietary supplement labeling, see S. McNamara, ''Structure/Function Claims in Dietary Supplement Labeling: Not All of These Claims Need to Be Submitted to FDA and Accompanied in Labeling by the DSHEA Disclaimer,'' *Food and Law Journal*, 1999; 54(1): 35–42.

2. FDA Proposal Re Use of Certain "Structure/Function" Claims in Dietary Supplement Labeling and Certain Prohibited "Disease Claims"

In the Federal Register of April 29, 1998 (63 Fed. Reg. 23624 et seq.), FDA has proposed a rule, to be codified at 21 C.F.R. § 101.93, that provides criteria to determine when a ''structure/function'' claim for a dietary supplement constitutes an impermissible ''disease claim.''

The proposed rule first defines ''disease'' as

> any deviation from, impairment of, or interruption of the normal structure or function of any part, organ, or system (or combination thereof) of the body that is manifested by a characteristic set of one or more signs or symptoms, including laboratory or clinical measurements that are characteristic of a disease.

FDA states in the preamble that ''laboratory or clinical measurements that are characteristic of a disease'' include, for example, ''elevated cholesterol fraction, uric acid, blood sugar, and glycosylated hemoglobin,'' and that ''characteristic signs of disease'' include ''elevated blood pressure or intraocular pressure.''

The agency then proposes the following 10 criteria for identifying ''disease claims'' that would be deemed to be impermissible for a dietary supplement (unless the product were to comply with drug requirements or with an applicable ''health claim'' regulation):

1. *Claimed effect on a specific disease or class of diseases*: FDA gives the following as examples of impermissible claims of an effect on a specific disease or class of diseases (''disease claims''): ''protective against the development of cancer''; ''reduces the pain and stiffness associated with arthritis''; ''decreases the effects of alcohol intoxication''; and ''alleviates constipation.'' The following are examples of acceptable claims that FDA acknowledges would *not* be ''disease claims'' for a dietary supplement: ''helps promote urinary tract health''; ''helps maintain cardiovascular function and a healthy circulatory system''; ''helps maintain intestinal flora''; and ''promotes relaxation.''
2. *Claimed effect on signs or symptoms*: The second type of ''disease claim'' identified by FDA is a claim of an effect on ''signs or symptoms that are recognizable to health care professionals or consumers as being characteristic of a specific disease or of a number of different specific diseases.'' Examples of these claims are: ''improves urine flow in men over 50 years old''; ''lowers cholesterol''; ''reduces joint pain''; and ''relieves headache.'' The following are examples of claims that FDA acknowledges are not ''disease claims'' because the signs or symptoms ''are not, by themselves, sufficient to characterize a specific disease or diseases'': ''reduces stress and frustration''; ''inhibits platelet aggregation'';

and ‘‘improves absentmindedness.’’ FDA also states that if ‘‘the context did not suggest treatment or prevention of a disease, a claim that a substance helps maintain normal function would not ordinarily be a disease claim.’’ The agency gives as examples of these appropriate claims ‘‘helps maintain a healthy cholesterol level’’ and ‘‘helps maintain regularity.’’ However, the agency is requesting comments on these ‘‘maintaining normal function’’ claims, because it could be that ‘‘the only reason for maintaining normal function is to prevent a specific disease or diseases associated with abnormal function.’’

3. *Claimed effect on a consequence of a natural state that presents a characteristic set of signs or symptoms*: These are claims about certain ‘‘natural states’’ (pregnancy, aging, menstrual cycle) that are not diseases but ‘‘are sometimes associated with abnormalities that are characterized by a specific set of signs or symptoms’’ that are ‘‘recognizable to health care professionals or consumers as constituting an abnormality of the body.’’ FDA gives as examples of these ‘‘abnormalities’’ ‘‘toxemia of pregnancy, premenstrual syndrome, or abnormalities associated with aging such as presbyopia, decreased sexual function, Alzheimer’s disease, or hot flashes.’’ Examples of claims that FDA acknowledges would not be ‘‘disease claims’’ are ‘‘for men over 50 years old’’ and ‘‘to meet nutritional needs during pregnancy.’’
4. *Claimed effect on disease through name of product, claims about ingredients in product, citation of publications, use of ‘‘disease’’ term, illustrations*: (1) Examples of names of products that FDA states constitute ‘‘disease claims’’ include: ‘‘Carpaltum’’ (carpal tunnel syndrome); ‘‘Raynaudin’’ (Raynaud’s phenomenon); and ‘‘Hepatacure’’ (liver problems). Names that FDA states do not imply an effect on disease include ‘‘Cardiohealth’’ and ‘‘Heart Tabs.’’ (2) A claim that a dietary supplement contains an ingredient that has been regulated primarily by FDA as a drug and is well known to consumers for its use in preventing or treating a disease (FDA gives aspirin, digoxin, and laetrile as examples) is deemed by FDA to be a ‘‘disease claim.’’ (3) A citation of a title of a publication or other reference ‘‘if the title refers to a disease use’’ is also deemed by FDA to be a ‘‘disease claim.’’ (4) Use of the term ‘‘disease’’ or ‘‘diseased’’ is deemed by FDA to be a ‘‘disease claim.’’ (5) Pictures, vignettes, symbols, or other illustrations that suggest an effect on disease are also said by FDA to be ‘‘disease claims.’’ FDA gives the following as examples: electrocardiogram tracings, pic-

tures of organs that suggest prevention or treatment of a disease state, the prescription symbol (Rx), or any reference to prescription use.

5. *Claim that product belongs to a class of products intended to diagnose, mitigate, treat, cure, or prevent disease*: This category includes identifying a product as ''antibiotic,'' ''antimicrobial,'' ''laxative,'' ''antiseptic,'' ''analgesic,'' ''antidepressant,'' ''antiviral,'' ''vaccine,'' or ''diuretic.'' In contrast, FDA states that acceptable identifiers would be ''energizer,'' ''rejuvenative,'' ''revitalizer,'' and ''adaptogen.''
6. *Claim that product is substitute for therapy product*: These include claims that a product has the same effect ''as that of a recognized drug or disease therapy'' (example: ''Herbal Prozac'').
7. *Claim that product augments a particular therapy or drug action*: These are claims that a product ''should be used as an adjunct to a recognized drug or disease therapy in the treatment of disease'' (e.g., ''use as part of your diet when taking insulin to help maintain a healthy blood sugar level'').
8. *Claim that product has a role in body's response to disease or to a vector of disease*: These are claims that a product augments the body's own disease-fighting capabilities (e.g., ''supports the body's antiviral capabilities''; ''supports the body's ability to resist infection''). This category also includes claims that a product is intended ''to affect the body's ability to kill or neutralize pathogenic microorganisms, or to mitigate the consequences of the action of pathogenic microorganisms on the body (i.e., the signs and symptoms of infection).'' In contrast, FDA states that an example of an acceptable claim would be ''supports the immune system.''
9. *Claimed effect on adverse events associated with disease therapy*: These are claims that a product treats, prevents, or mitigates adverse events that are associated with a medical therapy or procedure and manifested by a characteristic set of signs or symptoms. Examples of these ''disease claims'' identified by FDA are: ''reduces nausea associated with chemotherapy''; ''helps avoid diarrhea associated with antibiotic use''; and ''to aid patients with reduced or compromised immune function, such as patients undergoing chemotherapy.'' On the other hand, FDA acknowledges that ''helps maintain healthy intestinal flora'' would be an acceptable claim for a dietary supplement.
10. *''Catch-all'' provision*: FDA states that any claim that ''otherwise suggests an effect on a disease or diseases'' is also a ''disease claim.''

E. Claims for a Food (Other Than a Dietary Supplement)* About Impact on "Structure" or "Function" of the Human Body

1. The Basic Rules Concerning use of "Structure/Function" Claims for Foods Other Than Dietary Supplements

As described in Sec. I, the FDC Act provides that products that are ''intended to affect the structure or any function of the body'' generally are subject to regulation as ''drugs,'' but that this does not apply in the case of ''food'' (21 U.S.C. § 321(g)(1)(C)). Accordingly, it has long been recognized that a food may make labeling representations about its dietary impact on the structure or function of the human body provided that the particular claim used does not also represent that the food will cure, mitigate, treat, or prevent disease (which would create ''drug'' status), and provided further, that the claim does not trigger some other requirement for FDA preclearance (for example, if a particular claim about impact on structure or function is a claim that would also be regarded as a ''health claim,'' the claim would need to comply with ''health claim'' requirements, as described in Sec. II.A).

In practice, there are a few claims of this type that companies have made and that FDA generally has tolerated over the years, without asserting that the claim creates ''drug'' status or that the claim is a ''health claim'' that requires compliance with ''health claim'' requirements. For example, claims of the general type ''calcium helps build strong bones'' or ''protein helps build strong muscles'' have been made in food labeling and appear generally to have been tolerated by FDA as appropriate claims about the impact of a food on the ''structure'' or ''function'' of the body.

In principle, it would appear that this type of claim could be extended (assuming that a company possesses substantiating data that show that the claim is truthful and not misleading, of course). For example, it would appear to be proper to make a truthful and nonmisleading claim to the effect that a substance in a food ''helps maintain a normal, healthy cardiovascular system'' without triggering either ''drug'' status or requirements for approval of a ''health

* After enactment of DSHEA, at least some ''structure/function'' claims for dietary supplement products are regulated as ''statements of nutritional support'' under 21 U.S.C. § 343(r)(6) (see Sec II.D). It appears that FDA believes that a labeling claim about the effect of a dietary supplement on the normal, healthy structure or function of the human body must comply with the requirements of 21 U.S.C. § 343(r)(6) if the claim does not ''derive from'' ''nutritional'' or ''nutritive'' value, but that if the claim derives from ''nutritional'' or ''nutritive'' value, the supplement may be exempt from ''drug'' status because of 21 U.S.C. § 321(g)(1)(C) and need not comply with the requirements of 21 U.S.C. § 343(r)(6). (See 62 Fed. Reg. 49859 et seq., especially at 49860–49861 and 49863–49864 (September 23, 1997)).

claim.''* However, there is some uncertainty about ''how far'' this type of ''structure/function'' claim can be ''pushed'' before FDA will assert either ''drug'' status or ''health claim'' status.

In a preamble in the Federal Register of September 23, 1997 (62 Fed. Reg. 49860), FDA stated as follows:

> FDA points out that the claim that cranberry juice cocktail prevents the recurrence of urinary tract infections . . . is a claim that brings the product within the ''drug'' definition whether it appears on a conventional food or on a dietary supplement because it is a claim that the product will prevent disease. However, a claim that cranberry products help to maintain urinary tract health may be permissible on both cranberry products in conventional food form and dietary supplement form if it is truthful, not misleading, and derives from the nutritional value of cranberries. If the claim derives from the nutritive value of cranberries, the claim would describe an effect of a food on the structure or function of the body and thus fall under one exception to the

---

* For example, in two recent letters to manufacturers of margarine-type products, the agency has advised that claims of this type may appropriately be made as ''structure/function'' claims. In a letter dated April 30, 1999, to legal counsel for Lipton, FDA responded to a submission that had informed FDA of Lipton's view that ''vegetable oil sterol esters are generally recognized as safe (GRAS) for use in vegetable oil spreads . . . to supplement the nutritive value of the spread, and to help structure the fat phase and reduce the fat and water content of the spread.'' FDA responded not only that ''the agency has no questions at this time regarding Lipton's conclusion that vegetable oil sterol esters are GRAS under the intended conditions of use,'' but also that the agency regarded the claim, ''Helps promote healthy cholesterol levels as part of a diet low in saturated fat and cholesterol'' as a proper type of ''structure/function'' claim. (FDA letter dated April 30, 1999, from Alan M. Rulis, Ph.D., Director, Office of Premarket Approval, FDA Center for Food Safety and Applied Nutrition, to Daniel R. Dwyer re Food Master File 000625.)

Similarly, in a letter dated May 17, 1999, to McNeil Consumer Healthcare, in response to a submission that had informed FDA of ''McNeil's view that plant stanol esters are generally recognized as safe (GRAS) for use as a nutrient in spread,'' FDA replied both that the agency ''has no questions at this time regarding McNeil's conclusion that plant stanol esters are GRAS under the intended conditions of use'' and that the proposed claim, ''Helps promote healthy cholesterol levels'' was regarded as coming ''within the purview of structure/function claims.'' (FDA letter dated May 17, 1999, from Alan M. Rulis, Ph.D., Director, Office of Premarket Approval, FDA Center for Food Safety and Applied Nutrition to Vivian A. Chester and Edward B. Nelson, M.D., Ph.D., re Food Master File 000626.)

Interestingly, the record shows that both of these companies originally had intended to market their products as dietary supplements but subsequently were persuaded by FDA that the products should instead be marketed as conventional-type foods with ''structure/function'' claims in labeling (e.g., FDA memorandum of meeting on May 11, 1998, between FDA Food Center personnel and Lipton personnel concerning ''dietary supplement issues,'' and FDA memorandum of meeting dated October 16, 1998, between FDA personnel and McNeil personnel concerning ''Benecol''). Generally, a dietary supplement may not be ''represented as a conventional food''(21 U.S.C. § 321(ff)(2)(A)(ii), 350(c)(1)(B)(ii)) and also may not be ''represented for use as a conventional food'' (21 U.S.C. § 321(ff)(2)(B)). See also Sec. II.D.

> definition for the term ''drug''. . . . The claim is not a health claim because no disease is mentioned explicitly or implicitly. . . .

Clearly, there is considerable opportunity to make labeling claims about the favorable impact of a food on the normal, healthy structure or function of the human body.

2. Does a "Structure/Function" Claim Need to Derive from "Nutritional" Value?

As noted immediately above, FDA's Federal Register document of September 23, 1997, states that a food may include in its labeling a claim about the effect of the food on the ''structure'' or ''function'' of the human body (without triggering ''drug'' status) only if (in addition to being ''truthful'' and ''not misleading'') the described effect ''derives from the nutritional [or nutritive] value'' of the food. It appears, however, that FDA's insistence on derivation from ''nutritional'' or ''nutritive'' value may not be a correct statement of the law. Consider the following.

As discussed in Sec. I, the definition of ''drug'' in section 201(g)(1)(C) of the FDC Act includes the following provision: ''The term 'drug' means . . . articles (other than food) intended to affect the structure or any function of the body of man. . . .'' (21 U.S.C. § 321(g)(1)(C)). The clear meaning of this provision is that if an article is a ''food,'' and if the food is ''intended to affect the structure or any function of the body,'' such an intended effect does not create ''drug'' status for the article. Furthermore, it follows naturally that if an intended effect does not create ''drug'' status, then labeling statements about that effect also should not create ''drug'' status.

The exclusion from the ''drug'' definition in section 201(g)(1)(C) of the FDC Act applies broadly to ''food,'' not just to ''nutritional'' or ''nutritive'' components or aspects of a food. It appears that FDA infers that the ''food'' exception to the ''drug'' definition in section 201(g)(1)(C) applies only to ''nutritional'' or ''nutritive'' substances; however, that would appear to be a clearly unwarranted inference.

''Food'' is defined by the FDC Act to mean (1) articles used for food or drink for man or other animals, (2) chewing gum, and (3) articles used for components of any such article (section 201(f) of the FDC Act, 21 U.S.C. § 321(f)). In reviewing this definition, the U.S. Court of Appeals for the Seventh Circuit has stated: (*Nutrilab, Inc. versus Schweiker*, 713 F.2d 335, 338 (7th Cir. 1983)):

> When the statute defines ''food'' as ''articles used for food,'' it means that the statutory definition of ''food'' includes articles used by people in the ordinary way most people use food—primarily for taste, aroma, or nutritive value. To hold as did the district court that articles used as food are articles used solely for taste, aroma or nutritive value is unduly restrictive since

> some products such as coffee or prune juice are undoubtedly food but may be consumed on occasion for reasons other than taste, aroma, or nutritive value.

This interpretation of the meaning of ''food'' in the FDC Act has been accepted by other federal courts (*American Health Products Co. versus Hayes*, 574 F. Supp. 1498 (S.D.N.Y. 1983), aff'd, 744 F.2d 912 (2d Cir. 1984)).

Thus, the courts have recognized that the ''food'' exemption from the ''drug'' definition in 21 U.S.C. § 321(g)(1)(C) is not limited to ''nutritional'' or ''nutritive'' substances. Pursuant to the established case law cited above, an article may be deemed to be a ''food'' within the meaning of the FDC Act if it is used ''primarily'' for taste, or, for aroma, or, for nutritional value, and in addition sometimes a food—such as coffee or prune juice—will not even be used for any of these three purposes. Accordingly, the exclusion from ''drug'' status for a ''food'' in section 201(g)(1)(C) of the FDC Act is not properly to be limited by FDA only to products that are ''nutritional'' or ''nutritive''—since ''food'' is broader than that.

Since a food's effects need not be of a nutritional nature, there is no apparent reason why a valid ''food'' may not properly provide labeling information about its effects on the structure or function of the body that do not derive from ''nutritional value.'' Indeed, the U.S. District Court for the Southern District of New York has stated plainly (574 F. Supp. at 1507):

> . . . if an article affects bodily structure or function by way of its consumption as a food, the parenthetical [i.e., the ''(other than food)'' provision in 21 U.S.C. § 321(g)(1)(C)] precludes its regulation as a drug notwithstanding a manufacturer's representations as to physiological effect. . . . The presence of the parenthetical in [21 U.S.C. § 321(g)(1)(C)] suggests that Congress did not want to inhibit the dissemination of useful information concerning a food's physiological properties by subjecting foods to drug regulation on the basis of representations in this regard.

Thus, the courts have recognized that coffee may be used to help stay alert, or that prune juice may be used to help promote regularity, and that labeling claims about this type of physiological effect are appropriate for a food and do not create drug status—regardless of whether such effects and claims derive from the nutritional/nutritive value of the food.

Accordingly, it would appear that FDA's attempt to restrict ''structure/function'' claims for foods to claims about matters that ''derive from the nutritional (or nutritive) value'' of the food may be in error as a matter of law. The proper interpretation of the law would appear to be that insofar as a product is a food (whether a conventional food, a medical food, a dietary supplement, or any other type of food), it may properly make any claim in labeling that is truthful and nonmisleading about a ''physiological effect'' of the food, including a physiological effect of a component of the food, on the structure or function of the human body, provided that the claim does not represent that the product is intended to cure, treat, mitigate, or prevent disease (which would create ''drug'' status for the product), and provided also that the claim does not ''characterize the relationship'' between a ''substance'' and ''disease,'' ''damage,'' or ''dysfunction'' of the body (which would come within the definition of a ''health claim'' and therefore would require compliance with ''health claim'' requirements, or, in the case of a dietary supplement, would require compliance either with ''health claim'' requirements or with the requirements of section 403(r)(6) of the FDC Act, 21 U.S.C. § 343(r)(6)—see Sec. II.D).

3. Even If It Were True That a "Structure/Function" Claim for a Food Should Derive from Nutritional Value,* "Nutritional Value" Is a Broad Term That Encompasses Many "Structure/Function" Claims

It is far from clear just what FDA meant by ''nutritional'' or ''nutritive'' value. The agency did not explain what it meant in this particular context. There are at least three disparate observations to be made in this regard:

1. In the same Federal Register document, in the context of discussing the correct term to be used to describe the class of claims encompassed by section 403(r)(6) of the FDC Act, 21 U.S.C. § 343(r)(6), FDA states that even though the term ''statement of nutritional support'' was used by Congress in 21 U.S.C. § 343(r)(6) to describe this class of claims, FDA chooses not to use this term ''because many of the substances that can be the subject of this type of claim do not have nutritional value. Thus, the term 'statement of nutritional support' is not accurate in all instances.'' 62 Fed. Reg. at 49863. One might perhaps reply to FDA that it is Congress that has the authority to decide what is to be deemed to be ''nutritional'' for purposes of the labeling provisions of the FDC Act, and that this FDA fit of pique over semantics is in clear conflict with the intention of Congress to give a broad meaning to ''nutritional,'' and therefore contrary to law. Nevertheless, this FDA statement certainly suggests an FDA view that ''nutritional'' is a concept that should be interpreted critically and narrowly.
2. On the other hand, at another location in the same Federal Register document, in another context (determining the scope of a ''nutrient content claim''), FDA proceeds in the opposite direction and asserts

* To avoid triggering drug status in the case of a ''conventional''-type food, or, to avoid triggering the need to notify FDA and to use a ''section 403(r)(6) disclaimer'' in labeling in the case of a dietary supplement.

that the term ''nutrient'' is not narrow at all, but instead very broad and includes many substances that traditional nutritionists might not regard as ''nutritional.'' In this context FDA states that ''nutrient'' encompasses a long list of examples included in a discussion between Senators Metzenbaum and Symms before passage of the Nutrition Labeling and Education Act (NLEA) in 1990 (62 Fed. Reg. at 49859-49860). The quoted list of agreed-upon examples of ''nutritional'' substances includes the following:

> Primrose oil, black currant seed oil, coldpressed flax seed oil, ''Barley-green'' and similar nutritional powdered drink mixes, Coenzyme Q10, enzymes such as bromelain and quercetin, amino acids, pollens, propolis, royal jelly, garlic, orotates, calcium-EAP (colamine phosphate), glandulars, hydrogen peroxide (H_2O_2), nutritional antioxidants such a [sic, should be ''as''] superoxide dismutase (SOD), and herbal tinctures.

3. Moreover, unmentioned by FDA in either of the contexts described above is the definition of ''nutritive value'' that already appears in a final FDA regulation. This FDA regulation provides that ''[n]utritive value means a value in sustaining human existence by such processes as promoting growth, replacing loss of essential nutrients, or providing energy (21 C.F.R. § 101.14(a)(3)).*

In view of the dialogue between Senators Metzenbaum and Symms about Congress's understanding of the broad meaning of the term ''nutritional,'' a dialogue that FDA itself has accepted as both authoritative and correct, I believe that even if FDA were correct that a ''structure/function'' claim in labeling should ''derive from nutritional value,'' nevertheless, the meaning of ''nutritional'' in this context should be regarded as very broad and should encompass statements about the usefulness of the wide range of substances intended by the senators.

---

* It is instructive to note that when FDA published this regulation in the Federal Register of January 6, 1993 (58 Fed. Reg. 2478 et seq.), the agency included the following explanatory discussion (58 Fed. Reg. at 2488):

> FDA recognizes that certain substances can play a major role in reducing the risk of certain chronic diseases and may confer their benefits through a number of processes. Accordingly, the agency has worded the definition of ''nutritive value'' in new § 101.14(a)(3) to provide significant flexibility in determining whether a substance possesses such value. FDA used the phrase ''such . . . as'' in the definition to insure that the three referenced processes will be understood to be general examples of the ways in which a substance may legitimately confer nutritive value, rather than as an all-inclusive list.
>
> The agency believes that it is inappropriate to codify findings of nutritive value for specific substances. Such findings would only serve to undermine the intended flexibility of the definition because an extended listing of those substances that possess nutritive value could be interpreted as an exclusive list.

F. Claims About "Special Dietary Uses"

There has been a provision in the FDC Act since 1938 that has recognized that it can be proper for a food to be represented with claims "for special dietary uses" (21 U.S.C. § 343(j)). FDA is given authority to issue regulations that require additional informative labeling for foods that are represented for "special dietary uses."

In the past, FDA issued regulations requiring certain additional labeling information for certain types of foods for special dietary uses (21 C.F.R. Part 105). In particular, there continues to be a regulation of this type that governs the use of "hypoallergenic" labeling (21 C.F.R. § 105.62). This regulation provides that if a food is represented "for special dietary use by reason of the decrease or absence of any allergenic property or by reason of being offered as food suitable as a substitute for another food having an allergenic property," the label of the food must bear certain information, including the "quantity or proportion of each ingredient (including spices, flavoring, and coloring)."

FDA has said that if a claim that otherwise would require FDA approval as a "health claim" is already authorized by a regulation concerning foods for "special dietary use," FDA will not require that a new "health claim" regulation also be issued. (See, e.g., 58 Fed. Reg. 2478 et seq., at 2482 (January 6, 1993).) Accordingly, if a company is interested in making a new labeling claim that would fall within the definition of a "health claim," then instead of petitioning FDA to issue an approving "health claim" regulation, the company may be able to petition the agency to issue a "special dietary use" labeling regulation. However, this is a largely theoretical option. In practice, FDA has been avoiding issuance of new "special dietary use" regulations in recent years; indeed, the agency has been revoking some of these regulations.

G. General Freedom to Use Statements That Are Not "False or Misleading in Any Particular"

In addition to the various authorizations to use particular types of health-related claims (see Secs. II.A–F), it should also be remembered that there is no general requirement in the FDC Act that statements included in labeling of FDA-regulated foods must be approved by FDA prior to use. Instead, requirements for FDA preclearance are confined to certain specific types of labeling statements (e.g., "health claims"), and except for such specific requirements, food labeling generally may include any statement as long as it is truthful and not misleading in any particular (21 U.S.C. § 343(a)(1)).

H. A Word About "Functional Foods," "Nutraceuticals," and the Like

The reader will note that there has been no mention in this chapter until now about "functional foods," "nutraceuticals," "phytofoods," "vitafoods," or the like. These are terms that have come into use in the food industry to describe foods that have particular health-related benefits, but they are not terms that are recognized in the FDC Act or in FDA regulations. Just because, in industry parlance, a particular food product might be described as a "functional food" or "nutraceutical" does not mean that that food is subject to any special legal requirements or exemptions; instead, all of the general legal principles described above in this paper would potentially be applicable—i.e., insofar as a company wants to sell a food product that the company regards as a "functional food," "nutraceutical," or the like, the company must comply with all applicable requirements of law described here with respect to health-related claims that the company wants to include in labeling. Just because a food is regarded by the responsible company as a "functional food," "nutraceutical," or the like does not create any exemptions from, or additions to, the requirements of law that otherwise would be applicable to the use of health-related claims in labeling. For example, if such a food bears a label claim that comes within the definition of a "health claim," and the claim is not authorized under the applicable provisions of law concerning "health claims" (i.e., there is no FDA regulation that approves use of the claim, if the claim does not qualify for use under the exceptional provisions concerning "health claims" that are authorized by "authoritative statements," and [if the product is a dietary supplement] if the claim is not in compliance with the provisions of law applicable to use of "statements of nutritional support" in dietary supplement labeling), the food may be deemed to be either a misbranded/illegal food or an illegal drug. On the other hand, insofar as a company is selling a product that it regards as a "functional food," "nutraceutical," or the like, such a food may bear a health-related claim insofar as the claim does comply with applicable requirements of law described in this chapter.

III. CONCLUSION

As set forth above, existing law provides several different ways, each imposing certain critical restrictions, to make explicit health-related claims in labeling for food products. The current rules, and FDA's long-term intentions, are not always entirely clear, but in general there is little doubt that we are in the midst of a period that is moving toward greater opportunities to provide explicit health-related information in labeling for food products.

Index

ADM (age-related macular degeneration), 91, 96
Advanced glycation end products, 120
  see also Lipoic acid
Age-related macular degeneration (AMD), 91, 96
Allium, 8
Aloe vera gel, 10
α-tocopherol (*see* Vitamin E)
Alzheimer's disease, 2, 33, 35–36
Anthocyanidins, 195
Antioxidants (*see* Plant phenols; Vitamin E)
ATBC study, 21
Atherosclerosis, 104–105, 189–191

Beaberry, 9
Benecol, 308
β-carotene, 11, 281
  and skin protection, 11–17
    all-trans retinoic acid treatment, 13
    DNA damage, 12
    matrix-degrading metalloproteinases, 16
    ornithine decarboxylase, 12
    TBARS, 12
Black cohosh, 9
Black currant seed oil, 10
Body building, 178
Borage seed oil, 10

Caffeic acid, 193
Cancer-preventing agents, putative, 8
  in diet, 8
Cardiovascular disease (*see* β-carotene; Conjugated linoleic acid (CLA); Plant phenols; S-adenosylmethionine (SAMe); Vitamin E)
CARET study, 21
Carotenoids, 91–102
  acceptance by authorities, 99–100
Case-control study, 290
Cataract, 141
Cauliflower, 8
Chamomile, 9
CHAOS study, 34
Chaste tree berry, 110
Cigarette smoking, 17, 97–99
  effects of vitamins E and C, 17–20
  electron spin resonance, 18
  LDL oxidation, 17
  micronucleus test, 19–20
  TBARS, 17
Citrus, 8
Conjugated linoleic acid (CLA), 257–288
  activation of immunological functions, 280–281
  analytical methods, 262
  antiatherogenic effect, 271–277
  anticarcinogenic effect, 272–276
  biosynthesis and chemical synthesis, 260–261

[Conjugated linoleic acid (CLA)]
body fat, 277–279
food sources, 263–266
intake, 266–269
structure, 258
tissues and body fluids, 269–270
Coronary heart disease (CHD) (*see* β-carotene; Conjugated linoleic acid (CLA); Plant phenols; S-adenosylmethionine (SAMe); Vitamin E)
Cranberry, 9, 308
Creatine and exercise performance, 165–186
anti-inflammatory effect, 181
bioavailability, 170
body building, 178
body weight, 179
creatinine, 179
dose recommendations, 178
ergogenic aid, 182
exercise performance, 171–176
heart failure, chronic, 181
magnesium, 179
mode of action, 176
muscle metabolism, 167–168
renal function, 179–180
safety, 178
serum and urine, 169, 177
sources, 166
Creatine kinase, 168

Depression (*see* S-adenosylmethionine (SAMe))
Diabetes, 120–122, 138–141
Diet, factors linked to diseases, 2
Dietary Supplement Health and Education Act (DSHEA), 303
Dihydrolipoic acid, 114–117, 125
Doping, 180–181
Drug, FDA definition of, 293
DSHEA (Dietary Supplement Health and Education Act), 303

Echinacea, 9
Elcuthero, 9
Ellagic acid, 8
Ensure, 301
EPA (eicosapentaenoic acid), 104
Ephedra, 10
Epidemiology, 289–292
Evening primrose oil, 10

FDA, 293, 300
Ferrets, 97–99
see also β-carotene
Ferulic acid, 193
Feverfew, 9
Flavanols, 195
Flavones, 195
Flavonoids, 194–199
Flavonols, 195
Foam cell, 189
Folate (*see* Methylenetetrahydrofolate (MTHF))
Food, definition of, 309
Functional food, definition of, 1, 314

γ-butyrobetaine (*see* L-carnitine)
Garlic, 10
Ginger, 9
Ginkgo, 10
Ginseng, 9
Goldenrod, 9
Goldenseal, 10
Grapeseed, 10
Green tea, 8

Hawthorn, 10
Health claims, 293–314
by ''authoritative statement'' without FDA approval, 296, 299
''beneficial effects,'' 301
Dietary Supplement Health and Education Act (DSHEA), 303
freedom to use statements that are not false and misleading, 313
list of ''nutritional'' substances, 312
nutrient content claims, 298
prohibited disease claims, 304–306
requirements for FDA approval, 294–295
scientific proof, 295
structure/function claims, 303–314

Herbal products, 9–10
Homocysteine, plasma, 83–84, 88
Horehound, 10

Intervention trials, 97–99
  see also β-carotene
Isoflavones, 195

Lentago seed/psyllium, 9
L-carnitine,
  absorption, 221–222
  bioavailability, 233–234
  biosynthesis, 219–221
  deficiency syndromes, 227–231
  dietary sources, 232
  D,L-carnitine, 218
  enzymopathies, 230–231
  excretion, 224–225
  functions, 225–227
  γ-butyrobetaine as substitute, 239
  geriatric nutrition, 239
  in milk, 235
  mitochondria, 226
  myopathy, 229
  requirement in pregnancy and infancy, 234–235
  sports, 236–237
  tissue distribution, 222–223
  vegetarians, 235
LDL oxidation, 39, 190–199
Licorice, 9
Lifespan, 27–28
Lipoic acid, 113–163
  aging, 150
  analysis, 132
  antioxidant action, 114–118, 134–137
  bioavailability, 133
  diabetes, 120–122, 138–141
  diabetic polyneuropathy, 143–145
  modes of action, 125, 131–132
  polyol pathway, 120, 139–142
  racemate versus R-enantiomer, 122–125, 145–148, 152–155
  R-enantiomer, synthesis, 130
  repair of oxidative damage, 118–119
  structure, 114, 117
  vascular damage, 142
Longevity, 27–28
Lung emphysema, 118–119
Lutein, 91–102
  age-related macular degeneration, 96
  bioavailability, 95
  foods, 94
  interactions with other carotenoids, 95
Lycopene, 91–102
  foods, 92
  plasma half-life, 93
  prostate, 93–94
  stability, 92
  tissue distribution, 93

Margarine-type product, 308
Medical food, 300
Mediterranean diet, 207
Melissa, lemon balm, 10
Methylenetetrahydrofolate (MTHF), 75–89
  folate absorption, 75–76
  folate cofactors in nature, 75
  folate uptake by cells, 76
  folic acid, 84
  folic acid uptake by cells, 79
  homocysteine, 83–84, 88
  metabolic pathways, 77–79
  "methyl-trap hypothesis," 81
  natural S-isomer, 86–87
  neuropathy, 81
  pernicious anemia, 80, 88
  psychiatric illness, 89
  RDA for folate, 85
  structures of folates, 76
  supplement, 85–87
  vitamin B_{12}, 80–83
Milk thistle, 9
Minerals, 2–20
Myoglobinuria, 179–180

n-3-polyunsaturated fatty acids (n-3-PUFA), 7–112
  acute myocardial ischemia (AMI), 105–106
  angina pectoris, 106
  atherosclerosis, 104–105
  docosahexaenoic acid (DHA), 104

[n-3-polyunsaturated fatty acids (n-3-PUFA)]
eicosapentaenoic acid (EPA), 104
γ-linolenic acid, 104
restenosis after PTCA, 107
secondary prevention, 107
sudden cardiac death, 108
thrombosis, 105
Nurses' Health Study, 34
Nutraceuticals,
definition of, 1, 314
safety of, 20–23
products currently under development, 22–23

Observational study, 290
Osteoarthritis (*see* S-adenosylmethionine (SAMe))

p-coumaric acid, 193
Peppermint, 9
Phenolic acids (*see* Plant phenols)
p-hydrobenzoate, 193
Phytochemicals, 7, 9–10
see also Plant phenols
Pine bark, 10
Plant phenols, 187–215
and apoptosis, 205
and gene expression, 200–204
modulation of LDL oxidation, 190–199
phenolic acids, 193
Plant stanol esters, 308
Polymorphism, 6
Population survival curve, 28–29
Protokatechuic acid, 193
Pülant phenols, and modulation of cellular response, 200–201

Randomized study, 290
Relative risk, 291
Retinoic acid receptors, 98
Retinoid X receptor, 98
Rhabdomyolysis, 179–180

S-adenosylmethionine (SAMe), 47–58
blood–brain barrier, 50
clinical studies, 55–56
[S-adenosylmethionine (SAMe)]
depression, 54–56
health benefits, 56–57
metabolic role, 48–49, 63–68
oral absorption, 50
osteoarthritis, 68–71
pharmacokinetics, 49–51
tissues and biological fluids, 51–53, 67–68
transmethylations, 48, 64
Sage and pine bark, 198–199
Saw palmetto, 9
Senna, 9
Sinapic acid, 193
Skin, and vitamin E, 40–42
Slippery elm, 10
Smoking (*see* Cigarette smoking)
Soybean products, 198
St. John's wort, 9
Syringic acid, 193

Tea, 196
Tea tree oil, 10
Tocopherols (*see* Vitamin E)
Tocotrienols (*see* Vitamin E)
Tonalin, 279–280
Trace minerals, 2–20
Tumeric, 8

Valerian, 9
Vanillic acid, 193
Vegetable oil sterol esters, 308
Vitamin E, 27–42
antioxidant network, 32
chemical formula, 38
clinical conditions, 30
free radicals and oxidative stress, 28–30
LDL oxidation, 39
molecular basis of action, 36–37
prevention of disease, 34–36
tocotrienols, 37–40
Vitamins, 2–20

Willow bark, 9
Wine, 196
Witch hazel, 10